Case Studies in Bayesian Methods for Biopharmaceutical CMC

The subject of this book is applied Bayesian methods for chemistry, manufacturing, and control (CMC) studies in the biopharmaceutical industry. The book has multiple authors from industry and academia, each contributing a case study (chapter). The collection of case studies covers a broad array of CMC topics, including stability analysis, analytical method development, specification setting, process development and optimization, process control, experimental design, dissolution testing, and comparability studies. The analysis of each case study includes a presentation of code and reproducible output. This book is written with an academic level aimed at practicing nonclinical biostatisticians, most of whom have graduate degrees in statistics.

- First book of its kind focusing strictly on CMC Bayesian case studies
- Case studies with code and output
- Representation from several companies across the industry as well as academia
- Authors are leading and well-known Bayesian statisticians in the CMC field
- Accompanying website with code for reproducibility
- Reflective of real-life industry applications/problems

Chapman & Hall/CRC Biostatistics Series

Series Editors
Shein-Chung Chow, Duke University School of Medicine, USA
Byron Jones, Novartis Pharma AG, Switzerland
Jen-pei Liu, National Taiwan University, Taiwan
Karl E. Peace, Georgia Southern University, USA
Bruce W. Turnbull, Cornell University, USA

Recently Published Titles
Confidence Intervals for Discrete Data in Clinical Research
Vivek Pradhan, Ashis Gangopadhyay, Sandeep Menon, Cynthia Basu, and Tathagata Banerjee

Statistical Thinking in Clinical Trials
Michael A. Proschan

Simultaneous Global New Drug Development
Multi-Regional Clinical Trials after ICH E17
Edited by Gang Li, Bruce Binkowitz, William Wang, Hui Quan, and Josh Chen

Quantitative Methodologies and Process for Safety Monitoring and Ongoing Benefit Risk Evaluation
Edited by William Wang, Melvin Munsaka, James Buchanan and Judy Li

Statistical Methods for Mediation, Confounding and Moderation Analysis Using R and SAS
Qingzhao Yu and Bin Li

Hybrid Frequentist/Bayesian Power and Bayesian Power in Planning Clinical Trials
Andrew P. Grieve

Advanced Statistics in Regulatory Critical Clinical Initiatives
Edited By Wei Zhang, Fangrong Yan, Feng Chen, Shein-Chung Chow

Medical Statistics for Cancer Studies
Trevor F. Cox

Real World Evidence in a Patient-Centric Digital Era
Edited by Kelly H. Zou, Lobna A. Salem, Amrit Ray

Data Science, AI, and Machine Learning in Pharma
Harry Yang

Model-Assisted Bayesian Designs for Dose Finding and Optimization
Methods and Applications
Ying Yuan, Ruitao Lin and J. Jack Lee

Digital Therapeutics: Strategic, Scientific, Developmental, and Regulatory Aspects
Oleksandr Sverdlov, Joris van Dam

Quantitative Methods for Precision Medicine
Pharmacogenomics in Action
Rongling Wu

Drug Development for Rare Diseases
Edited by Bo Yang, Yang Song and Yijie Zhou

Case Studies in Bayesian Methods for Biopharmaceutical CMC
Edited by Paul Faya and Tony Pourmohamad

For more information about this series, please visit: https://www.routledge.com/Chapman--Hall-CRC-Biostatistics-Series/book-series/CHBIOSTATIS

Case Studies in Bayesian Methods for Biopharmaceutical CMC

Edited by
Paul Faya
Tony Pourmohamad

CRC Press
Taylor & Francis Group
Boca Raton London New York

CRC Press is an imprint of the
Taylor & Francis Group, an **informa** business
A CHAPMAN & HALL BOOK

First edition published 2023
by CRC Press
6000 Broken Sound Parkway NW, Suite 300, Boca Raton, FL 33487-2742

and by CRC Press
4 Park Square, Milton Park, Abingdon, Oxon, OX14 4RN

CRC Press is an imprint of Taylor & Francis Group, LLC

ISBN: 978-1-032-18548-4 (hbk)
ISBN: 978-1-032-18550-7 (pbk)
ISBN: 978-1-003-25509-3 (ebk)

DOI: 10.1201/9781003255093

Publisher's note: This book has been prepared from camera-ready copy provided by the authors.

Access the data and code for this book at https://github.com/BayesCMC/Book

To our families:
Erin, Quintin, and Owen
Josie, Vincent, and Ava

Contents

Foreword

Statistical inference problems that naturally arise in Chemistry and Manufacturing Control (CMC) experiments are rather varied and sometimes quite challenging. Proper solutions often do not fit into common categories of two-sample t-tests or simple linear regression. In fact, I would say that in my consulting experience in the CMC area, I was driven to embrace Bayesian statistical methods simply as a way to adequately solve some of these statistical problems. The first CMC problem that struck me as awkward to formulate within the frequentist realm of inference was that of ICH Q8 design space. The solution seemed to fall elegantly into place, however, when taking a Bayesian approach to the problem. But, as time passed, I could see from my own work and that of other Bayesians, that this methodology was also a natural and effective tool for many other CMC statistical problems, such as specification setting, shelf-life estimation, dissolution testing, and assay optimization and validation. The Bayesian approach has the added benefit that solutions to multiple-response generalizations of these problems are obtained within this methodological framework in a straightforward manner. In addition, the Bayesian paradigm allows for the use of informative priors (e.g., built using historical data) to bring in much-needed supporting information in small sample size situations. I believe that a good acronym for Bayesian methods, particularly within the CMC and Quality-by-Design areas is FIT. In addition to being "FIT for use," a well-known quality definition, I like to think of FIT methodology as standing for "Flexible, Informative, Technology." It is clearly flexible for handling tricky inferential problems of the type that arise in CMC situations. It is informative for the scientific way it quantifies information, both current and historical. It is also clearly a technology with clever algorithms and software for powerful implementation.

This book takes us through a tour of using this FIT system on a wide variety of CMC statistical problems. The first three chapters give practical motivation for the reader through explaining the industry and regulatory need for Bayesian statistics, followed by technical discussions of Bayesian methods implementation. The case studies that follow give substantial evidence that Bayesian methods can successfully tackle all of the CMC inferential challenges presented. Currently, this is critical in that "the quality, safety, and efficacy of the final drug product are ultimately defined through CMC results and statistical tools to evaluate them" (Chapter 1). Soon, this FIT methodology will also be important as pharmaceutical manufacturing is expected to fold into the manufacturing 4.0 industrial environment (i.e., the smart factory of the future). Here, the statistical challenges will only grow in complexity. Such an environment may generate a multitude of quality responses, measured at many points in time. Here, I believe Bayesian methods will continue to be an effective and much-needed approach. I wish to thank the editors, Paul Faya and Tony Pourmohamad, and all of the chapter authors for making this important and timely work possible.

John J. Peterson, Ph.D.
PDQ Research & Consulting
Birdsboro, PA 19508
June, 2022

Preface

The use of Bayesian methods to support biopharmaceutical drug development has grown in recent years. In the clinical space, the drive to provide patients with faster access to medical treatments has led to a heightened focus by the industry and regulatory authorities on embracing innovative clinical trials designs, including those that apply Bayesian methods. Outside of clinical trials, the chemistry, manufacturing, and control (CMC) area has the greatest impact on the speed of medicines to patients, yet the same level of attention to, and acceptance of, Bayesian methods has not been given to this area of drug development. This book brings together multiple perspectives across several leading companies in pharma, as well as academics active in CMC research, to shed light on the benefit of applying Bayesian methods in CMC for biopharmaceutical drug development.

The impetus for this book was born out of many meetings of the ASA-DIA Bayesian Nonclinical Working Group, which is a partnership between the Nonclinical Biostatistics Working Group of the American Statistical Association Biopharm Section and the Drug Information Association Bayesian Scientific Working Group. In particular, in 2020, the ASA-DIA Nonclinical Bayesian Working Group conducted a broad survey of nonclinical statisticians in the biopharmaceutical industry. The survey results were recently published in the journal Pharmaceutical Statistics (Faya et al., 2021). One of the key findings from the survey was the need for more Bayesian case study examples for practicing nonclinical statisticians. Responders expressed the need for examples (with code) to provide them with a starting place to learn about Bayesian methods. This book is a culmination of the efforts to address this need. Each chapter of the book focuses on a unique area of CMC biopharmaceutical drug development and provides in-depth analyses of real case studies encountered in practice. Moreover, in each chapter, all analyses are accompanied by reproducible code that should allow readers to understand how to implement the Bayesian paradigm practically. Although most chapters are completely self-contained in terms of reproducibility, additional computer code and data sets for each chapter can be found freely available at `https://github.com/BayesCMC/Book`.

The book will serve as a useful companion to anyone working in the field of CMC and drug development. Geared toward CMC statisticians, Chapters 2 and 3 will be of most use to statisticians with little to no experience in implementing Bayesian methodology in general. Readers who are fully competent in the use of Bayesian methods will find Chapters 2 and 3 to be a useful review but will likely be able to jump right into the subsequent chapters with no difficulty in understanding the materials. Additionally, statisticians with a background in Bayesian statistics, but with little to no background in CMC, should find the book an interesting case study of the applicability of Bayesian methods to biopharmaceutical drug development. We expect that CMC scientists and engineers will also gain insight from the case studies in this book. Indeed, we find that the probabilization of risk inherent in the Bayesian paradigm permits scientists to make decisions in a manner that is intuitive to them. Moreover, the scientific process inherently weighs prior evidence in the design of future studies; the Bayesian approach naturally aligns with this process through the quantification and synthesis of prior knowledge with new evidence.

We are grateful for everyone who has enabled and supported us in this work. The fantastic staff at Chapman & Hall/CRC, especially Senior Editor David Grubbs, helped bring the idea of this book to fruition. People who provided early stimulating discussion and inspired us to work on this include Steven Novick, Dwaine Banton, Percy Sondag, John Peterson, Yanbing Zheng, John Seaman Jr., and Dave LeBlond. A special thank you to all of the chapter authors who provided the terrific content that made this book possible. We are also grateful for the statistics leadership at Eli Lilly and Company and Genentech for encouraging us in this effort and giving us the time and space to make it happen. And finally, we appreciate the support and forbearance of our families as we worked on this book.

Indianapolis, IN — *Paul Faya*
South San Francisco, CA — *Tony Pourmohamad*

May, 2022

Contributors

Misbah Ahmed
Early Development Statistics, GSK
Stevenage, United Kingdom

Stan Altan
Janssen R&D, LLC
Raritan, New Jersey

Dwaine Banton
Labcorp Clinical Development
Solna, Sweden

Aili Cheng
Pfizer
Andover, Connecticut

Hans Coppenolle
Janssen Pharmaceutical R&D, LLC.
Beerse, Belgium

Mike Denham
CMC Statistics, GSK
Ware, United Kingdom

Hesham Fahmy
Data and Statistical Sciences, AbbVie Inc.
North Chicago, Illinois

Paul Faya
Eli Lilly and Company
Indianapolis, Indiana

Katherine E.D. Giacoletti
Merck & Co., Inc.
West Point, Pennsylvania

Buffy Hudson-Curtis
Research Statistics, GSK
Philadelphia, Pennsylvania

Mark Johnson
Data and Statistical Sciences, AbbVie Inc.
North Chicago, Illinois

David J. Kahle
Department of Statistical Science, Baylor University
Waco, Texas

Ji Young Kim
Merck & Co. Inc.
West Point, Pennsylvania

Martin Kovarik
Janssen-Cilag s.r.o., Pharmaceutical Companies of Johnson & Johnson
Prague, Czechia

David LeBlond
Robert Singer Consulting
Wadsworth, Illinois

Richard Lewis
Fellow, American Society for Quality
Cary, North Carolina

Guillermo Miro-Quesada
AstraZeneca
Gaithersburg, Maryland

Laurent Natalis
PharmaLex Belgium SA
Frankfurt, Germany

Steven Novick
Data Sciences and Quantitative Biology, Discovery Sciences, Biopharmaceuticals R&D, AstraZeneca
Gaithersburg, Maryland

Martin Otava
Janssen-Cilag s.r.o., Pharmaceutical Companies of Johnson & Johnson
Prague, Czechia

Tony Pourmohamad
Genentech, Inc.
South San Francisco, California

Adam Rauk
Eli Lilly and Company
Indianapolis, Indiana

James Reynolds
Data and Statistical Sciences, AbbVie Inc.
North Chicago, Illinois

Robert Richardson
Department of Statistics, Brigham Young University
Provo, Utah

Tara Scherder
SynoloStats LLC
Flemington, New Jersey

Christian Schmid
Pennsylvania State University
University Park, Pennsylvania

John W. Seaman Jr.
Department of Statistical Science, Baylor University
Waco, Texas

Robert Singer
Robert Singer Consulting
Union City, California

Perceval Sondag
Novo Nordisk Inc.
Plainsboro Township, New Jersey

James D. Stamey
Department of Statistical Science, Baylor University
Waco, Texas

Man Tang
Data and Statistical Sciences, AbbVie Inc.
North Chicago, Illinois

Chris Thompson
AstraZeneca
Gaithersburg, Maryland

Ke Wang
Pfizer
Groton, Connecticut

Lu Xu
PRAV Biosciences
San Francisco, California

Harry Yang
Fate Therapeutics, Inc.
San Diego, California

Rong Zeng
Amador Bioscience
Pleasanton, California

Yanbing Zheng
Data and Statistical Sciences, AbbVie Inc.
North Chicago, Illinois

1

Introduction

Paul Faya

Eli Lilly and Company

Tony Pourmohamad

Genentech, Inc.

CONTENTS

1.1 Motivation

Nonclinical biostatistics can be broadly defined as statistical methods applied to areas in the pharmaceutical/biotechnology industries that do not include clinical studies (Zhang and Su, 2016). These areas include preclinical discovery, nonclinical development, translational science, safety, pharmacology, and chemistry, manufacturing and controls (CMC).

CMC studies and data are focused on the development, characterization, and control of biopharmaceutical products, processes, and analytical methods. They represent an integral part of the drug development life-cycle and are required for market approval. New Drug Application (NDA) and Biologics License Application (BLA) submissions include many lengthy sections devoted to CMC aspects. Indeed, the quality, safety, and efficacy of the final drug product are ultimately defined through CMC results and the statistical tools used to evaluate them.

CMC data describe the manufacturing process and associated control measures, as well as detail the capability of measurement systems to adequately characterize the critical quality attributes of the drug substance and drug product. For example, CMC scientists must propose and justify lot release and shelf-life specifications for the quality attributes of future manufactured lots. They must demonstrate the robustness, precision, and accuracy of analytical methods used to measure the quality attributes as well as describe and justify process control measures. They must also demonstrate the long-term chemical and biological stability of the molecule throughout the supply-chain and proposed shelf-life. And they must provide evidence of comparability of the drug throughout its various stages of the process and product development. When changes are made to analytical methods or manufacturing processes, comparability or bridging studies must be performed to demonstrate the continuity of the measurement system and quality attributes of the drug. For biosimilar development, CMC scientists must demonstrate analytical similarity between the proposed and reference products. Analytical similarity is foundational for providing the totality-of-evidence of biosimilarity to regulatory agencies. Comparative analytical data

DOI: 10.1201/9781003255093-1

influence decisions about the type and amount of animal and clinical data needed to support a demonstration of biosimilarity.

As a candidate molecule advances to late-stage development, CMC studies become more complex and undergo greater scrutiny by health authorities. Moreover, the sponsor is expected to achieve greater understanding of how CMC aspects impact the quality, safety, and efficacy of the drug. In this way, CMC studies are ideally suited for the application of Bayesian methods. Knowledge regarding the product, process, and measurement systems accumulates and improves as molecules move from early to late-phase development. For example, early screening studies of critical manufacturing process parameters evolve into process characterization and optimization studies in late phase. Novick et al. (2021) and Faya et al. (2022) also illustrate the application of Bayesian methods to a "continuous" learning approach to method validation. Moreover, it is common for biopharmaceutical manufacturers to adopt "first-to-try" or "platform" manufacturing processes and analytical methods, particularly for proteins of similar structure (e.g., monoclonal antibodies). Knowledge from such platform processes and methods can naturally be quantified across molecules using Bayesian methods. As such, high-quality and carefully collected prior information can be available from the current project as well as from similar molecules. There are also benefits to using Bayesian statistics that extend beyond using prior knowledge. These include the probabilistic quantification of uncertainty, the clarity and coherence of posterior-based inference (Robert, 2007), and the ability to analyze complex models directly instead of relying on approximations, as can be common in frequentist methods.

1.2 Regulatory Considerations

Regulatory reviewers of new drug and biologic applications insist that CMC studies for new molecular entities and biosimilars meet the highest of standards. The current guidance documents governing CMC practice (from Food and Drug Administration (FDA), European Medicines Agency (EMA), International Council for Harmonisation (ICH), and United States Pharmacopeia (USP)) are silent on the use of Bayesian methods, not even mentioning them as alternatives to traditional approaches. This is curious given the enormous emphasis on risk control in pharmaceutical development and quality metrics (see ICH Q8 (2005) and ICH Q9 (2005)). In contrast, as far back as 1998, ICH E9 (1998), which governs statistical principles for clinical trials, noted that "the use of Bayesian and other approaches may be considered when the reasons for their use are clear and when resulting conclusions are sufficiently robust."

Demonstrating equivalence of biosimilars is similarly bereft of Bayesian guidance. This is despite the natural suitability of Bayesian approaches for such studies. Bayesian posterior and predictive distributions can be used to make probabilistic (i.e., risk-based) conclusions regarding the similarity of the physiochemical and functional properties of two products. However, in the most recent FDA draft guidance (2019) for the development of therapeutic protein biosimilars, only frequentist equivalence testing is proposed, with no mention of the potential for Bayesian methods.

In a recent cover article of the American Institute of Chemical Engineers Journal, Tabora et al. (2019) called for chemical engineers to adopt Bayesian-based approaches, which quantify risk more effectively and meet the FDA's vision for robust pharmaceutical manufacturing. They argued that Bayesian methods are exceptionally effective at characterizing variability from limited data and anticipate a much wider adoption across the pharmaceutical industry. However, the authors also noted that regulatory agencies need to encourage the use of such probabilistic risk-based methods.

At a broader level, the FDA's vision for Pharmaceutical Quality for the 21st Century – A Risk Based Approach (FDA, 2004) has been around for nearly 20 years. One of the key pillars of the initiative was the concept of "Quality by Design" (QbD). QbD involves developing a thorough understanding of the product and process along with a knowledge of the risks involved in manufacturing the product. Extensive research has been published by the industry (see for example, Peterson (2008), Peterson and Yahyah (2009), Peterson and Lief (2010), Rozet et al. (2013)) on how Bayesian methods are ideally suited for QbD applications. Yet, in the years since the launch of the FDA QbD initiative, no regulatory document has been revised to reflect this fact.

We can also learn from the "least burdensome" provisions of the Center for Devices and Radiological Health (CDRH), which are linked to the FDA Modernization Act of 1997. Although written from the perspective of medical device clinical trials, the spirit of the provisions is completely relevant to other spheres such as CMC. Principles such as using only necessary (minimum required) information, acceptance of alternative approaches, the efficient use of resources, the use of alternative sources of data, leveraging existing data, and considering the "most efficient means" of obtaining scientific evidence are important in CMC, and in many ways, can be realized through Bayesian statistics. The current draft guidance documents for ICH Q2(R2) (2022) and ICH Q14 (2022) published in 2022 make encouraging steps toward a "least burdensome" principle applied to analytical method validation. For example, the draft Q2(R2) explicitly allows for the use of pre-existing knowledge in addition to, or in lieu of, a formal validation study to provide evidence of the validated state of a method. The draft Q14 notes that prior knowledge can come from internal or external sources and that existing platform procedures can be leveraged to evaluate the attributes of a specific molecule without conducting additional method development. In addition, Q2(R2) introduces a predictive approach to method performance assessment, combining the evaluation of accuracy and precision into a measure of total error. Despite the fact that Bayesian methods are naturally suited for the new validation strategies offered in the draft Q2(R2) and Q14, there still remains an inherent frequentist method bias, with a focus on confidence interval-based inference and no mention of Bayesian techniques.

In sum, adopting Bayesian methods in CMC has the potential to enhance decision-making and improve the quality, safety, and efficacy of biopharmaceutical products. Modernizing CMC regulatory guidance will open new paths for CMC scientists, engineers, and statisticians to properly and fruitfully apply Bayesian principles throughout the product development and manufacturing life-cycle. The clinical space has already paved the way with guidance documents and examples of industry-regulatory collaborative efforts that the nonclinical community can learn from and leverage. The need for initiative, clarity, and collaboration from the CMC regulatory community on both the industry and government sides is high. For further discussion on some of the reasons for the slower uptake of Bayesian methods in the CMC space, see Faya and Berry (2022).

1.3 Objectives and Organization of the Book

The following chapters offer examples of Bayesian methods motivated by real case studies in traditional CMC areas. The contributing authors include current and former CMC statisticians with extensive experience in the field as well as academics who have collaborated in CMC research projects. In selecting the authors and topics for this book, our goal was to provide as diverse a set of perspectives as possible. Many of the contributors to this book are members of the DIA-ASA Nonclinical Bayesian Working Group. While some case studies are presented with simulated data (for the sake of data anonymity), the Bayesian methodologies proposed in each chapter are those that have been used by the authors to support CMC decision-making. In addition, a variety of software applications and packages are used to demonstrate the implementation of Bayesian inference throughout the book. We view one of the main bottlenecks to the adoption of Bayesian methods in the CMC space as the lack of available easy-to-understand resources for implementing Bayesian techniques practically (see industry survey results in Faya et al. (2021)). Our hope is that the numerous practical examples and reproducible code will alleviate this bottleneck.

Recent advances in computational tools have reduced the barriers to the adoption of Bayesian methods for many practitioners. However, the need for simulation methods to derive inference for most problems means that there is a learning curve for those unfamiliar with computational techniques. Chapters 2 and 3 of this book provide an overview of Bayesian computational strategies and model checking. While the content in these chapters is not a pre-requisite for understanding the subsequent case studies, the concepts, theoretical foundations, and mathematical derivations offer readers a sound foundation for simulation-based Bayesian modeling. Of particular value are the "quick-kill" and "due diligence" lists in Chapter 3, which provide practical checks for diagnosing convergence of posterior distributions.

One of the primary aims of this book is the reproducibility of the statistical methods presented. As such, each chapter contains code chunks and details integrated within the body of the text. While some chapters may be reproduced by beginners, others are more advanced and require a sound understanding of Bayesian ideas and methods. Our hope is that regardless of the level of Bayesian training, CMC statisticians, scientists, and engineers can find scenarios that will motivate, challenge, and equip them to use Bayesian inference in their work. We also hope that this book will provide material to fill a gap in teaching biostatistics, a field that extends beyond the design and analysis of clinical trials.

2

An Overview of Bayesian Computation

David J. Kahle, John W. Seaman Jr., and James D. Stamey

Baylor University: Department of Statistical Science

CONTENTS

2.1 Bayesian Computation – A Conceptual Perspective

2.1.1 The Importance of Computation in the Bayesian Paradigm

Every domain of modern statistical practice relies heavily on computation. This is especially true for Bayesian statistics, where even the most basic of inferential strategies requires – or at least in practice almost always involves – computations using very powerful algorithmic tools with complex mathematical underpinnings. While the algorithms may be complex, the basic problem is easily identifiable. Every Bayesian inferential method relies on the posterior distribution $p(\boldsymbol{\theta}|\mathbf{y})$, a multivariate distribution over the parameter space of a statistical model conditional on the observed data $\mathbf{y}$. Here, $\boldsymbol{\theta}$ denotes a vector of unknown parameters taken from a set $\boldsymbol{\Theta}$ and $\mathbf{y}$ denotes a vector of observations. The posterior distribution, in turn, depends exclusively on the likelihood $l(\boldsymbol{\theta}|\mathbf{y})$, which is the data model $p(\mathbf{y}|\boldsymbol{\theta})$ viewed as a function of the parameter $\boldsymbol{\theta}$ for fixed $\mathbf{y}$, and the prior distribution $p(\boldsymbol{\theta})$ through the relationship characterized by Bayes' theorem:

$$p(\boldsymbol{\theta}|\mathbf{y}) = \frac{p(\mathbf{y},\boldsymbol{\theta})}{p(\mathbf{y})} = \frac{p(\mathbf{y},\boldsymbol{\theta})}{\int_{\boldsymbol{\Theta}} p(\mathbf{y},\boldsymbol{\theta})\,d\boldsymbol{\theta}} = \frac{l(\boldsymbol{\theta}|\mathbf{y})p(\boldsymbol{\theta})}{\int_{\boldsymbol{\Theta}} l(\boldsymbol{\theta}|\mathbf{y})p(\boldsymbol{\theta})\,d\boldsymbol{\theta}} \propto l(\boldsymbol{\theta}|\mathbf{y})p(\boldsymbol{\theta}) =: \tilde{p}(\boldsymbol{\theta}|\mathbf{y}) \tag{2.1}$$

Here $\tilde{p}(\boldsymbol{\theta}|\mathbf{y}) = l(\boldsymbol{\theta}|\mathbf{y})p(\boldsymbol{\theta})$ represents the un-normalized posterior distribution, a function we use often as it is always available. Although we have depicted the unknown parameters and observations as vectors, it is often more helpful to think of $\mathbf{y}$ as simply "the data" and $\boldsymbol{\theta}$ "the parameters." In real applications these are usually a collections of vectors and matrices with complex structures.

Statistical analyses typically involve assessments of $\boldsymbol{\theta}$ or some subset thereof given $\mathbf{y}$. For example, we may want interval estimates for components of $\boldsymbol{\theta}$ or posterior probabilities

DOI: 10.1201/9781003255093-2

of attaining some critical value. Such assessments can almost always be written in the form of expectations taken with respect to the posterior.[1] For example, the Bayes estimator $\hat{\boldsymbol{\theta}}$ of $\boldsymbol{\theta}$ is the mean of the posterior distribution, $\mathbb{E}_{p(\boldsymbol{\theta}|\mathbf{y})}[\boldsymbol{\theta}]$.[2] The probability that $\boldsymbol{\theta}$ falls in some subset $\boldsymbol{\Theta}_0 \subset \boldsymbol{\Theta}$ is $\Pr_{p(\boldsymbol{\theta}|\mathbf{y})}[\boldsymbol{\theta} \in \boldsymbol{\Theta}_0] = \mathbb{E}_{p(\boldsymbol{\theta}|\mathbf{y})}[1(\boldsymbol{\theta} \in \boldsymbol{\Theta}_0)]$, i.e. the expected value of the indicator function over $\boldsymbol{\Theta}_0$. Regions of high probability can be determined through the iterative computation of such probabilities. Thus, almost all Bayesian analyses can be reduced to computing expectations with respect to the posterior of the form $\mathbb{E}_{p(\boldsymbol{\theta}|\mathbf{y})}[g(\boldsymbol{\theta})]$ for some function g, and this is generally the approach taken when conducting Bayesian inference. Note that g can be and often is vector-valued.

In this chapter, we will loosely refer to both of these computations–computing $p(\boldsymbol{\theta}|\mathbf{y})$ and computing $\mathbb{E}_{p(\boldsymbol{\theta}|\mathbf{y})}[g(\boldsymbol{\theta})]$ for a given g–as "computing the posterior." Notice that the computations are similar: both involve evaluation of integrals of the form $\int_{\mathcal{R}} \tilde{p}(\boldsymbol{\theta}|\mathbf{y})\, d\boldsymbol{\theta} = \int_{\mathcal{R}} l(\boldsymbol{\theta}|\mathbf{y})p(\boldsymbol{\theta})\, d\boldsymbol{\theta}$. When $\mathcal{R} = \boldsymbol{\Theta}$, this constant goes by various names, including the marginal, the prior predictive, and the partition function; it is the expected value of the likelihood with respect to the prior. For convenience, we write $Z(\mathbf{y}) = \int_{\boldsymbol{\Theta}} \tilde{p}(\boldsymbol{\theta}|\mathbf{y})\, d\boldsymbol{\theta}$, so Bayes' theorem can alternatively be written $p(\boldsymbol{\theta}|\mathbf{y}) = \tilde{p}(\boldsymbol{\theta}|\mathbf{y})/Z(\mathbf{y})$.

Once the model and prior are specified, doing Bayesian data analysis is equivalent to computing the posterior. Although there are important exceptions, most modeling scenarios involve parameter spaces $\boldsymbol{\Theta}$ that are "continuous," "nice" subsets of a real Euclidean space, as distinct from "discrete." Consequently, the expectations are integrals against the posterior: $\mathbb{E}_{p(\boldsymbol{\theta}|\mathbf{y})}[g(\boldsymbol{\theta})] = \int_{\boldsymbol{\Theta}} g(\boldsymbol{\theta})p(\boldsymbol{\theta}|\mathbf{y})\, d\boldsymbol{\theta}$. Unfortunately, in all but the nicest of circumstances these integrals are intractable: we do not have closed-form antiderivatives with which to apply the fundamental theorem of calculus, and alternative approaches are required.

Several approaches are routinely used for this purpose. We break these into two major categories: approaches that approximate computations with respect to the exact posterior and approaches that perform exact computations on approximations to the posterior. Myriad strategies exist for each of these situations. We limit ourselves to those most commonly seen in practice. Most notably, in this chapter, we do not consider variational methods or (sequential) importance sampling (particle filters).

To facilitate our discussion, we focus on a familiar example, the estimation of the normal mean and variance. To that end, consider an independent and identically distributed (*iid*) sequence of random variables $Y_1, \ldots, Y_n \overset{iid}{\sim} \mathcal{N}(\mu, \sigma^2)$ with n a fixed known constant. For observed values $y_1, \ldots, y_n$, the likelihood is

$$l(\boldsymbol{\theta}|\mathbf{y}) = l(\mu, \sigma^2|\mathbf{y}) = (2\pi\sigma^2)^{-n/2} \exp\left\{-\frac{1}{2\sigma^2}\sum_{i=1}^{n}(y_i - \mu)^2\right\}, \tag{2.2}$$

over the parameter space $\boldsymbol{\Theta} = \mathbb{R} \times \mathbb{R}_+$. The y_i are known, and the likelihood is a function of $\boldsymbol{\theta} = (\mu, \sigma^2)$ over $\boldsymbol{\Theta}$. We will use this data model with reference to different prior structures throughout this chapter.

Sections 2.1.2 and 2.1.3 focus on more technical details of Bayesian computing. If you are primarily interested in more applied aspects of Bayesian computation, we encourage you to skip them and proceed to Section 2.2. From there, you can proceed to Chapter 3, which provides an overview of practical diagnostic criteria to assess whether the computational strategies you use are functioning properly.

[1] Or marginal distributions derived from the posterior; however, we always discuss the former as it makes the mathematics simpler and only trivially affects the prevailing computational strategy, Monte Carlo methods.

[2] The notation $\mathbb{E}_{p(\boldsymbol{\theta}|\mathbf{y})}[\boldsymbol{\theta}]$ means the expected value of $\boldsymbol{\theta}$, viewed as a random variable, where $\boldsymbol{\theta}$ has the distribution $p(\boldsymbol{\theta}|\mathbf{y})$, the posterior distribution.

2.1.2 Approximate Computations of the Exact Posterior

2.1.2.1 Deterministic Strategies

Deterministic strategies are methods for computing the posterior that yield the same result for a given likelihood and prior specification. Their implementations may differ in detail, but if two statisticians use the same deterministic approach they obtain the same posterior. We describe three such approaches: symbolic integration, conjugate priors, and numerical integration. A closely related approach, discretization, is discussed in Section 2.1.3.

Symbolic integration. The most obvious approach to computing the posterior is to try to use symbolic methods to find an antiderivative of the integrand and appeal to the fundamental theorem of calculus.

Suppose that prior information leads us to believe with certainty that $\sigma^2 \leq 4$ and $-2 \leq \mu \leq 2$, and we place a bivariate uniform prior of $p(\mu, \sigma^2) = 1/16$ over this range. Notice that restricting the support of the prior to a subset of the parameter space also limits the support of the posterior to the same range. This is a very stringent assumption since no amount of contrary data will take the posterior outside of that support. By Bayes' theorem, the posterior distribution is

$$p(\mu, \sigma^2|\mathbf{y}) = \frac{l(\mu, \sigma^2|\mathbf{y})p(\mu, \sigma^2)}{\int_0^4 \int_{-2}^2 l(\mu, \sigma^2|\mathbf{y})p(\mu, \sigma^2)\, d\mu\, d\sigma^2} = \frac{l(\mu, \sigma^2|\mathbf{y})\frac{1}{16}}{\int_0^4 \int_{-2}^2 l(\mu, \sigma^2|\mathbf{y})\frac{1}{16}\, d\mu\, d\sigma^2}, \tag{2.3}$$

where $l(\mu, \sigma^2|\mathbf{y})$ is as presented in (2.2). The integrand in the denominator is itself a Gaussian integral: it has no closed form in terms of elementary expressions (Conrad, 2005). Similarly, the Bayes estimator of $\boldsymbol{\theta} = (\mu, \sigma^2)$, which is the vector $\hat{\boldsymbol{\theta}} = (\hat{\mu}, \hat{\sigma}^2) = \left(\mathbb{E}_{p(\mu,\sigma^2|\mathbf{y})}[\mu], \mathbb{E}_{p(\mu,\sigma^2|\mathbf{y})}[\sigma^2]\right)$, also has no closed form antiderivative. The symbolic strategy fails: we cannot compute the integral using elementary means, even with this very simple prior structure.

Unfortunately, this is typically the case. Notice that the intractability of $p(\boldsymbol{\theta}|\mathbf{y})$ is derived from the intractability of $\int \tilde{p}(\boldsymbol{\theta}|\mathbf{y})\, d\boldsymbol{\theta}$, which appears in the denominator of Bayes' theorem. That is to say: the inability to normalize the posterior is closely related to the inability to compute integrals with respect to the posterior even in the event that the normalization constant were known, i.e. compute posterior probabilities. While in some rare circumstances we can directly compute integrals like this using the elementary methods of calculus, in almost all real-world problems this strategy fails.

Conjugacy and conjugate priors. One approach to trying to make the problem more tractable is to select a prior $p(\boldsymbol{\theta})$ that combines with the likelihood $l(\boldsymbol{\theta}|\mathbf{y})$ in such a way as to make the overall integrand $\tilde{p}(\boldsymbol{\theta}|\mathbf{y})$ recognizable as the un-normalized kernel of a common well-known distribution. The normalizing constant can then be determined without integration.

As an example, suppose that we select a prior of the form $p(\mu, \sigma^2) = p(\mu|\sigma^2)p(\sigma^2)$, where $p(\mu|\sigma^2)$ is chosen to be a normal distribution and $p(\sigma^2)$ is chosen to have an inverse-gamma distribution. The joint prior is said to have a normal-inverse-gamma distribution. Remarkably, it can be shown that the posterior $p(\mu, \sigma^2|\mathbf{y})$ also has a normal-inverse-gamma distribution with different parameters, and no integration is necessary (Gelman et al., 2013, ff.67). This phenomenon is known as conjugacy.

A family of distributions is said to be conjugate for a given likelihood if members of the family, when used as prior distributions, result in posterior distributions that are also members of the family. These are called conjugate priors. Many likelihoods of simple data models admit conjugate families that are well-known parametric distributions, and in these cases the posterior parameters are typically simple functions of the data and the parameters identifying the prior in the conjugate family, in this context called hyperparameters. Examples include the binomial, Poisson, normal, gamma, and multivariate normal data models. These are so common that tables are made associating common likelihoods with their conjugate families and formulas for the posterior parameters; these can be found in most textbooks on Bayesian data analysis as well as popular online encyclopedias. Unfortunately, conjugacy tends to not scale well to larger modeling contexts, e.g. generalized linear or survival models, and so cannot be used as a general purpose tool for Bayesian inference. Nevertheless, recognizing conjugacy where it exists and taking advantage of it is an important device in many samplers used for the stochastic methods presented in Section 2.1.2.2.

Numerical integration. Numerical integration involves using strategies from numerical analysis to approximate definite integrals, typically using a linear combination of the values the function assumes at various points in the domain of integration. It relies on the observation that, while $\tilde{p}(\boldsymbol{\theta}|\mathbf{y})$ is hard to integrate, it is typically easy to evaluate for a given value of $\boldsymbol{\theta}$. This is usually done on the log scale in order to both keep it numerically stable as well as take advantage of the decoupling of the product.

Consider again the posterior distribution for the normal model when the prior distribution is uniform on the region $\mathcal{R} = (-2, 2) \times (0, 4)$. While the volume $Z(\mathbf{y})$ under the bivariate surface $\tilde{p}(\mu, \sigma^2|\mathbf{y})$ over $\mathcal{R}$ cannot be determined using the standard techniques from calculus, it can be determined with numerical integration with a high degree of accuracy and precision. Probabilities and expectations with respect to the posterior can usually be computed using the same strategy.

As a simple form of numerical integration, consider the use of Riemann sums based on a mesh of $N+1$ points in both the μ and σ^2 dimensions illustrated in Figure 2.1. The mesh yields N^2 rectangles over the region $\mathcal{R}$, each of area $\frac{2-(-2)}{N} \times \frac{4}{N} = \frac{16}{N^2}$. Using a midpoint rule to evaluate the density at the center of each rectangle, the un-normalized posterior $\tilde{p}(\mu, \sigma^2|\mathbf{y})$ is evaluated at N^2 locations of the form $\tilde{p}_{ij} = \tilde{p}\big(-2 + (i + \frac{1}{2})(\frac{2-(-2)}{N}), 0 + (j + \frac{1}{2})(\frac{4-0}{N})|\mathbf{y}\big)$ where $i, j = 0, \ldots, N-1$. The corresponding rectangular prisms are of volume $\frac{16}{N^2}\tilde{p}_{ij}$, and summing these yields an approximation $Z_N(\mathbf{y}) = \sum_{i=1}^{N}\sum_{j=1}^{N}\frac{16}{N^2}\tilde{p}_{ij}$ of the partition function $Z(\mathbf{y})$. Of course, as $N \to \infty$, $Z_N(\mathbf{y}) \to Z(\mathbf{y})$, and N can be chosen to be arbitrarily large. Bounds for the integral can be derived using mean value theorems, but such technical details are not needed here.

One way to think of Riemann sums created in this way is that they subdivide the domain of integration via the partition $\mathcal{R} = \bigcup_{i,j=1}^{N}\mathcal{R}_{ij}$, decompose the integral $\int_{\mathcal{R}}\tilde{p}(\boldsymbol{\theta}|\mathbf{y})\,d\boldsymbol{\theta} = \sum_{i,j=1}^{N}\int_{\mathcal{R}_{i,j}}\tilde{p}(\boldsymbol{\theta}|\mathbf{y})\,d\boldsymbol{\theta}$ as a sum of integrals over the partition, and approximate each of these integrals by using a constant approximation to $\tilde{p}(\boldsymbol{\theta}|\mathbf{y})$ over each subdomain. As an alternative, if the gradient $\nabla_{\boldsymbol{\theta}}\tilde{p}(\boldsymbol{\theta}|\mathbf{y})$ is available, linear approximations to $\tilde{p}(\boldsymbol{\theta}|\mathbf{y})$ can be constructed over each sub-region in a manner similar to the trapezoid rule in one dimension, and the volumes of the trapezoidal prisms can be summed to approximate $Z(\mathbf{y})$. While these are more accurate, there is a trade-off in computational complexity: should one use higher-degree approximations, or simply more rectangular prisms? In general, these are called Newton-Cotes rules and are only one form of numerical integration.

There are two problems with this kind of numerical integration. The first is that while numerical integration is helpful in computing integrals over nice rectangular domains, it may not be as helpful for non-rectangular ones that some probabilities require, e.g. $\Pr_{p(\mu,\sigma^2|\mathbf{y})}[\mu \leq \sigma^2]$. (For a closely related strategy that doesn't suffer from this problem, see Section 2.1.3.) The second, more serious problem with this kind of numerical integration is that it does not scale well. For two parameters, N^2 evaluations of $\tilde{p}(\boldsymbol{\theta}|\mathbf{y})$ are required; for three parameters, N^3 evaluations are required; and for p parameters, N^p evaluations are required. Griding simply does not scale well and quickly becomes infeasible. For example, a trivariate normal data model has $p = 9$ parameters: three for the mean, and 6 for the covariance matrix. If one uses even $N = 10$ boxes in each dimension, this requires 10^9 evaluations $\tilde{p}(\boldsymbol{\theta}|\mathbf{y})$. Worse, care must be taken when griding the parameter space of the covariance matrix, as it is not rectangular.

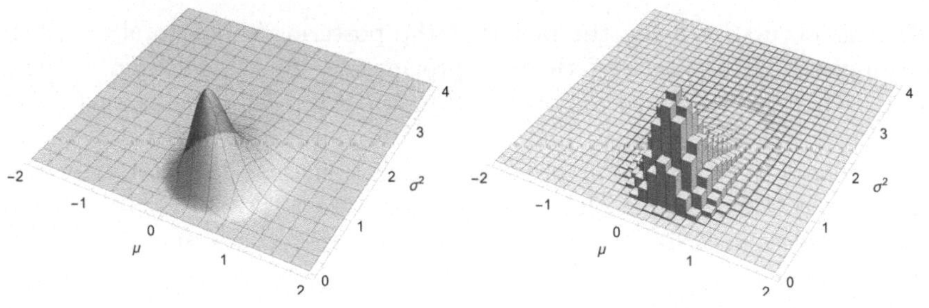

FIGURE 2.1
Numerical approximations to the partition function (the integral of the un-normalized posterior) can be obtained via numerical integration. This is shown here for $\tilde{p}(\mu, \sigma^2|\mathbf{y}) = l(\mu, \sigma^2|\mathbf{y})p(\mu, \sigma^2)$ assuming the uniform prior given a sample of size $n = 10$ from a standard normal distribution using $N = 30$ boxes in each dimension.

2.1.2.2 Stochastic Strategies

While deterministic approaches provide straightforward and satisfying solutions to computing the posterior, their inability to scale up to more complex models frequently seen in practical Bayesian data analysis limits their use. Instead, stochastic, or "Monte Carlo," approaches are typically used. Monte Carlo algorithms are numerical algorithms that fundamentally rely on randomness.

Most Monte Carlo strategies in statistics rely on two fundamental results: the law of large numbers (LLN) and the central limit theorem (CLT). These two probabilistic results exist in both univariate and multivariate forms. The LLN essentially says that under very general conditions, the sample mean of a collection of n *iid* observations approaches the mean of the population as $n \to \infty$. The CLT says that under slightly more restrictive yet still very general conditions, for a fixed sample size n the sample mean has an approximate normal distribution that is centered at the population mean and has a variance that depends on the sample size and the (co)variance of the underlying population. Both the LLN and CLT have been studied extensively and have many well-known variants, for example that accommodate autocorrelation in the observations.

Monte Carlo methods are the standard strategy used in practice to compute the posterior. They do so by side-stepping the problem of computing the partition function $Z(\mathbf{y})$ and integrals of $p(\boldsymbol{\theta}|\mathbf{y})$ entirely. Instead, they use random draws from the posterior distribution along with the LLN to approximate the desired expectation $\mathbb{E}_{p(\boldsymbol{\theta}|\mathbf{y})}[g(\boldsymbol{\theta})]$. Mathematically, if $\boldsymbol{\theta}_1, \ldots, \boldsymbol{\theta}_N \sim p(\boldsymbol{\theta}|\mathbf{y})$ can be simulated for some large number of Monte Carlo draws N (also called iterations), the desired expectation can be approximated as

$$\bar{g}_N = \frac{1}{N}\sum_{i=1}^{N} g(\boldsymbol{\theta}_i) \approx \mathbb{E}_{p(\boldsymbol{\theta}|\mathbf{y})}[g(\boldsymbol{\theta})], \tag{2.4}$$

which, as $N \to \infty$, converges to the desired expectation $\mathbb{E}_{p(\boldsymbol{\theta}|\mathbf{y})}[g(\boldsymbol{\theta})]$ by the LLN. Furthermore, its accuracy can be gauged via the CLT if desired.

In a sense, the use of Monte Carlo methods in Bayesian statistics swaps one hard problem for another. Instead of computing multidimensional integrals, they rely on the statistician's ability to simulate draws from the desired posterior distribution. Thus, the question becomes: how does one generate/simulate draws from the posterior distribution when it is unknown?

Usually this occurs by using the fact that the posterior is not totally unknown; it is simply incompletely known. Bayes' theorem provides the functional form of the posterior distribution up to some unknown constant: $\tilde{p}(\boldsymbol{\theta}|\mathbf{y}) = l(\boldsymbol{\theta}|\mathbf{y})p(\boldsymbol{\theta})$. Perhaps surprisingly, there is an entire class of sampling algorithms that accommodate simulating draws from an un-normalized probability distribution based on Markov chains. The resulting strategy for computing the posterior is called Markov chain Monte Carlo (MCMC). To understand how MCMC works, however, it first helps to understand a more basic sampling scheme called rejection sampling.

Rejection sampling. Rejection sampling relies on a simple, powerful fact that applies to any distribution: if we are able to sample from the uniform distribution on the volume under the probability density function (PDF), we can convert those draws to draws from the PDF by marginalizing out the height, a nuisance quantity referred to as an "auxiliary" variable (Robert and Casella, 2004, p.47). This is most commonly achieved by sampling from a surrogate proposal distribution whose density $f(\boldsymbol{\theta})$ dominates the target density $p(\boldsymbol{\theta}|\mathbf{y})$ in the sense that there exists an $M \in \mathbb{R}$ such that $p(\boldsymbol{\theta}|\mathbf{y}) \leq Mf(\boldsymbol{\theta})$ for all $\boldsymbol{\theta}$. Since M is arbitrary, the posterior can be replaced with the un-normalized posterior $\tilde{p}(\boldsymbol{\theta}|\mathbf{y})$. To obtain a draw from the target, first draw $\boldsymbol{\theta}' \sim f(\boldsymbol{\theta})$, then $u \sim \text{Unif}(0, Mf(\boldsymbol{\theta}'))$, and assess whether $(\boldsymbol{\theta}', u)$ lies in the volume under $\tilde{p}(\boldsymbol{\theta}|\mathbf{y})$. If so, $\boldsymbol{\theta}' \sim p(\boldsymbol{\theta}|\mathbf{y})$, and if not repeat the process. Thus, "rejection" sampling. This is illustrated in Figure 2.2 using a uniform distribution as the proposal distribution.

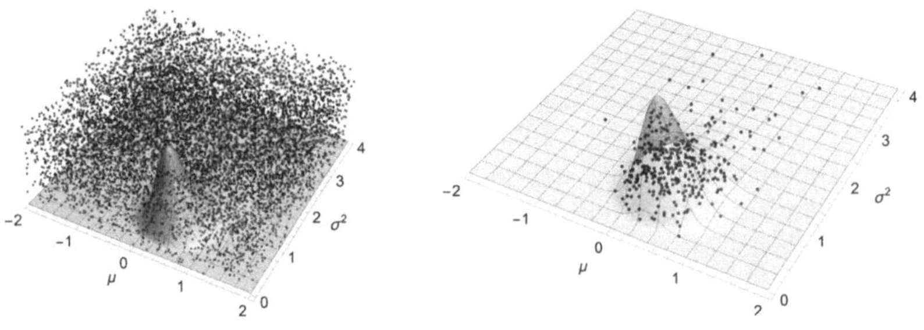

FIGURE 2.2
Rejection sampling is achieved by sampling from the uniform distribution on the volume under $\tilde{p}(\boldsymbol{\theta}|\mathbf{y})$. (Left) $N = 10{,}000$ proposal draws from the uniform distribution over $[-2, 2] \times [0, 4] \times [0, m]$ are illustrated, where $m = \tilde{p}(\hat{\boldsymbol{\theta}}_{MAP}|\mathbf{y})$ is the largest value $\tilde{p}(\boldsymbol{\theta}|\mathbf{y})$ assumes over $\boldsymbol{\Theta}$. (Right) The points that fall under the surface $\tilde{p}(\boldsymbol{\theta}|\mathbf{y})$ are retained. Of these, the (μ, σ^2) components are distributed according to the posterior $p(\mu, \sigma^2|\mathbf{y})$. At less than 4% of draws, this is a very inefficient sampler.

The general problem with rejection sampling is its inefficiency. Unless $f(\boldsymbol{\theta})$ is very similar to $p(\boldsymbol{\theta}|\mathbf{y})$, the algorithm will reject a large proportion of draws, as in Figure 2.2. Worse, as the dimensionality of $\boldsymbol{\theta}$ increases, it becomes increasingly difficult to choose a $f(\boldsymbol{\theta})$ sufficiently similar to $p(\boldsymbol{\theta}|\mathbf{y})$. Thus, the inefficiency of the sampler tends to grow with the number of parameters. As a result rejection sampling is ill-suited for most Bayesian problems. However, rejection sampling is important in two ways. First, it lays a conceptual foundation for many sampling strategies that do not require the target distribution to be normalized. Second, it can be expanded to adaptive rejection sampling (ARS), significantly improving its performance for some target densities (Gilks and Wild, 1992). ARS is particularly helpful in situations where evaluating the target density, here $\tilde{p}(\boldsymbol{\theta}|\mathbf{y})$, is computationally expensive.

Slice sampling. Another strategy used to generate draws from the uniform distribution under the PDF goes by the name slice sampling (Neal, 2003). Slice sampling uses a completely different strategy to sample uniformly under the PDF, one based on a kind of random walk on that space. We begin by describing an algorithm that is not a slice sampler but shares with it the underlying motivation of randomly moving under the surface to sample uniformly from it.

Starting from some initial position $(\boldsymbol{\theta}_0, u_0)$ in the interior of the volume, suppose that we were to obtain a new position under the surface by adding a mean-zero multivariate normal draw with a reasonably small variance. If the point falls outside the volume, we simply discard it and add a different draw, and if it remains inside, we do it again and again to move around under the surface $\tilde{p}(\boldsymbol{\theta}|\mathbf{y})$. Under mild conditions, if we do this for many steps and stop the process, the last position is roughly equally likely to be observed anywhere under the surface. As a consequence, one strategy might be to construct a Markov chain in this way, run it for a long time, and sub-sample the list of visited positions.

Unfortunately this strategy doesn't work well in practice because the proposal distribution that is generating the steps is not well tailored to the target distribution: if the variance is too small, it hardly moves, and if it's too big, it doesn't fit into the tails well and yields draws outside the volume under the surface. It is therefore very inefficient. However, a modification actually works quite well: at each step, simply sample one coordinate at a time from a uniform distribution over the range of possible values holding the others fixed.

For example, starting at a point $(\boldsymbol{\theta}_0, u_0) = (\mu_0, \sigma_0^2, \tilde{p}(\boldsymbol{\theta}_0|\mathbf{y})/2)$, draw μ_1 from the uniform distribution on its range of possible values, which can be determined by solving univariate root finding problems on $h(\mu) = \tilde{p}(\mu, \sigma_0^2|\mathbf{y}) - u_0$. Then do the same on σ^2 for fixed μ_1 and u_0; and do the same for u for fixed μ_1 and σ_1^2. At each step of this sampling scheme the task is equivalent to randomly selecting a point on a line segment in three dimensions: a line segment because two of the dimensions are fixed and the other ranges as much as it can while keeping the segment under the surface. This sampling strategy is called slice sampling; it is illustrated in Figure 2.3. Notice that by construction the sampler will never go outside the volume bounded by the surface and, to an extent determined by the particular shape of the region, is likely to move around it quite efficiently.

Gibbs sampling. Gibbs sampling, one of the most powerful tools for inference for the Bayesian statisticians, can be seen to be a kind of variant and simplification of slice sampling (Geman and Geman, 1984; Gelfand and Smith, 1990; Casella and George, 1992; Gelfand, 2000). It is also the default form of computation used in many Bayesian software platforms.

The slice sampler generally works by iteratively sampling each of the parameters given all the others and the auxiliary variable u in turn. Thus, in our example we sampled from the uniform distributions over $[\mu|\sigma^2, u]$, $[\sigma^2|\mu, u]$, and $[u|\mu, \sigma^2]$ over and over to ultimately obtain uniform draws under the surface $\tilde{p}(\mu, \sigma^2|\mathbf{y})$. The Gibbs sampler takes advantage of two facts: first, that for the long-run behavior, the order of the sampling really doesn't matter; and second, that a clever choice of order admits a nice simplification. The first point is quite clear: in the long run, for sampling uniformly under the surface it doesn't matter whether you sample $(\mu, \sigma^2, u), (\mu, \sigma^2, u), \ldots$, or, say, $(\mu, u), (\mu, u), \ldots, (\sigma^2, u), (\sigma^2, u), \ldots, (\mu, u), \ldots$, the end result will be the same.

And this motivates the second point. Consider the first sequence of steps in the second sampling scheme: $(\mu, u), (\mu, u), \ldots$. One way to think of these is as sampling along the

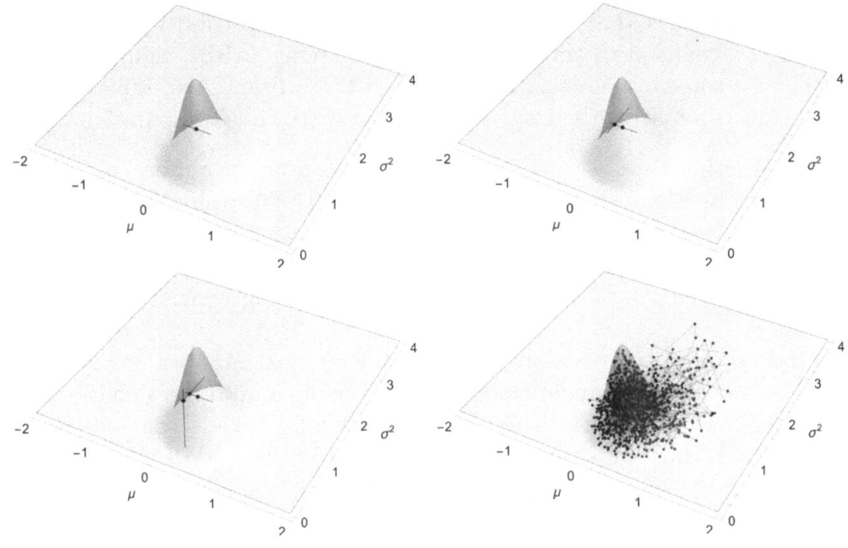

FIGURE 2.3
Slice sampling is performed by iteratively sampling uniformly over the support of each parameter (and u) given the others to generate a Markov chain under the surface $\tilde{p}(\boldsymbol{\theta}|\mathbf{y})$. This is illustrated for the two parameters of our example, along with the auxiliary variable u, along with a collection of $N = 1{,}000$ draws initialized at $\hat{\boldsymbol{\theta}}_{MAP}$ with $u_0 = \tilde{p}(\hat{\boldsymbol{\theta}}_{MAP}|\mathbf{y})/2$.

$\mu - u$-plane leaving σ^2 fixed. Ultimately, u is discarded, so in the end, the resulting draw taken from this, the last μ, can be seen as one draw from the conditional distribution of $[\mu|\sigma^2]$. And similarly for the other sequence: $(\sigma^2, u), (\sigma^2, u), \ldots$ ultimately results in one draw from $[\sigma^2|\mu]$. These distributions are referred to as "full conditionals": they are either one parameter given all the others, or a block of parameters given all of the others. The result is that one iterates oversampling from these full conditionals, reducing a multivariate problem into a sequence of univariate ones or smaller block sampling problems. This is known as Gibbs sampling.

Many cases of practical interest have closed-form full conditionals recognizable as distributions of a particular type, e.g. normal. This significantly simplifies sampling from the full conditionals as one can use off-the-shelf samplers designed for that distribution. In fact, the present scenario is in this category when the prior $p(\boldsymbol{\theta}) = p(\mu, \sigma^2) = p(\mu)p(\sigma^2)$ with $p(\mu)$ normal and $p(\sigma^2)$ inverse-gamma. While these marginal priors are conjugate for their corresponding parameters in the one-parameter case, they are not jointly conjugate, and in fact, the joint posterior does not admit a closed-form. However, the posterior $p(\boldsymbol{\theta}|\mathbf{y}) = p(\mu, \sigma^2|\mathbf{y})$ *can* be sampled from efficiently via Gibbs sampling by iteratively sampling a normal distribution dependent on $\mathbf{y}$ and σ^2 and an inverse-gamma distribution dependent on $\mathbf{y}$ and μ (Lunn et al., 2013, p.67). This is illustrated in Figure 2.4. More generally, in the event that one or more of the full conditionals is not known, that component can be sampled using any other available strategy, such as slice sampling or ARS (Robert and Casella, 2004).

Hamiltonian Monte Carlo. One of the challenges posed by slice and Gibbs sampling for multivariate distributions is that every intermediate transition occurs parallel to the coordinate axes. If the distribution of interest (the posterior) is not aligned with the coordinate axes, the samplers are very inefficient because their intermediate steps are necessarily very

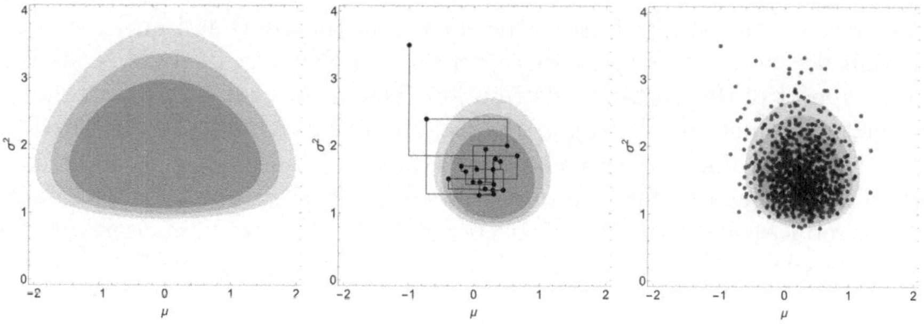

FIGURE 2.4
Gibbs sampling generates draws by iteratively sampling from the full conditional distributions $[\mu|\sigma^2]$ and $[\sigma^2|\mu]$. From left to right: the 80%, 90%, and 95% highest density regions of the independent normal-inverse-gamma prior; the posterior along with 20 draws and the Gibbs paths; and the posterior with 1000 draws. The priors were selected such that $\mathbb{E}_{p(\mu)}[\mu] = 0$ and $\Pr_{p(\mu)}[-2 \leq \mu \leq 2] = .99$, and $\mathbb{E}_{p(\sigma^2)}[\sigma^2] = 1$ and $\Pr_{p(\sigma^2)}[\sigma^2 \leq 4] = .99$, similar to the flat prior.

small. This happens for posteriors with large correlations or strong nonlinear associations, for example.

Both the slice and Gibbs samplers use Markov chains. While both of these are MCMC algorithms, they do not exhibit a signature feature generally associated with MCMC algorithms: proposal of a candidate next value and probabilistic acceptance/rejection of that proposal, similar to rejection sampling. Most MCMC algorithms consist of (1) a starting point $\boldsymbol{\theta}_0$ indicating a particular location in the support of the target posterior distribution $p(\boldsymbol{\theta}|\mathbf{y})$, and (2) a transition kernel K that provides a probability distribution with which to move to from $\boldsymbol{\theta}_0$. The algorithm then advances in two stages: first, the kernel and current location are used to draw a new proposed location in the support, and second, the candidate location is accepted or rejected probabilistically using a criterion that depends on the relative likelihood of the current and proposed locations and each's ability to swap positions. This probabilistic criterion, called the Metropolis or Metropolis-Hastings (MH) probability, guarantees certain technical conditions that are needed for the long-term behavior of the chain to sample from the target (posterior) distribution of interest.[3] This general formulation of the algorithm is called the Metropolis or Metropolis-Hastings algorithm.

Hamiltonian Monte Carlo (HMC) is an MH-style MCMC algorithm that generates proposals based on a kind of physics simulation that uses Hamiltonian dynamics (Duane et al., 1987; Neal, 1995). While the mathematics grows difficult quickly (Betancourt et al., 2017), the basic ideas are surprisingly intuitive, and there are a number of free high-quality expository introductions to the topic, e.g. (Betancourt, 2017; Neal, 2011). HMC simulates Hamiltonian dynamics to generate proposal draws in high probability regions of the posterior. The simulation is equivalent to monitoring the position of a puck imparted with a randomly generated momentum and sliding on a frictionless surface whose height is proportional to the negative log of the target density. The momentum is typically sampled from a tuned multivariate Gaussian. Regions of high probability density are low regions on the surface, and so the puck tends to stay in them even as it slides around the irregularly (but smoothly) shaped surface. After some time, the puck is stopped, and its location is used as the proposed value. Then the standard MH probability is computed, and the draw is

[3]See Casella and Robert (2004) or Roberts and Rosenthal (2004) for a more in-depth perspective.

accepted or rejected in the phase space (position + momentum) and projected back down into the original space, the position space, which in a Bayesian analysis is the parameter space – the support of the posterior distribution. This is illustrated in Figure 2.5.

Under general conditions, as long as the Hamiltonian dynamics are simulated carefully, this process leads to a Markov chain whose stationary distribution is indeed the distribution of interest. Where slice sampling introduces a single auxiliary variable for the sampling process, HMC introduces one auxiliary variable per variable (parameter) of interest representing the momentum of the puck in that dimension, doubling the dimension of the chain's sample space. The momenta variables are discarded at the conclusion of the simulation, resulting in draws from the marginal distribution that is the posterior, just as in slice sampling.

Mathematically, the physics simulation itself is simply a system of ordinary differential equations (ODEs) that evolve in time. These are Hamilton's equations. To generate a proposal, the ODEs are solved numerically using a numerical integrator, with a simple variant of Euler's method known as the leap-frog method sufficient for many problems. The solution is projected forward for some time, stopped, and the proposed value is used.

Like any MCMC algorithm, various tuning parameter values are required in the process, e.g. the fineness of the discretization of the numerical integrator, length of time to project into the future, etc. The No-U-Turn Sampler (NUTS) is a HMC variant that runs the algorithm forward and backward in time to try to avoid inefficient cyclic behavior (Hoffman and Gelman, 2014). Figure 2.5 illustrates HMC for our normal example using the independent normal-inverse-gamma prior used in the Gibbs sampling example.

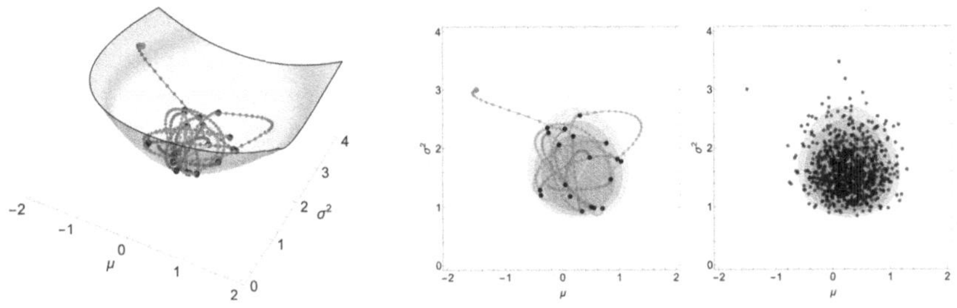

FIGURE 2.5
Hamiltonian Monte Carlo is a Metropolis-Hastings style MCMC algorithm that generates its transitions via a physics simulation of a frictionless puck sliding around on the surface defined by $-\log \tilde{p}(\boldsymbol{\theta}|\mathbf{y})$ after having been imparted with a randomly generated momentum. Using the posterior in the Gibbs sampling example, from left to right we have 3D and 2D plots of $-\log \tilde{p}(\boldsymbol{\theta}|\mathbf{y})$ with 20 draws with their numerically calculated paths initialized at the red point, and 1,000 draws.

2.1.3 Exact Computations of Posterior Approximations

Discretization. The simplest approximation to the posterior is one obtained via discretization. In this scheme, the un-normalized posterior $\tilde{p}(\boldsymbol{\theta}|\mathbf{y}) = l(\boldsymbol{\theta}|\mathbf{y})p(\boldsymbol{\theta})$ is evaluated on a mesh over $\boldsymbol{\Theta}$ (or some subset thereof, if the support is restricted by the prior) and the points are renormalized into a proper discrete multivariate probability mass function; this is illustrated in Figure 2.6 for the flat prior's posterior. Computing probabilities with probability mass functions is a good deal easier than with probability density functions (PDFs), owing to the fact that sums are easier than integrals. Moreover, discretization accommodates complex joint probability statements more easily because sums accommodate implicitly described regions more easily than integration: it is easier to test whether a point is in a region of space than modify an integral's domain of integration.

Computing probabilities with respect to discrete approximations is a matter of brute force and computational power. This method is similar to the Riemann sum strategy described above in numerical integration, but in fact, it is simpler in at least two ways: first, the area of the base need not be determined; and second, the strategy accommodates expectations directly by computing them with respect to the discrete approximation, instead of first approximating $Z(\mathbf{y})$ and then using it in the computation of $\mathbb{E}_{p(\boldsymbol{\theta}|\mathbf{y})}[g(\boldsymbol{\theta})]$. Nevertheless, discretization shares the same drawback as the Riemann sum strategy: it doesn't scale well. It is, however, an interesting reversal of the common statistical strategy of approximating large discrete computations with integrals, such as with the normal approximation to the binomial. In low-dimensional problems with nice parameter spaces, discretization can be an easy, convenient way to get good resolution into low-probability regions of a posterior.

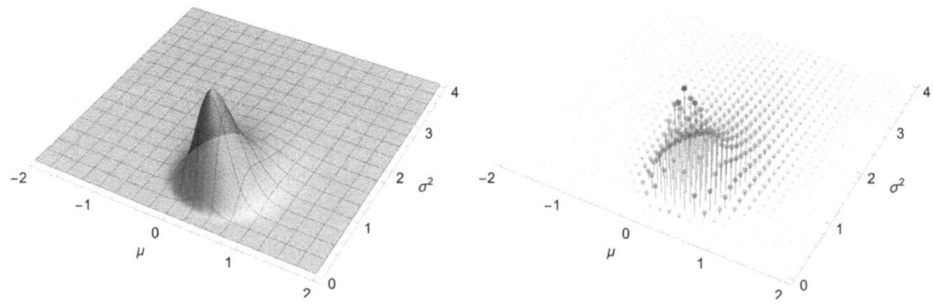

FIGURE 2.6
Discrete approximations to the posterior are easily computed in low-dimensions by gridding the parameter space, evaluating the un-normalized posterior, and renormalizing to obtain a discrete probability distribution. The model, prior, and data are the same as Figure 2.1, making this plot comparable. $N = 30$ points are used in each dimension, and alpha aesthetics are used to improve visibility.

Laplace approximation. Under general regularity conditions, as the sample size n grows, the posterior distribution will be dominated by the data, and the asymptotic behavior of likelihood theory prevails to ensure that the posterior distribution tends to normality. Laplace approximation provides a convenient strategy to approximate the posterior through the following clever trick. In many cases, the maximum value of the posterior, the maximum a-posteriori (MAP) estimator $\hat{\boldsymbol{\theta}}_{MAP} = \arg\max_{\boldsymbol{\theta}\in\boldsymbol{\Theta}} p(\boldsymbol{\theta}|\mathbf{y}) = \arg\max_{\boldsymbol{\theta}\in\boldsymbol{\Theta}} l(\boldsymbol{\theta}|\mathbf{y})p(\boldsymbol{\theta})$ can be obtained using standard strategies from numerical optimization.

Consider the second-order Taylor approximation to the log-posterior at the MAP estimator:

$$\begin{aligned}\log p(\boldsymbol{\theta}|\mathbf{y}) \approx & \log p(\hat{\boldsymbol{\theta}}_{MAP}|\mathbf{y}) + \nabla_{\boldsymbol{\theta}} \log p(\hat{\boldsymbol{\theta}}_{MAP}|\mathbf{y})'(\boldsymbol{\theta} - \hat{\boldsymbol{\theta}}_{MAP}) \\ & + (\boldsymbol{\theta} - \hat{\boldsymbol{\theta}}_{MAP})'\mathbf{D}(\hat{\boldsymbol{\theta}}_{MAP})(\boldsymbol{\theta} - \hat{\boldsymbol{\theta}}_{MAP}),\end{aligned} \tag{2.5}$$

where $\nabla_{\boldsymbol{\theta}} \log p(\hat{\boldsymbol{\theta}}_{MAP}|\mathbf{y})$ is the vector of first derivatives of the log posterior evaluated at $\hat{\boldsymbol{\theta}}_{MAP}$ and $\mathbf{D}(\hat{\boldsymbol{\theta}}_{MAP})$ is the matrix of second derivatives (the Hessian) of the log posterior evaluated at $\hat{\boldsymbol{\theta}}_{MAP}$. Since $\hat{\boldsymbol{\theta}}_{MAP}$ occurs at a critical point of the log-posterior, the linear term vanishes to yield

$$\log p(\boldsymbol{\theta}|\mathbf{y}) \approx \log p(\hat{\boldsymbol{\theta}}_{MAP}|\mathbf{y}) + \frac{1}{2}(\boldsymbol{\theta} - \hat{\boldsymbol{\theta}}_{MAP})'\mathbf{D}(\hat{\boldsymbol{\theta}}_{MAP})(\boldsymbol{\theta} - \hat{\boldsymbol{\theta}}_{MAP}), \tag{2.6}$$

and exponentiating both sizes reveals that

$$p(\boldsymbol{\theta}|\mathbf{y}) \mathrel{\overset{\approx}{\propto}} \exp\left\{\frac{1}{2}(\boldsymbol{\theta} - \hat{\boldsymbol{\theta}}_{MAP})'\mathbf{D}(\hat{\boldsymbol{\theta}}_{MAP})(\boldsymbol{\theta} - \hat{\boldsymbol{\theta}}_{MAP})\right\}, \tag{2.7}$$

where $\overset{\approx}{\propto}$ means "is approximately proportional to." Note that this is the exponential of a quadratic form: $\mathbf{D}(\hat{\boldsymbol{\theta}}_{MAP})$ is simply a constant matrix. Multiplying the leading $\frac{1}{2}$ and the matrix $\mathbf{D}(\hat{\boldsymbol{\theta}}_{MAP})$ by -1, and recognizing the latter to be the observed Fisher information of the posterior reveals that the approximating distribution is, in fact, multivariate normal centered at the MAP estimate $\hat{\boldsymbol{\theta}}_{MAP}$ and with a covariance matrix equal to the inverse of the observed Fisher information of the posterior. This is illustrated in Figure 2.7. Of course, this is a very convenient distribution to deal with, because many things are known about it, in particular exact formulas for marginal and conditional distributions.

Laplace approximation suffers from a few drawbacks. First, the method effectively assumes the posterior is multivariate normal, and thus is unable to capture features of the distribution that the multivariate normal cannot manifest: nonlinear associations, skewness and other forms of asymmetry, etc. Second, the approximated posterior is not parameterization invariant, so selecting a different parameterization may lead to different results. Third, if the strategy is to compute Gaussian probabilities and expectations using properties of Gaussians and related high-quality algorithms, this strategy will fail when considering questions about functions of parameters, as these will transform the questions of interest away from normality. In practice, computing probabilities and expectations with Laplace approximation tends to use Monte Carlo methods, alleviating this concern. Putting these drawbacks aside, Laplace approximation (and its modern variants) can be a fast, effective tool for Bayesian inference.

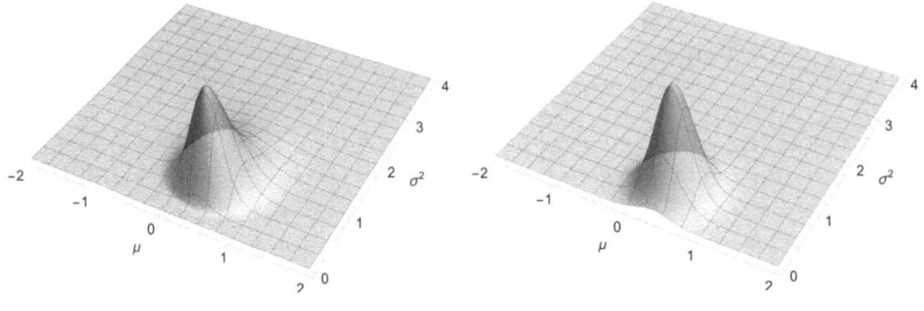

FIGURE 2.7
The Laplace approximation (right) to the posterior (left) is a multivariate normal distribution centered at the posterior mode $\hat{\boldsymbol{\theta}}_{MAP}$ with covariance matrix equal to inverse of the observed Fisher information matrix, i.e. the matrix obtained by taking the Hessian of the log of $\tilde{p}(\boldsymbol{\theta}|\mathbf{y})$. The model, prior, and data are the same as in Figures 2.1 and 2.6, making this plot comparable. Note that the normal distribution cannot model asymmetry in the posterior. In this case, the tail behavior in σ^2 is not captured well and the normal distribution does not respect the boundary constraint that $\sigma^2 > 0$, albeit slightly.

2.2 Bayesian Computation – An Applied Perspective

In this section, we provide very brief descriptions of software implementations commonly used in practice to perform Bayesian data analysis. We begin with coding environments in which one typically conducts Bayesian data analysis and then transition into the software that actually performs the computations.

2.2.1 Generic Coding Environments

Software that enables users to compute the posterior via the previously described methods requires much more than implementations of those methods. In practice, we require an entire ecosystem of tools that can be used to load data, manipulate it, view it, visualize it, modify and transform it, and so on. There are several coding environments that currently play this role.

R. The most popular platform among Bayesian statisticians is R (`https://cran.r-project.org`). A natively interactive computing environment and language, R grew out of the statistical programming language S developed by Bell Labs in the 1970s. It is centrally managed by a core team of developers distributed across the globe and has a collection of modular add-ons called packages distributed on the Comprehensive R Archive Network (CRAN) in a similar fashion to software developed by the GNU project and TEX. CRAN also hosts curated lists of packages called task views oriented toward particular application domains. Bayesian statistics is one of these domains, and the list can be found at `https://cran.r-project.org/web/views/Bayesian.html`. We only describe some of these packages below; the full list of tools is significantly larger.

While R is natively distributed with a simple graphical user interface (GUI), most users interact with R though an integrated development environment (IDE) such as RStudio (`https://www.rstudio.com`) or Visual Studio Code (VSCode, `https://code.visualstudio.com`) that facilitates coding by providing syntax highlighting, linting (light code checking) and styling, and a host of other useful features that help put thought onto the screen. These IDEs are typically distributed under freemium business models that offer free non-commercial use and paid versions with more advanced features through a subscription software as a service (SaaS) model. Traditionally R users have interacted with it via a scripting window and console interface, although that is changing to some extent with the advent of R Markdown (`https://rmarkdown.rstudio.com`), a literate programming document preparation system for creating documents that include R analyses, and R notebooks. Inside R, the `tidyverse` suite of packages provides broad support for most data science tasks (Wickham et al., 2019; Wickham and Grolemund, 2016).

Python. The most popular data science platform overall is powered by the programming language Python (`https://www.python.org`). With a syntax and feel similar to other object-oriented languages (e.g. C++ or Java), Python generally appeals to a broader audience of programmers and, as a useful over-generalization, is popular among data scientists with a more general coding background. It is popular among computer scientists, for example. Developed in the early 1990s, Python is a general purpose programming language, so where R has native data structures and methods for linear algebra and linear models (for example), in Python these come as add-ons called modules such as `NumPy` analogous to R's packages (Harris et al., 2020). Nevertheless, these are very well established and high-quality software, and the two platforms are considered to be more or less equivalent in quality and stature, but not necessarily in capabilities in the sense that the two are used by different communities with interests that overlap substantially but not completely.

Python was originally intended to be used as a scripting language where one would write a `.py` text file containing Python code that would be evaluated top-to-bottom source-style by the Python interpreter, much like shell scripting. Now IDEs enabling interactive use of Python abound, including Jupyter (`https://jupyter.org`), Spyder (`https://www.spyder-ide.org`), and VSCode, and it is common to see both notebook-style programming and scripting window and console-style workflows. RStudio can also be used as an IDE for Python, and this is a common platform for bilingual R-Python users who are using both languages in the same project using the R package interface `reticulate` (Ushey et al., 2021). As its developer base is more decentralized, the Python community does not have a direct equivalent to CRAN, but the Python Package Index (PyPI, `https://pypi.org`) generally fills this role. Because of this disparity, R users often find installing and managing Python modules challenging due to incompatibility of different software versions. Data science distributions, pre-bundled software including the Python interpreter as well as a collection of common modules, such as Anaconda (`https://www.anaconda.com`), exist to try to streamline doing data science with Python, and these are generally a good place to start.

Julia. First released in 2012, Julia (`https://julialang.org`) is another technical computing language growing in popularity among computational scientists in diverse areas, including Bayesian statisticians (Bezanson et al., 2017). While it is still small compared to the large ecosystems of software R and Python have amassed over time, Julia has achieved the kind of "exit velocity" needed for a platform to be considered a long-term viable option for statistical science and Bayesian computing.

Interpreted and interactive like R and Python, Julia prides itself on being both high-level and fast, with performance near compiled languages such as C++, much faster than one could achieve in R or Python for many tasks. As a result, one can program MCMC algorithms in Julia without ever having to leave to a more performant language, and thus the whole code pipeline is more transparent. Indeed, some high-quality Bayesian engines are implemented in Julia itself, but Julia also has bindings to some of the mainstream platforms such as Stan (see below). Like Python, there is not a single IDE that captures most Julia users; Jupyter, VSCode, Atom (`https://atom.io`), and others are common, in addition to some IDEs specifically designed for Julia such as Pluto (`https://github.com/fonsp/Pluto.jl`). Both notebook and scripting window and console workflows are common. Add-on packages are available through a built-in package manager that integrates with the JuliaRegistries General repository on GitHub (`https://github.com/JuliaRegistries/General`), which functions as its dissemination platform.

Others. There are a few other languages/platforms of note in this exposition. SAS (`https://www.sas.com`) has been an industry-leading computing environment for statistical science for 50 years. It is widely considered to provide robust, industry-grade implementations of statistical algorithms, and in fact, has its own suite of sampling software described below. Other computational platforms, smaller by user base among Bayesian statisticians, include Mathematica (Wolfram; `https://www.wolfram.com/mathematica/`), a closed-source, proprietary computer algebra system with very broad capabilities for symbolic computing and data visualization, and Matlab (`https://www.mathworks.com/products/matlab.html`), a closed-source, proprietary computing platform that excels at robust, efficient numerical computing, particularly at scale.

2.2.2 Probabilistic Programming Languages and Other Abstractions

To implement an MCMC procedure yourself, you would need to write a `for()` loop, often a very large `for()` loop, that implements the random walk-like behavior of the procedure. This can become very complicated quickly, is prone to error, and requires a moderate level of expertise to do correctly, so most Bayesian statisticians don't code MCMC algorithms themselves. Instead, they use probabilistic programming languages and other higher-level abstractions that allow them to specify their models without coding the sampling procedures themselves.

A *probabilistic programming language (PPL)* is a kind of domain-specific programming language that is developed specifically for sampling from the distributions of unknowns of a Bayesian model, in most cases its unknown parameters. It is a higher-level language than most other programming languages, which means that it relies heavily on abstraction in order to enable you to express your model in a very simple way and let the computer do the hard work of translating the simple specification into more complex code to do the sampling. Ideally, with a PPL you can focus exclusively on the model itself and leave the sampling details to the PPL. In this section, we discuss a few commonly used PPLs and package/module abstractions used in practice. The list is not intended to be exhaustive but rather a background on the topic and a guidepost to where to learn more.

BUGS and variants. Perhaps the first and most important PPL historically was BUGS ("Bayesian inference using Gibbs sampling"). Initiated in 1989, BUGS was the first mainstream, general purpose platform used for Bayesian modeling (Lunn et al., 2009). This version is now referred to as "ClassicBUGS." It was written in the now-antiquated Modula-2 language, which allowed it to be compiled into a command-line tool that could be run Windows and on some Unix platforms. One of the most important contributions of ClassicBUGS was the language that it used to specify Bayesian models, now simply called BUGS. The BUGS language is a simple declarative language, syntactically similar to the R language, that is used to specify a Bayesian model that can be converted into a directed acyclic graph (DAG). This representation is helpful in conceptualizing the model and implementing the sampler. In the DAG representation, the nodes of the graph represent either data or parameters, and the edges communicate dependencies.

ClassicBUGS used expert systems to analyze a BUGS model specification and automatically create a posterior sampler based on Gibbs sampling. The software classified the full conditional distributions of each node in the DAG according to how it should be sampled/"updated". The sampling strategies were originally quite limited: inverse transform sampling (applying the quantile function to uniform draws), conjugate sampling, and adaptive rejection sampling (ARS).

ClassicBUGS was eventually superseded by two other software projects by the same general group of developers: WinBUGS in 1997 and OpenBUGS in 2005 (`https://www.mrc-bsu.cam.ac.uk/software/bugs/`), both written in Component Pascal (Lunn et al., 2000; Spiegelhalter et al., 2014). The transition from Classic- to Win- to OpenBUGS was essentially an evolution of the same system, the BUGS Project, over time as the developers learned more in an environment that was rapidly changing technologically and expanding theoretically in a context of shifting use cases (Lunn et al., 2009). As the names suggest, one of the prevailing early concerns was portability: the ability to use the same platform on many different kinds of computers in a way that allowed for modular add-ons. OpenBUGS is the most "open" of the three, having an open code base and working cross platform, a feat accomplished with Wine on a Mac. In addition to various programmatic changes, the underlying samplers improved over time as well, notably with the incorporation of the slice sampler and Metropolis-Hastings (MH) algorithm.

Both Win- and OpenBUGS have standalone GUIs; they also have R packages that enable users to perform complete Bayesian analyses without leaving the R ecosystem. The most common of these are the `R2WinBUGS`, `R2OpenBUGS`, and `BRugs` R packages (Sturtz et al., 2005; Thomas et al., 2006). These packages allow you to specify the BUGS code either in a separate file or in the body of an R function[4] along with other sampling parameters to run and monitor the sampler directly from R. It is common to see these packages used in concert with the R package `coda` ("convergence diagnosis and output analysis"), a tool that has been used alongside BUGS implementations since the mid-1990s to analyze the output of the Markov chains.

ClassicBUGS, WinBUGS, and OpenBUGS are no longer maintained, but it is not uncommon to find the latter two still used in practice and in Bayesian literature. A more modern variant, MultiBUGS (`https://www.multibugs.org`), has been proposed by members of the same team with the key new feature of running chains in parallel (Goudie et al., 2020). In the meantime, however, other software packages have developed that offer viable alternatives.

JAGS and NIMBLE. More modern implementations of engines that accept BUGS model specifications are JAGS ("Just Another Gibbs sampler"; `https://mcmc-jags.sourceforge.io`) and NIMBLE ("Numerical Inference for statistical Models using Bayesian Likelihood Estimation"; `https://r-nimble.org`), both designed to be run through R (Plummer, 2003; de Valpine et al., 2017). JAGS and NIMBLE use extensions of BUGS for their specification languages, but the sampling part of the software is different. We refer to the actual sampling part, as opposed to the code you use to specify the model, as the *Bayesian engine.* JAGS and NIMBLE can be thought of as Bayesian engines that use the BUGS specification language, but it is not incorrect or uncommon to refer to JAGS/NIMBLE as both a PPL and a Bayesian engine, and in most cases, the line between the two is blurred.

Originally a self-described clone of WinBUGS, JAGS is written in C++ and was intended to provide better modularity and experimentation, similar goals that OpenBUGS would try to address (Plummer, 2003). First released in the early 2000s, the last major release of JAGS was in 2017 (4.3.0), and the latest patch in 2022 (4.3.1) suggests that it is in the maintenance-only phase of its software life cycle. JAGS is typically used via R through one of a few packages, such as `rjags` and the more flexible `runjags` (Plummer, 2021; Denwood, 2016). While relatively simple, JAGS is a flexible platform that has surprisingly good performance and is a good PPL for those just getting started.

Along with MultiBUGS, the most recent of the BUGS-based implementations that can be considered to be in some sense successors to the older BUGS platforms is NIMBLE. Accessed through R as the package `nimble`, in its basic usage NIMBLE feels very much like a more modern `R2WinBUGS`, `R2OpenBUGS`, or even `rjags`/`runjags`, although it is actually quite a bit more substantial than those packages. NIMBLE decouples the model specification, basic model parsing and querying, and computational inference stages (e.g. the type of sampler used). Model specification is done in an extension of the BUGS language, and the sampling can be done in R or compiled into C++, which performs the sampling stage much faster after an up-front compilation time cost.

Stan. Named after the famous 20th-century physicist and Monte Carlo pioneer Stanislaw Ulam, Stan is perhaps the current standard for high-quality Bayesian computation (`http://mc-stan.org/`). First released in 2012, Stan is a cross-platform software system written in C++ that generally is used as a NUTS-HMC-based sampling engine, but it can also be used for variational inference and penalized maximum likelihood estimation. Key

[4] The basic syntax of BUGS and R code is sufficiently similar for the parser to accept this.

to Stan's success is a novel C++ library for automatic differentiation, an essential tool for efficient and accurate computation of gradients in a manner different than symbolic or numerical differentiation.

A native and perhaps the first HMC-based engine, Stan has many benefits over its competitors: it is older than most current PPLs and so benefits from more extensive use; it has a larger collection of modeling tools, such as numerical integrators for modeling with differential equations; it has a comprehensive set of documentation (more below); and it is has a large active community of developers sufficient to hold an annual conference. It also has some disadvantages. Unlike the BUGS software, it does not support discrete parameter spaces, which can make certain models challenging to implement, notably some model selection problems. It also has to be compiled, but to understand that aspect it helps to first understand its basic workflow.

Like BUGS platforms, Stan works by accepting a model specification, data, and various other parameters (e.g. initial values) and returning draws from the corresponding posterior. Its specification language is also called Stan; it is syntactically similar to C++ but does not require knowing C++. Unlike BUGS, Stan makes a new sampling executable for every new model analysis. That is to say, every time Stan encounters a new model, it down-compiles that model into a machine code executable program that draws samples from the posterior. As a consequence, run-time sampling in Stan is very fast, since it can take advantage of low-level code and model- and machine-specific compiler optimizations. However, the first time a model is run, there is a non-trivial startup cost in compiling the model, usually 15 seconds to a minute or so, maybe more for larger models.

Like other recent PPLs, Stan does not have its own user interface. Instead, it connects to many other computational platforms: R, Python, Julia, bash (i.e. a Linux command-line version), Matlab, Stata, Mathematica, and Scala. It has a surprisingly large support ecosystem, especially for R users: syntax-highlighting and linting in IDEs such as RStudio and VSCode for standalone `.stan` files, and Emacs and VIM plugins. It has a very comprehensive collection of documentation, including a user guide, language reference manual, functions reference, and several volumes of case studies all freely available online. R has an increasingly large number of support packages for Stan developed by the Stan team such as `posterior` and `bayesplot` (Bürkner et al., 2021; Gabry and Mahr, 2021); many of these support the output of other sampling platforms as well. And, like other recent PPLs, Stan is open-source, version controlled with Git on GitHub, free, and has a permissive license.

R abstractions. In addition to the PPL interfaces described above, R has a number of packages that enable and facilitate Bayesian model fitting without having to code in a PPL directly and that more generally support the Bayes paradigm. Two such packages are `brms` ("Bayesian regression models using Stan," `https://paul-buerkner.github.io/brms/`) and `rstanarm` ("applied regression modeling," `https://mc-stan.org/rstanarm/`), both of which accept a model formula syntax similar to the built-in `lm()` and `glm()` functions familiar to R users (Bürkner, 2017; Goodrich et al., 2020). Both use Stan to draw posterior samples for the model in question and summarize them into coefficient estimates with credible intervals. Both are designed for fitting multilevel/hierarchical models and use the base-R formula specification extension provided by `lme4` to express those models (Bates et al., 2015). While there are a number of differences between the two, one of the most direct differences is that `rstanarm` modeling functions come pre-compiled, whereas `brms` functions are first translated into Stan code and then compiled and run with Stan. `rstanarm` makes this possible by providing suites of functions that are named according to their counterparts that are typically used to fit the model using maximum likelihood. For example, instead of base-R's `glm()`, `rstanarm` provides `stan_glm()`.

In addition to these, two other packages are worth noting: `bayesplot` and `posterior`. `bayesplot` accepts a model fit using the packages listed above to create various kinds of visualizations of the posterior using the `ggplot2` plotting system, such as those presented in Chapter 3 (Gabry and Mahr, 2021). `posterior` allows users to extract the draws output from a sampler into a convenient R object such as a data frame. This is useful for generating custom graphics as well as more hands-on manipulation of the sampler's output.

Another interesting addition in the R's Bayesian computation ecosystem is `greta` (`https://greta-stats.org`). `greta` is an R package that provides the same functionality of a PPL, e.g. model specification. Unlike the previously mentioned PPLs, `greta` is entirely implemented in the R language itself, so there is no separate model specification language apart from what is written in R (Golding, 2019). Like Stan, `greta` is an HMC-based sampler. To compute gradients and distribute computations (potentially very significantly distribute computations), it uses the high-quality TensorFlow and TensorFlow Probability engines through Python's interface using the `tensorflow` and `reticulate` R packages (Abadi et al., 2015; Dillon et al., 2017; Allaire and Tang, 2022; Ushey et al., 2021). The result is an interesting and novel approach to Bayesian sampling within R, but as it is quite new, it is not clear how widespread its use will be.

While stochastic strategies are the standard in Bayesian computing currently, a sophisticated variant of Laplace approximation called integrated nested Laplace approximation (INLA) is also available for hierarchical models via the R package `INLA` (Rue et al., 2009; Martins et al., 2013). The methods involve Monte Carlo computations, and so are not fully deterministic but can, in some cases, provide significant speed-ups over MCMC approaches.

Python abstractions. Python also has a substantial Bayesian data analysis community and consequently a corresponding ecosystem of tools for Bayesian computations. Apart from `PyStan`, Python's port to Stan, perhaps the most popular library for Bayesian computation in Python is `PyMC3` (`https://docs.pymc.io/en/v3/`) (Salvatier et al., 2016). `PyMC3` uses a NUTS-HMC-based sampling engine that computes gradients via automatic differentiation with `aesara`, formerly `theano`, similar to how `greta` uses TensorFlow. Also similar to `greta`, `PyMC3`'s implementation is entirely in Python, so users don't need to leave their working environment. Unlike Stan and `greta`, `PyMC3` supports distributions with discrete support using slice and Metropolis-Hastings samplers, and for some projects this presents a significant advantage. To visualize `PyMC3` output, as well as output from other Bayesian computation platforms in Python or Julia, you can use the `ArviZ` module (`https://www.arviz.org`) (Kumar et al., 2019).

Julia abstractions. In addition to the Stan Julia port `Stan.jl`, Julia has several packages for Bayesian computation at various stages of development. Probably the most advanced at the time of this writing is `Turing.jl` (`https://turing.ml`), the flagship package of a suite of packages called `TuringLang` (`https://github.com/TuringLang`). Like `greta` and `PyMC3`, `Turing.jl` is a PPL situated inside another language's environment, here Julia (Ge et al., 2018). `Turing.jl` supports many advanced sampling schemes, including Gibbs sampling, NUTS-HMC, and others, and can support discrete distributions in addition to continuous ones.

SAS abstractions. SAS provides an alternative to the platforms previously discussed for fitting Bayesian models (Chen, 2014; Stokes et al., 2014). The MCMC procedure was initially introduced in SAS/STAT 9.2 in 2009 as an experimental procedure and has been continuously developed since then. While not the only procedure that supports Bayesian computation, it is the most flexible and allows for a diverse collection of sampling algorithms, including Gibbs, Metropolis-Hastings, (NUTS-)HMC, and more, and supports myriad modeling scenarios such as time series, survival, and differential equations. The syntax for PROC

MCMC is similar to PROC NLMIXED. Priors are specified with the `prior` statement, while the model is specified with the model statement. Common families of distributions are included for the model statement, but the user can input their own log-likelihood and use the `general` command to specify new probability distributions.

3

Basic Bayesian Model Checking

John W. Seaman Jr., David J. Kahle, and James D. Stamey
Baylor University: Department of Statistical Science

CONTENTS

3.1 Overview

The Bayesian paradigm affords a remarkably flexible framework for statistical inference. While posterior inference can make use of prior information and avoids the need for large sample approximations required by much of frequentist modeling, there are other practical burdens to bear. Prior distributions must be constructed and justified, requiring acquisition of historical data, elicitation from subject-matter experts, or both. Posterior sensitivity to prior choices must be examined carefully. Iterative simulation methods such as Markov chain Monte Carlo (MCMC) algorithms allow the practitioner to obtain posterior distributions and examine their features with relative ease, but raise questions of convergence. In what follows we provide concise guidelines for checking convergence and questioning prior choices with suggestions for further reading. These items correspond to a subset of what should be reported in a Bayesian analysis. For an extensive discussion about such guidelines see Kruschke (2021) and the literature cited therein.

In Section 3.2 we begin with a "quick kill" list of items allowing a rapid assessment of convergence and a list of "due diligence" checks on model features. Each item in these lists refers to a more elaborate discussion in subsequent sections. In Section 3.3 we consider convergence issues in more detail. Posterior accuracy and suitability are discussed in Section 3.4. The justification of prior distributions and prior-to-posterior sensitivity is covered in Section 3.5. We conclude with a brief look at model performance assessment in Section 3.6.

3.2 "Quick Kill" and "Due Diligence" Checks

We have found the following items to be essential in assessing convergence. The list can be used by the modeler, or in evaluating a model constructed by others. Often, a lack of

DOI: 10.1201/9781003255093-3

convergence can be spotted very quickly. The "quick kill list" can be used to rapidly detect a lack of convergence for the MCMC algorithm. If any of them do not hold, then failure to converge to a stable distribution, model identifiability, or other problems should be investigated. The "due diligence" list details key model features that should always be examined carefully. We consider each in more detail in subsequent sections. The numbers cited below indicate numbered comments within each section.

Quick Kill Checklist:

1. Kernel density plots of the posterior marginals should be relatively "smooth". See 3, Section 3.3.
2. History or trace plots should exhibit good "mixing". See 2, Section 3.3.
3. Autocorrelation plots should dampen quickly. See 6, Section 3.3.
4. Brooks-Gelman-Rubin diagnostic plots should approach 1. See 8, Section 3.3. This assumes the modeler employed at least two chains. (Multiple chains are recommended, starting from "overdispersed" initial values.)
5. For fully identified models, prior-to-posterior comparisons (as in 3, Section 3.3, and comment 4 in Section 3.5) should reveal change from the prior to the posterior. That is, the prior should be "updated" by the data. Models that are not fully identified, such as purposefully over-parameterized measurement error models, are exceptions.
6. Interval estimates for parameters of interest should be sufficiently narrow to be of practical use. See 3, Section 3.4.
7. For priors with interval support, the corresponding posterior density plot should not exhibit mass "piling up" near either endpoint without reason. See 4d of Section 3.5.

Due Diligence Checklist:

1. Prior choices should be justified, whether based on expert opinion or historical data. Commensurability of the current data with historical data sets used in constructing the prior should be examined. Independence assumptions in prior construction should be justified. See Section 3.5.
2. If informative priors are used, the prior equivalent sample size and prior predictive probability of success should be reported. If either is "too large," then the prior might be too influential. See 5 in Section 3.5.
3. Prior-to-posterior sensitivity should be examined. See 4b and 4c in Section 3.5.
4. Where "diffuse" or "non-informative" priors are used on parameters, induced priors on functions of those parameters should be examined, as they may be unintentionally informative. See 7 in Section 3.5.
5. Model characteristics such as the use of fixed vs random effects, constant error variances, exchangeability assumptions, and identifiability should be noted and justified. See 4a of Section 3.5.
6. The model should be tested using simulated data representing various truth scenarios. The prior predictive distribution is particularly useful for this purpose. See Section 3.6.

3.3 Basic Convergence

Before MCMC samples can be used for inference, the chains from which they are drawn must be checked for convergence. By "convergence" we mean that the chain has progressed sufficiently that subsequent draws can be considered approximately distributed as the target posterior. To help assess convergence of the MCMC algorithm for a model, there are several things to consider.[1]

1. The number of chains, their initial values, burn-in length, and subsequent chain length should be noted. How the initial values were chosen should be detailed. See Lunn et al. (2013), p. 70ff, or Carlin and Louis (2008), pp. 158-159.[2] Attempts to dampen autocorrelation such as thinning should be noted, as discussed in 6 below. The use of over-relaxation to speed convergence should be indicated.
2. Trace (history) plots including all chains should be provided for each parameter. These plots can indicate problems with convergence. Chain lengths needed for convergence may vary across parameters and starting values. Examples for good and bad single chains are shown in Figures 3.1 (left) and 3.2. Figure 3.3 exhibits trace plots for multiple chains. Trace plots suggest a sufficient number of iterations for convergence if they "mix". That is, the plots of the individual chains merge after convergence.[3]
3. Histograms and kernel density estimates of all marginal priors and corresponding marginal posteriors should be examined.[4] Functions of model parameters (e.g. hazard ratios or ED50's) will require computation of induced priors via separate simulation. The "smoothness" of a kernel-density estimate (KDE) can suggest the extent of convergence, as illustrated in Figure 3.1. This is a subjective assessment and will depend on graphics options, such as features of the KDE. We recommend that histograms be examined as well because kernel density smoothers can yield misleading results, especially where there are large probability concentrations in a relatively small subset of the support.
4. To gauge the prior's influence on the posterior, it helps to make comparisons to a posterior obtained with a relatively diffuse prior on the same parameter. Alternatively, the maximum likelihood estimate of the parameter can be indicated on the posterior plot. This is approximately the posterior mode under a very diffuse prior for that parameter and suggests what the data "says" without prior influence.
5. Estimates of posterior means and quantiles should stabilize with increasing chain length. To check this, plot the posterior mean and, say, two quantiles of interest, as depicted in Figure 3.4. See Rosner et al. (2021), p. 104ff and Section 3.4.
6. MCMC algorithms produce correlated iterates, by construction. Thus, autocorrelation plots for each parameter should be examined. As autocorrelation in the chain increases, requisite chain-lengths required for convergence and subsequent inference also increase. That is, the effective sample size from the posterior is

[1]For a more detailed development, see Gelman and Shirley (2011).

[2]For an alternate view on the use of multiple chains see, for example, Geyer (2011), who recommends the use of single, very long chains.

[3]See Rosner et al. (2021), Section 4.4.5 for a thorough discussion of this and other aspects of convergence diagnostics. See also Gelman et al. (2013), Section 11.4, and Carlin and Louis (2008), p. 156ff.

[4]Such plots may be problematic if the prior is extremely diffuse compared to the posterior; that is, the relative maxima of prior and posterior densities may make plotting difficult.

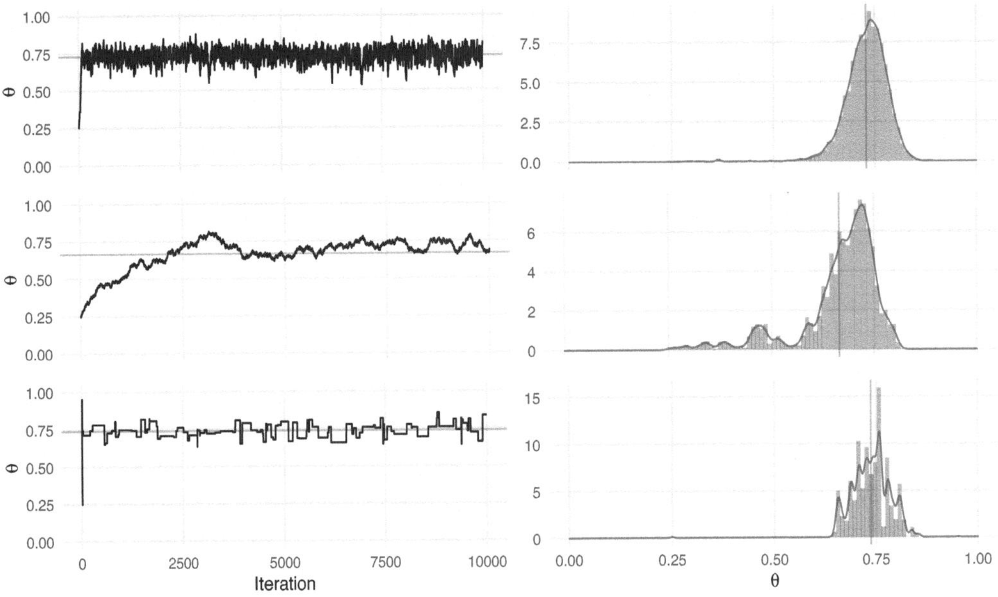

FIGURE 3.1
Trace plots along with histograms and KDEs for three different chains. At the top, a well-behaved chain yields a relatively smooth KDE. The poor convergence depicted in the middle and bottom trace plots results in correspondingly rough KDEs.

reduced as autocorrelation in the chain increases. It is often helpful to center continuous covariates. Autocorrelation can be alleviated by thinning, that is, retaining only every kth iterate, where k is typically similar to the lag required to dampen autocorrelation evident in plots such as these. Such thinning should be reported. However, thinning necessarily decreases the amount of information in the MCMC sample. See Figure 3.5 for an illustration.

7. Parameters can be dependent *a posteriori* even when corresponding priors are constructed to be independent. If parameters are highly dependent, using posterior marginals for inference can be problematic. See, for example, Carlin and Louis (2008), p. 159. Thus, it is prudent to examine bivariate plots for each pair of the parameters. This can be done, for example, by exporting the chains to R and use the `pairs()` function in the `GGally` package, which employs `ggplot2` graphics. See Figure 3.6.

8. In general, multiple chains should be run starting at over-dispersed initial values. After convergence, the within-chain variability should resemble the between chain variability. The Brooks-Gelman-Rubin (BGR) diagnostic assesses between- and within-chain variability and should be plotted. The R package `coda` computes this diagnostic using the `gelman.diag` function and plots can be constructed with `gelman.plot`. Figure 3.7 provides an illustration. See, for example, Rosner et al. (2021), p. 108ff,

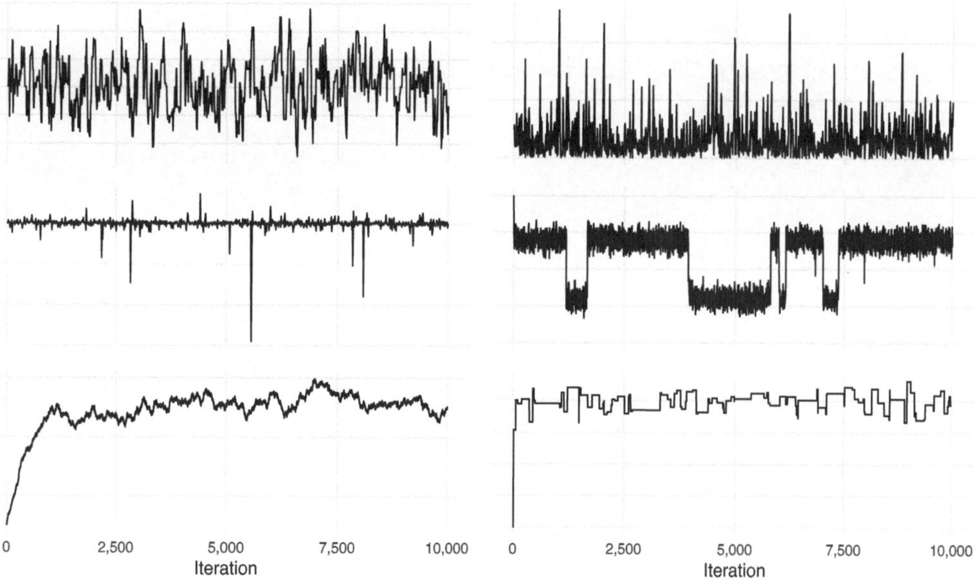

FIGURE 3.2
History (trace) plots for a hypothetical parameter. Top left: The chain appears to have converged to a symmetric stable distribution; Top right: This chain appears to have converged to a positively skewed distribution; Middle left: The chain has converged to a heavy-tailed distribution; Middle right: This chain exhibits poor mode switching from a bimodal target distribution; Bottom left: Here, burn-in values (the "tail" on the left) should be discarded and high autocorrelation is slowing convergence. Bottom right: This trace suggests an inefficient sampler due to a proposal distribution with an overly large variance. This is a frequent problem when using standard Metropolis-Hastings algorithms in Bayes problems for which probability mass is concentrated around a relatively low-dimensional subset of a high-dimensional space.

3.4 Posterior Accuracy and Suitability

Markov chain Monte Carlo algorithms produce a Markov chain from which posterior samples can be drawn. However, the chain length must be sufficient to adequately represent its stationary distribution. How we recognize adequate chain length is as much of an art as a science. In fact, we must manage a compound approximation here. The chain must be long enough that new iterates may be considered as sampled from the posterior (the stationary distribution) and the number of subsequent iterates must be large enough to adequately approximate the posterior feature of interest. That is, once "convergence" obtains, we must run the chain long enough to obtain a good approximation of the posterior feature of interest.

1. To assess such approximation goals, the Monte Carlo standard error (MCSE) and the posterior standard deviation should be included for each parameter. A rule of thumb is that the chain should extend beyond convergence long enough to

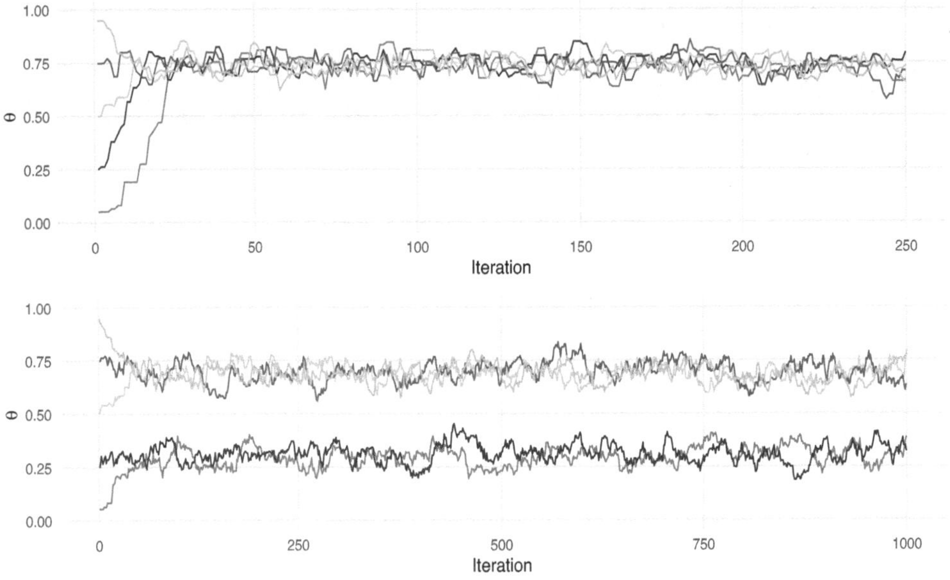

FIGURE 3.3
History (trace) plots for multiple chains from the posterior of a parameter. Top: These five chains exhibit good mixing after a burn-in of about 50 iterations. Bottom: Poor mixing of the plots is evident for these five chains, even after burn-in iterations.

render the MCSE no more than 5% of the posterior standard deviation for the parameter. See Cowles (2013), pp. 137-138, and Lunn et al. (2013), p. 77ff.[5]

2. For a visual assessment, plot posterior summary values (mean, standard deviation, percentiles) as a function of chain-length. Once all such summaries have stabilized within prescribed boundaries, chain length adequate for accuracy can be said to have been attained. This is illustrated in Figure 3.8. See, for example, Lunn et al. (2013), p. 79. The chain lengths you utilize should be at least that required by the most "demanding" parameter.
3. Interval estimates for parameters of interest should be sufficiently narrow for practical purposes. For a fixed sample size, this need must be carefully balanced against the justifiability of informative priors. Priors can usually be made sufficiently informative as to render credible sets arbitrarily narrow. However, doing so may result in unreasonably high prior probability of study success, or unrealistically large prior effective sample size. For more on justification of priors, see Section 3.5.

3.5 Prior Justification and Prior-to-Posterior Sensitivity Analysis

The posterior distribution clearly depends on both the choice of data model and the joint prior distribution. The former is an issue for any approach to modeling. The latter is

[5]A more extensive discussion is provided in Flegal et al. (2008).

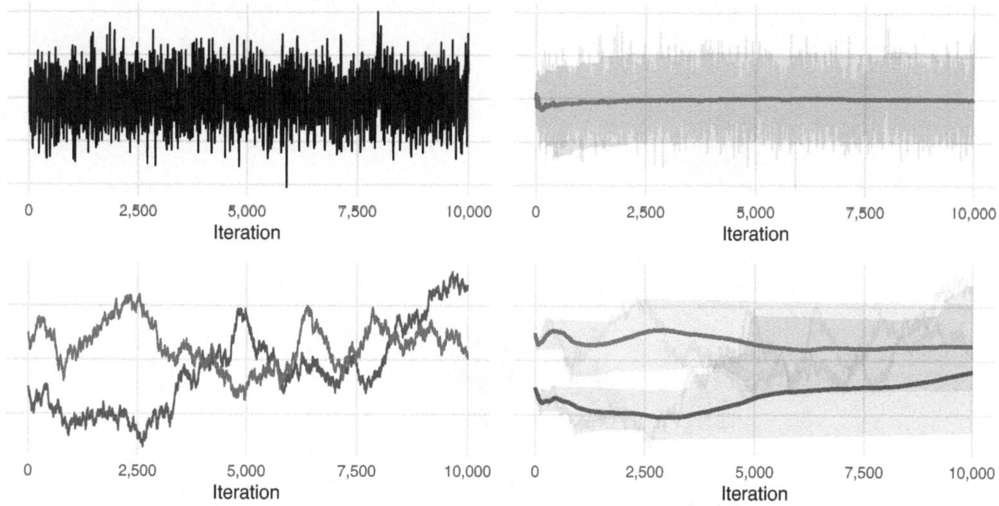

FIGURE 3.4
History (trace) plots of two chains that start at different values along with their mean and quantile plots. Top left: The trace of two well-behaved chains. Top right: The corresponding history plot of posterior means and quantiles, all well-behaved. Bottom left: Two chains exhibiting poor mixing and high autocorrelation. Bottom right: The corresponding badly behaved mean and quantile plots.

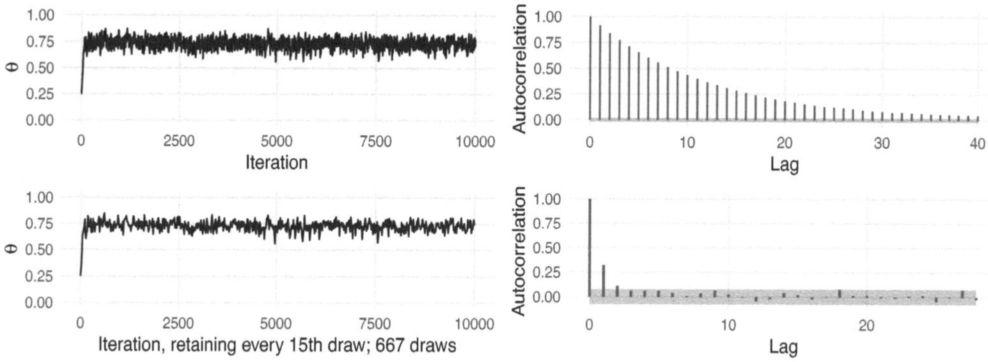

FIGURE 3.5
The trace displayed in the upper left plot exhibits possibly problematic correlation, as revealed in the autocorrelation function plot at top right. Thinning at $k = 15$ or or so will render the autocorrelation negligible, as seen in the autocorrelation function plot depicted bottom right. However, such thinning reduces the effective sample size to 667 draws for inference, down from 10,000.

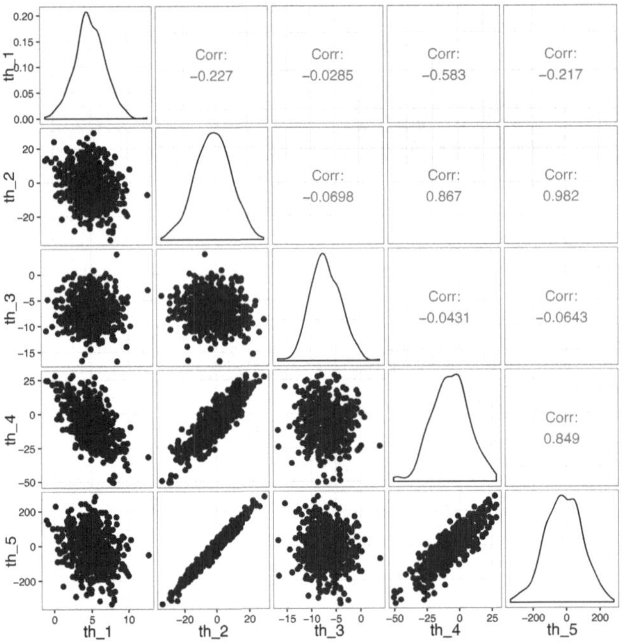

FIGURE 3.6
Scatter plots of posterior samples from pairs of five parameters. Parameter pairs $(\theta_1, \theta_4), (\theta_2, \theta_4), (\theta_2, \theta_5)$, and (θ_4, θ_5) are evidently dependent.

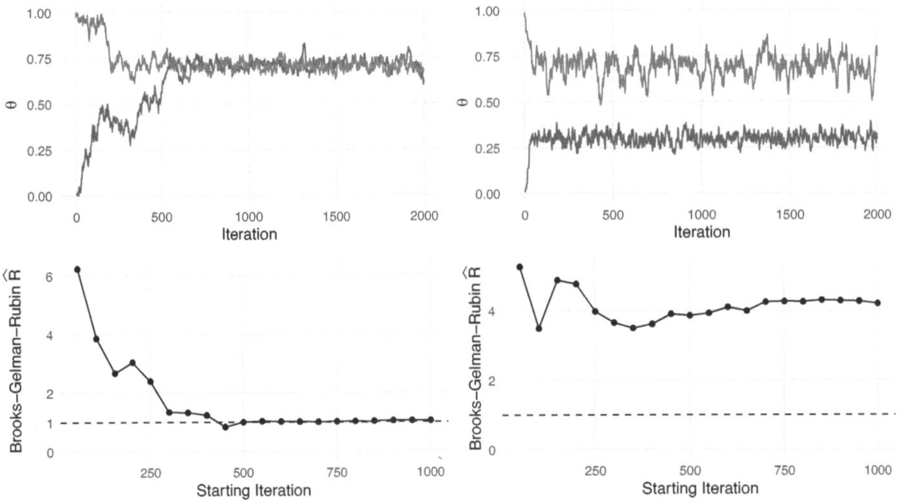

FIGURE 3.7
Brooks-Gelman-Rubin plots for two chains. The left column exhibits two chains with good mixing as indicated by the BGR plot, which converges to 1 at about the 500th iteration. The right column also shows two chains, however mixing does not occur within the depicted chain length. Note that the BGR plot does not apporach 1.

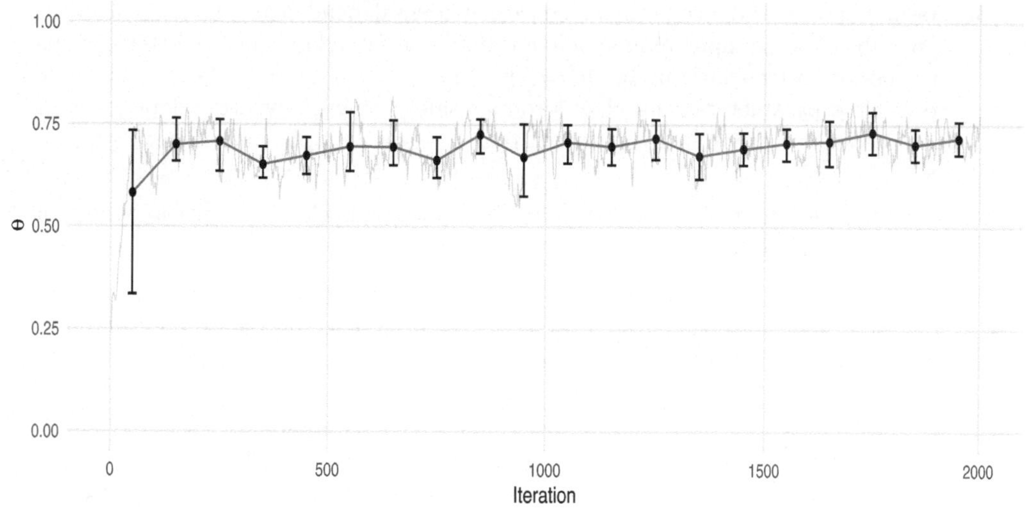

FIGURE 3.8
Posterior means plotted as a function of iterations.

unique to Bayesian methods. Priors should be carefully justified, even if using relatively non-informative priors. Furthermore, posterior results should be reasonably robust with respect to prior choices. That is, "small" changes in the joint prior structure should not produce "large" changes in posterior results. Thus, checking the sensitivity of focal posterior results to changes in the prior structure is a necessary task in Bayesian model building. The list below provides guidance for prior-to-posterior sensitivity analyses.[6]

1. The choice of each prior distribution should be justified.
   (a) Justification is needed even for relatively non-informative (diffuse) priors on parameters, especially if functions of those parameters are of interest, as their induced priors may, in fact, be informative. See 7 below.
   (b) Furthermore, priors intended to be relatively non-informative can be chosen to be unnecessarily diffuse, sometimes resulting in convergence problems. For example, suppose a relatively non-informative prior is desired for the mean shelf-life (in years) of a drug product. A normal prior with a standard deviation of 100 years is surely overly diffuse. For more on this, see 4d and 4e below.
2. Parameters are often given independent priors for convenience, especially if relatively non-informative priors are desired. Assuming independent priors for a normal mean and variance may be quite plausible in many situations, for example, as might modeling variance components as independent. Of course, *a priori* independence need not yield *a posteriori* independence. Examining posterior plots of pairs of parameters can be revealing, even when independent priors are used, as we saw in 7 of Section 3.3. Strong posterior bivariate relationships suggest that modeling dependency in the joint prior might have afforded more efficient use of the data.

[6] More formal approaches have been considered in the literature. Such methods are beyond the scope of this document. For a good brief overview of formal methods see Roos et al. (2015). In addition, they offer a relatively practical approach to formal sensitivity analysis that has the virtue of reproducibility.

3. Assuming independence in the presence of evident dependencies should be avoided if possible. For example, monoclonal antibodies are well known to be heterogenous because of postranslational modifications (Yang, 2017). It would be unreasonable to assume parameters related to product safety or efficacy are independent of parameters corresponding to variants that have distinct pharmacokinetic properties.

4. Gauging the influence of the prior on the posterior is clearly a critical aspect of Bayesian inference.

   (a) It may be that the posterior is little changed from the prior for some parameters. Indeed, in the absence of MCMC convergence problems, identifiability issues manifest themselves in the failure of a prior to be updated *a posteriori*.

      i. That is, the posterior for the unidentified parameter looks pretty much like the prior, with the same location and dispersion. In effect, as Robert (2007)(page 24) notes, "An important aspect of the Bayesian paradigm in non-identifiable settings is ... that the prior distribution can be used as a tool to *identify* the parts of the parameter that are not covered by the likelihood, even though the choice of prior may have a bearing on the identifiable part."

      ii. An important consequence of a lack of identifiability when implementing iterative simulation methods like the Gibbs sampler is the possibility of "drifting". If the prior on a parameter is not informative, then trajectories of the Markov chain for components of that parameter may drift to extreme values. The diffuse prior structure offers no centering effect. This can compromise convergence assessment and yield inaccurate estimates.

      iii. There is nothing about the mechanics of Bayesian inference that requires indentifiability in models. In fact, no statistical methodology is immune from its consequences. In Bayesian inference, nonidentifiability may cause convergence issues with MCMC methods, as noted above. One area in which Bayesian methods provide a considerable advantage in the presence of nonidentified parameters is models with mismeasured variables. Gufstafson (2004)(page 55) notes that

         "An interesting facet of Bayesian inference is that in one sense it 'works' whether or not one has parameter identifiability. That is, the mechanics of forming a posterior distribution and obtaining parameter estimates from this distribution can be carried out equally well in nonidentifiable situations, modulo some technical concerns about MCMC... Of course in another sense no form of inference can work in a nonidentifiable model, as estimators which tend to true parameter values do not result. One intuitive way of thinking about Bayesian inference in the absence of parameter identifiability is that the prior distributions play more of a role than usual in determining the posterior belief about the parameters having seen the data."

   (b) Small changes in prior location or scale should result in small corresponding posterior changes. In particular, slightly altering the prior should not change decisions based on the posterior.

   (c) The effect of substantial changes in the prior should also be examined. It can be useful to compare posterior results under vague ("relatively non-informative" or "diffuse"), skeptical, enthusiastic, clinical (i.e., expert-elicited), and just-significant (i.e., barely meeting success criteria). For

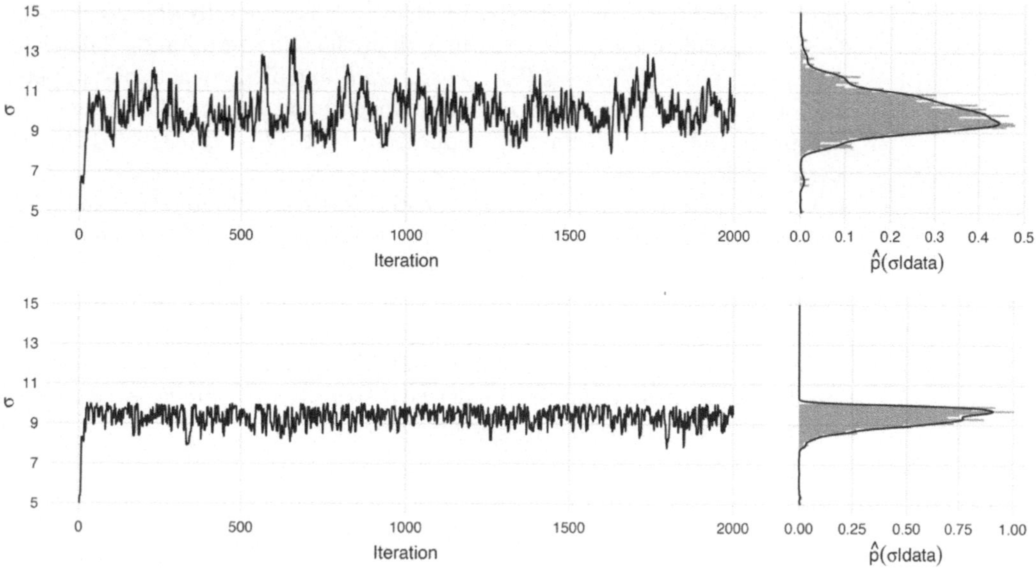

FIGURE 3.9
Posterior plots for a standard deviation with a $U(0, B)$ prior. The KDEs are approximate marginal posteriors for the standard deviation. In the lower plot, $B = 10$, resulting in a "pile-up" of probability mass at that bound. In the upper plot, $B > 14$, resulting in a reasonable posterior plot.

examples of such "archetypal" priors see Lesaffre and Lawson (2012) and Lunn et al. (2013). The latter illustrates use of skeptical priors in two clinical trials, and an enthusiastic prior for another. Spiegelhalter et al. (2004) discuss the use of skeptical priors at length.

(d) Assumptions made about variance components can greatly affect posterior results. Choosing priors on such parameters is highly problem-dependent. Gamma priors for precision and inverse-gamma priors for variances, both with very small shape parameters (e.g., 0.001), were once widely used. However, they are now known to be problematic (Gelman, 2006; Gelman et al., 2013). Alternatives, such as half-normal, half-t, or uniform distributions on standard deviations are often preferable. Placing a uniform prior with support $(0, B], B > 0$, on a standard deviation requires specification of the upper bound, B. This choice should be large enough to prevent probability mass from "piling up" at B. See Figure 3.9 for an illustration.

(e) Justification of priors on variance components should be done in terms of standard deviations, arguing from operational scales.

i. As an example, for prediction of shelf-life in accelerated studies, a log-linear regression model for reaction rate can be used. Faya et al. (2016) suggest a Bayesian approach to fitting such models, employing a uniform prior on the error standard deviation, σ_L, with support $(0, B]$. Suppose the stability-limiting drug characteristic is potency loss, and the aim is to estimate the time required for 10% degradation at 25°C.

ii. It is typically expected from a prudent drug manufacturer that the process tolerance is inside the time-zero release limits. That is, $(URL - LRL) > 6\sigma$ or $(URL - LRL)/6 > \sigma_L$, where URL and LRL denote the upper and lower release limits, respectively. Moreover, it is generally the case that shelf-life specification limits are wider than the time-zero limits. That is, $(USL - LSL) > (URL - LRL)$, where USL and LSL denote the upper and lower shelf-life limits, respectively Murphy and Hofer (2002). Thus, a reasonable choice for B for this application is $(USL - LSL)/6 = (110 - 90)/6 = 3.33$.

iii. As another illustration, suppose the posterior feature of interest is an 80% credible interval on some parameter for which a Uniform$(0, B)$ must be specified. It is straightforward, if computationally intensive, to perform a sensitivity analysis *a posteriori* to verify that the choice of B has not impacted posterior inference. We illustrate this in Figure 3.10. To aid in choosing B, a similar examination might be performed *a priori* using samples drawn from the prior predictive distribution. A similar sensitivity analysis can be performed for any prior parameter.

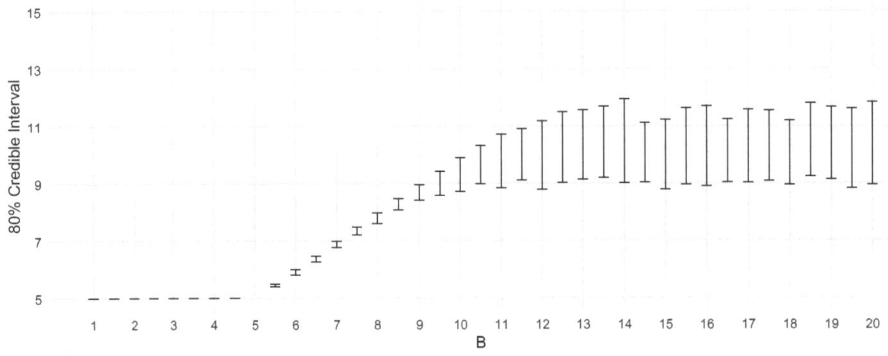

FIGURE 3.10
Prior-to-posterior sensitivity analysis for a parameter with a Uniform$(0, B)$ prior. The model is refit for each value of B, so this is a potentially computationally intensive task. The widths appear to stabilize beyond $B \approx 13$.

5. The prior effective sample size (ESS) is an important and intuitive measure of prior informativeness. See Morita et al. (2008, 2010, 2012) and the R code referred to therein. This ESS approximates the sample size that would be necessary to achieve similar posterior results if a vague prior structure had been used. Following the FDA (2010) guidance on the use of Bayesian methods in device trials, the prior probability of study success should be carefully considered.

6. The use of large historical studies in prior construction can yield inappropriately small prior variances with correspondingly high posterior influence. Methods such as power priors can be used to attenuate this influence (see, for example, Ibrahim et al. (2015) and Neuenschwander et al. (2009)). Power priors effectively attenuate the variance of the resulting prior. In the normal sampling case, for example, attenuation is by a factor of $1/a_0$, $0 < a_0 < 1$. Clearly, a_0, known as the power parameter, must be very carefully chosen. One can plot the prior probability of study success against values of a_0 to assess the power parameter's influence. Computing the prior ESS as a function of a_0 is another approach. See Figure 3.11 for illustrations. Again see the papers by Morita et al. (2008, 2010, 2012). See

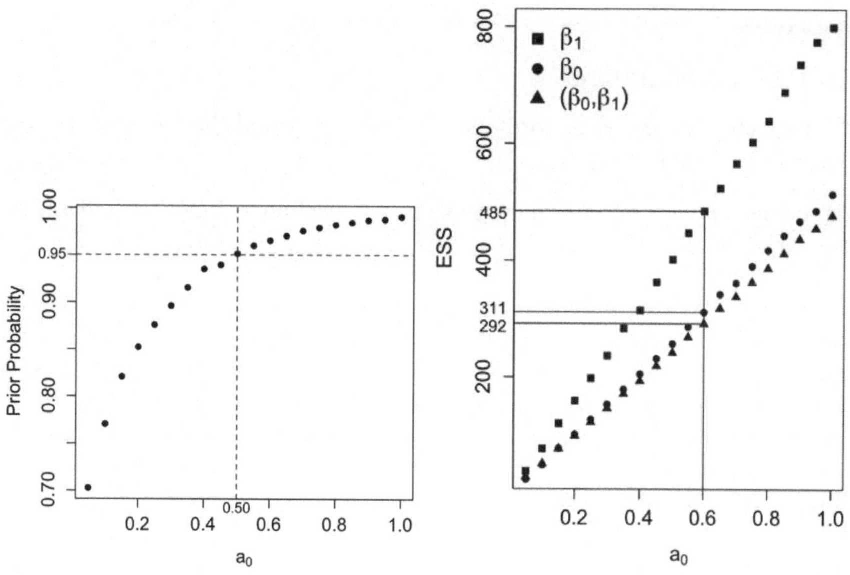

FIGURE 3.11
Two methods for justifying the choice of a fixed power parameter, a_0, when using power priors. In the plot at left, the prior probability of success for some model is plotted against values of the power parameter, a_0. The value of a_0 can be chosen so as to achieve a prior probability of success no larger than some specified value. In this case, all values of a_0 yield relatively large values for the prior probability of study success. In the plot at right, we have illustrated selection of a_0 with respect to prior ESS. Here, prior ESS is computed for each parameter, as well as the joint parameter, for a hypothetical two-parameter model. Selection of $a_0 = 0.6$ corresponds to a prior ESS of approximately 292 for the vector parameter.

also FDA (2010), pp. 26, 39. Thompson et al. (2021) introduce a new measure of similarity between the current and historical data that limits similarity by a pre-specified margin.[7]

7. Induced priors should be examined carefully. Suppose you construct a joint prior on a parameter vector $\boldsymbol{\theta} \in \Theta$. Let $\varphi(\boldsymbol{\theta})$ be a function of interest. If φ is a linear function, and the elements of $\boldsymbol{\theta}$ are given, say, independent diffuse normal distributions, then $\varphi(\boldsymbol{\theta})$ can be expected to be diffuse. However, if $\varphi(\boldsymbol{\theta})$ is nonlinear, the induced prior may be very, and unintentionally, informative. See Seaman, J. III et al. (2012).

8. If several models are under consideration, sensitivity analyses should precede model selection. Model choice involves deciding which among several models is most appropriate.[8] Candidates may differ in both their data models (likelihood functions) and corresponding prior structures.·The candidate models should each have been subjected to a sensitivity analysis *before* the selection process.

---

[7]Many other methods for handling a_0 have been proposed. The R package `BayesPPD` (Shen et al., 2022) facilitates use of the normalized power prior and computation of power and type I error rates. For an overview, see Shen et al. (2021).

[8]Or the use of more sophisticated methods such as Bayesian model averaging or mixture models.

3.6 Model Performance

A thorough treatment of model performance analysis is beyond the scope of this guide, but here are some brief comments.

1. A Bayesian model requires specification of a likelihood function, $l(\boldsymbol{\theta}|\mathbf{x})$, for parameter vector $\boldsymbol{\theta} \equiv (\theta_1, \ldots, \theta_p)$ and data $\mathbf{x}$, as well as a joint prior structure, $p(\boldsymbol{\theta})$. The joint probability distribution, $f(\mathbf{x}|\boldsymbol{\theta})$, associated with the likelihood function can be used to simulate data sets, with parameter values generated using a joint "design prior," $p_D(\boldsymbol{\theta})$, analogous to Bayesian sample size determination.[9] Location of the design prior is chosen to reflect θ_i values of interest. Dispersion parameters for $p_D(\boldsymbol{\theta})$ are chosen to reflect uncertainty about which values of the θ_i's will obtain in an experiment. For each generated data set, the model is fit using the joint prior, $p(\boldsymbol{\theta})$. More than one design prior can be chosen to represent different scenarios, e.g., optimistic or skeptical.
2. Testing a model under various truth scenarios (values of $\boldsymbol{\theta}$) in the fashion described above can result in hundreds or even thousands of MCMC runs. Clearly not all can be checked for convergence, but we recommend doing so for a small subset of such runs, chosen to represent the range of parameters generated by the design prior.
3. Summarizing the results of testing a model across multiple model characteristics (diffuse priors vs informative priors, for example) and/or truth scenarios can be done compactly with graphical tools. A particularly useful graphical summary can be constructed like that illustrated in Figure 3.12.

[9] See, for example, Brutti et al. (2008) for more detail.

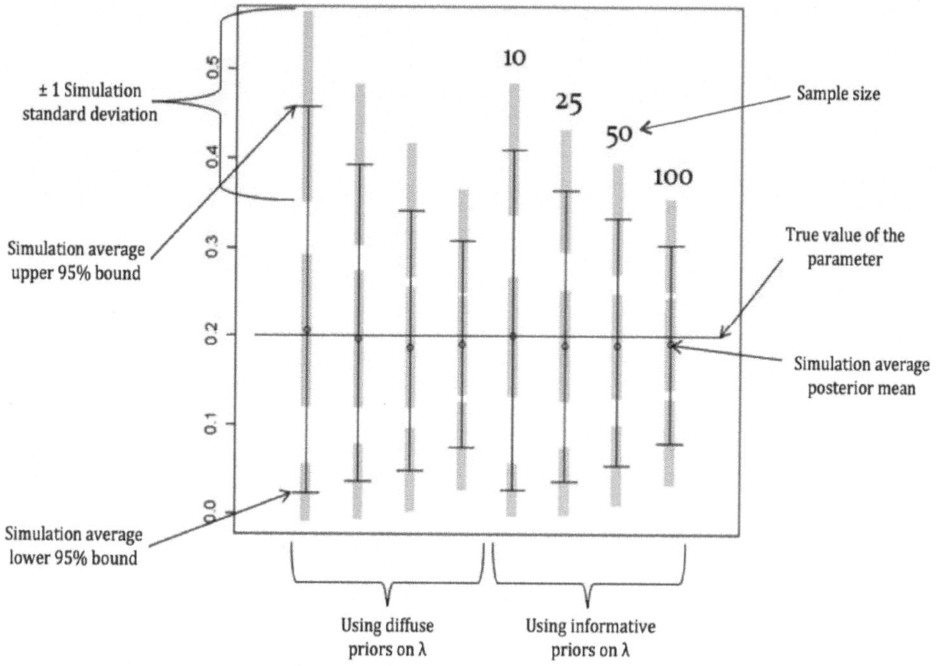

FIGURE 3.12
Simulation summary plot for 500 samples simulated to study model performance under a single truth scenario, indicated by the horizontal line at 0.2. In this case, the plot compares model performance for a diffuse prior structure to an informative prior structure for a hypothetical parameter, λ, at various simulated sample sizes. Each vertical bar summarizes the results of multiple simulations. Included are the average of 500 posterior means, 500 upper and lower 95% credible set bounds, and associated ± 1 simulation standard deviation bars (in gray). In some cases, simulation and/or posterior medians or other measures may be preferred to simulation averages.

4

Quantitative Decision-Making, a CMC Application to Analytical Method Equivalence

Misbah Ahmed

Early Development Statistics, GSK

Mike Denham

CMC Statistics, GSK

CONTENTS

4.1 Introduction

In-vitro analytical methods are developed and validated in Research and Development (R&D) in order to ensure the identity, strength, quality, purity, and potency of the drug substance and drug product. During drug development, sufficient information is required at each phase to demonstrate the above for each batch used in clinical studies. When submitting an application for approval by a regulatory authority, the applicant must detail the analytical methods necessary to demonstrate that the commercially manufactured product meets prescribed standards. Before the launch of the asset these validated methods are typically transferred out to manufacturing sites via a transfer study. The quality control laboratories at the manufacturing sites use these methods to measure the product quality of every manufactured commercial batch in order to release the batch into the community. It's crucial to ensure these analytical methods are (1) successfully transferred from R&D to the manufacturing site, and (2) once at the manufacturing site, they can still perform well. If a transfer study is unsuccessful, this could potentially delay the launch of an asset. If the method is transferred but does not achieve an acceptable level of performance, this also has potential negative implications such as medicines not getting to people who need them because of wrongly rejected batches.

DOI: 10.1201/9781003255093-4

4.2 Assurance for Method Transfer Studies

Transfer studies usually require a formal statistical assessment to demonstrate that the methods perform in an equivalent way at both the transferring and receiving sites. Typically, a Two One-Sided Tests (TOST) equivalence test (see for example, Schuirmann (1987); Limentani et al. (2005); Borman et al. (2009)) is used to show that the means of the two sites do not differ by more than a small amount, called the margin of equivalence. We let μ_T and μ_R denote the true mean laboratory measurement at the transferring and receiving sites respectively. The null hypothesis of non-equivalence is that the actual difference in means ($\Delta = \mu_T - \mu_R$) is either $\geq E_U$ or $\leq E_L$, where E_L is the lower equivalence limit, and E_U is the upper equivalence limit. The alternative hypothesis of equivalence is then $E_L < \Delta < E_U$. The null and alternative hypotheses can be deconstructed into the following sets of null and alternative hypotheses representing separate one-sided tests.

$$\begin{array}{lcl} H_{0L}: \Delta \leq E_L & \text{vs} & H_{1L}: \Delta > E_L \\ H_{0U}: \Delta \geq E_U & \text{vs} & H_{1U}: \Delta < E_U \end{array} \tag{4.1}$$

Both null hypotheses must be rejected to demonstrate equivalence.

In the case of an equivalence study using two independent groups of measurements and assuming equal method variances the test is carried out using two t statistics of the form:

$$T_L = \frac{\bar{X}_T - \bar{X}_R - E_L}{s_p\sqrt{1/n_T + 1/n_R}} \qquad \text{and} \qquad T_U = \frac{\bar{X}_T - \bar{X}_R - E_U}{s_p\sqrt{1/n_T + 1/n_R}} \tag{4.2}$$

where $\bar{X}_T$, s_T, n_T, $\bar{X}_R$, s_R, and n_R are the sample mean, sample standard deviation, and sample size for the transferring and receiving sites respectively and s_p is the pooled estimate of standard deviation given by

$$s_p = \sqrt{\frac{(n_T - 1)s_T^2 + (n_R - 1)s_R^2}{n_T + n_R - 2}}. \tag{4.3}$$

The null hypothesis is rejected in favor of equivalence if T_L and $-T_U$ equal or exceed $t_{1-\alpha,\nu}$, the $1 - \alpha$ quantile of the t distribution with degrees of freedom equal to $\nu = n_T + n_R - 2$. The value of α is chosen to control the Type I error, i.e. the maximal probability of falsely rejecting the null hypothesis when the sites are not equivalent. It is possible to generalise this TOST approach to allow for different variances at the two sites by replacing the t statistics given above with ones based on Welch's t statistic (Welch, 1947) however in what follows we will assume that the variances are the same at the two sites.

Statistical power is typically used to help define a suitable sample size for an upcoming transfer study via an equivalence assessment. For specified "true" values of the difference in means Δ, common measurement variability σ^2, sample sizes n_T, n_R and type I error α, the power to reject the null hypothesis in favor of equivalence is given by

$$\text{Power}(\Delta, \sigma, n_T, n_R, \alpha) = \Pr(T_L \geq t_{1-\alpha, n_T+n_R-2} \text{ and } T_U \leq -t_{1-\alpha, n_T+n_R-2}). \tag{4.4}$$

Owen (1965) showed that the joint distribution of (T_L, T_U) is given by a bivariate non-central t distribution and derived methods for efficiently evaluating probabilities of the form given above. The R package `PowerTOST` (Labes et al., 2022) includes functions for obtaining power and sample size for the equal variance TOST.

Traditionally, to calculate an appropriate sample size for an equivalence study that has a target power of say at least 90%, assumptions must be made about the measurement variability and the true site difference between the "equivalent" sites. We can use the function `sampleN.TOST` within the `PowerTOST` package to obtain the total number of measurements required based on assumed values of Δ and σ for a given target power, type I error and equivalence limits. Because the functions in `PowerTOST` were developed for bioequivalence studies, see for example Chow (2014), their use can feel rather cumbersome. We therefore define a wrapper function for `sampleN.TOST` as follows:

```
sampleN.TOST.equiv <- function(Delta=0, Sigma=1,
                               TargetPower=0.9, alpha=0.05,
                               UpperLimit=1,
                               LowerLimit=-UpperLimit){
if (!requireNamespace("PowerTOST")) {
stop("Please install the PowerTOST package prior to
      using this function.")
}
out <- PowerTOST::sampleN.TOST(logscale=FALSE,
                               targetpower=TargetPower,
                  theta1=LowerLimit, theta2=UpperLimit,
                   alpha=alpha, theta0=Delta, CV=Sigma,
                       design="parallel", print=FALSE)[-1]

names(out) <- c("alpha", "Sigma","Delta", "LowerLimit",
                "UpperLimit", "SampleSize",
                "AchievedPower", "TargetPower")
return(out)
}
```

The function returns the minimum sample size in total assuming equal numbers of measurements are taken at both sites. For example, to find the minimum total number of measurements needed to achieve 90% power when $\Delta = 0, \sigma = 1, -E_L = E_U = 2$ and the type I error is 0.05 we use the following:

```
sampleN.TOST.equiv(Delta=0, Sigma=1, UpperLimit=2, TargetPower=0.9,
                   alpha=0.05)
##   alpha Sigma Delta LowerLimit UpperLimit SampleSize AchievedPower
##    0.05     1     0         -2          2         14     0.9391631
##   TargetPower
##           0.9
```

We see that we need a total of at least 14 measurements, i.e. 7 measurements per site to achieve 90% power and that our actual power will be nearly 94%.

For a given sample size, we can obtain the power for any assumed true difference in means using `power.TOST`. The following code defines a wrapper function for `power.TOST`.

```
power.TOST.equiv <- function(Delta=0, Sigma=1, SampleSizes,
                             alpha=0.05, UpperLimit=1,
                             LowerLimit=-UpperLimit){
 if (!requireNamespace("PowerTOST")) {
     stop("Please install the PowerTOST package prior to
        using this function.")
}
 PowerTOST::power.TOST(alpha=alpha, logscale=FALSE,
                      theta1=LowerLimit, theta2=UpperLimit,
                      theta0=Delta, CV=Sigma, n=SampleSizes,
                      design="parallel", method="exact")
}
```

We can use this wrapper function to produce a plot of the power curve for a TOST based on $n_T = n_R = 7, \sigma = 1, -E_L = E_U = 2$ and $\alpha = 0.05$ as follows:

```
data <- tibble(Delta=seq(-2.5, 2.5, length.out=101),
               Power=power.TOST.equiv(Delta=Delta,
                     Sigma=1, UpperLimit=2,
                     SampleSizes=rep(7,2)))

ggplot() +
    xlab(expression(Delta)) +
    ylab("Power (%)") +
    scale_y_continuous(expand=c(0,0), breaks=seq(0,100,10),
                       limits=c(0,100)) +
    scale_x_continuous(expand=c(0,0),
          breaks=seq(-2.5,2.5,by=0.5), limits=c(-2.5,2.5)) +
    geom_path(data=data, aes(x=Delta, y=100*Power)) +
    geom_segment(aes(x=-2, y=95, xend=2, yend=95),
                 colour="darkgrey",
                 arrow=arrow(ends="both",
                 length=unit(0.1,"inches"))) +
    geom_hline(yintercept=5, colour="darkgrey", lty=2) +
    geom_text(aes(x=-2.4, y=6, label="5%"), hjust=0, vjust=0,
              colour="darkgrey") +
    geom_segment(aes(x=c(-2,2),y=c(0,0), xend=c(-2,2),
                 yend=c(95,95)), colour="darkgrey") +
    geom_text(aes(x=0, y=98, label="Equivalence Region"),
              colour="darkgrey")
```

The resulting plot is reproduced in Figure 4.1. We can clearly see that when the true difference (Δ) is at the boundary of the equivalence region $(-2, 2)$ the power to demonstrate equivalence is just 5% (the Type I error). We also see that maximal power occurs when the true difference is zero. In this example, the maximal power is 94% which is consistent with the results from the `sampleN.TOST` function.

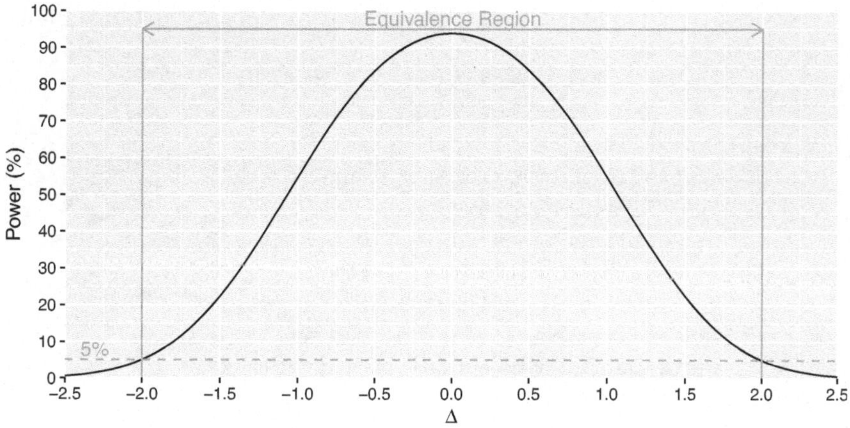

FIGURE 4.1
Power of equal variance TOST ($-E_L = E_U = 2$, $n_T = n_R = 7$, $\sigma = 1$, $\alpha = 0.05$).

In the preceding power analysis, assumptions had to be made about the measurement variability and the true site difference between the "equivalent" sites. Hence, the calculated power is conditional on these assumed (fixed) but unknown values. Crisp et al. (2018) discuss that whilst historically statisticians have focused on power as the probability of statistical success (PoS) for a study, use of assurance (O'Hagan et al., 2005) as a broader and more relevant measure of PoS has grown in recent years. In fact, Crisp et al. (2018) as well as Temple and Robertson (2021) describe how GSK routinely use assurance as a measure of PoS in clinical development. Assurance is a Bayesian alternative to a power calculation where in the context of a transfer study, it effectively averages the power over the possible true site differences weighted by their associated probabilities. If Δ is the true site mean difference, $\pi(\Delta)$ is the prior distribution for the true site mean difference, and $S1$ denotes the event of achieving a successful outcome (i.e. concluding equivalence based on the TOST), then assurance can be defined as the following:

$$\text{Assurance} = \Pr(S1) = \int_{\Delta} \Pr(S1|\Delta, \sigma, n_T, n_R, E_L, E_U, \alpha)\pi(\Delta)d\Delta. \tag{4.5}$$

Figure 4.2 illustrates the above calculation graphically using the same equivalence study information used to obtain the power curve in Figure 4.1 together with an assumed uniform prior distribution over the interval [−2,2] for the true site difference Δ. The associated code is as follows:

```
data <- data %>%
    mutate(Prior=dunif(Delta, min=-2, max=2),
           Product=Power*Prior)
ggplot() +
    xlab(expression(Delta)) +
    ylab("Power/Density") +
    scale_y_continuous(expand=c(0,0), breaks=seq(0,1,by=0.1),
                       limits=c(0,1)) +
```

```
scale_x_continuous(expand=c(0,0),
                   breaks=seq(-2.5,2.5,by=0.5),
                   limits=c(-2.5,2.5)) +
geom_area(data=filter(data, abs(Delta)<=2),
          aes(x=Delta, y=Prior), colour="black",
              fill="lightgrey",
              outline.type="full", lwd=.5, lty=3) +
geom_path(data=data, aes(x=Delta, y=Power),
                         color="black", lty=1) +
geom_area(data=filter(data, abs(Delta)<=2),
          aes(x=Delta, y=Product), color="black",
              fill="darkgrey",
              outline.type="upper", lwd=.5, lty=2)
```

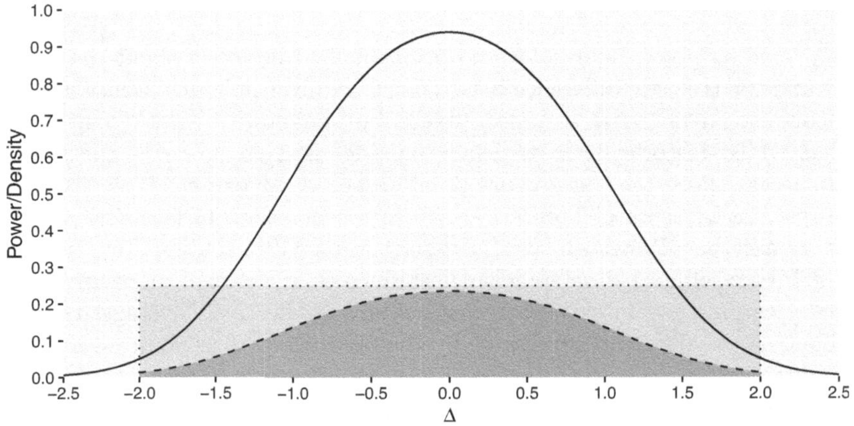

FIGURE 4.2
Assurance of Equal Variance TOST ($-E_L = E_U = 2$, $n_T = n_R = 6$, $\sigma = 1$, $\alpha = 0.05$) with a uniform prior for Δ over $[-2, 2]$. The solid line represents $\Pr(S1|\Delta, \sigma, n_T, n_R, E_L, E_U, \alpha)$, the power curve for the TOST. The dotted line and light gray shaded region represent $\pi(\Delta)$, the prior density for Δ. The dashed line represents the product of the power and prior, whilst the area of the associated dark gray region gives $\Pr(S1)$, the assurance, which equals 53%.

To obtain the assurance requires us to perform some numerical integration. There are multiple ways of achieving this in R. Here, we have used direct calculation based on the trapezoidal rule.

```
AssuranceData <- filter(data, abs(Delta)<=2)
Assurance <- 0.5*sum(diff(AssuranceData$Delta)*
                    (AssuranceData$Product[-1] +
        AssuranceData$Product[-length(AssuranceData$Delta)]))
```

```
Assurance
## [1] 0.5275533
```

In this example, the assurance is 53%. This low level of assurance reflects our uncertainty about the true value of the difference in means between the sites and the associated low power over a range of differences that we have a reasonable probability of encountering.

It is clear that if on the basis of the TOST assessment we conclude that the transferring and receiving sites are equivalent (i.e. we deem the method transfer to be successful), this does not mean that there is no true analytical bias between the sites. It is important to understand the potential impact this true bias could have when measuring the product quality (at the transferring site) since this, in turn, will determine whether the batch is successfully released onto the market. Therefore, when designing the analytical method transfer study, we wish to ensure any potential bias following a successful transfer has minimal impact on the measurement of product quality. To understand this impact we also need to know how capable the manufacturing process is of producing product of the required quality.

Let $S2$ denote the event that a future batch meets the required quality criteria for commercial release when tested using our analytical method of interest. A useful measure to aid decision making at the planning of the transfer study would be to calculate the conditional assurance of achieving $S2$ given $S1$, i.e. $\Pr(S2|S1)$. Note that this assessment is done before we have conducted the method transfer study so that $\Pr(S2|S1)$ is evaluated based on $\pi(\Delta)$, the prior distribution of Δ.

To obtain $\Pr(S2|S1)$, we note that

$$\Pr(S2|S1) = \int_{\Delta} \Pr(S2|\Delta)\pi(\Delta|S1)d\Delta \tag{4.6}$$

where

$$\pi(\Delta|S1) = \frac{\Pr(S1|\Delta)\pi(\Delta)}{\int_{\Delta} \Pr(S1|\Delta)\pi(\Delta)d\Delta} = \frac{\Pr(S1|\Delta)\pi(\Delta)}{\Pr(S1)}. \tag{4.7}$$

We can therefore obtain the conditional assurance of a future batch meeting the quality standard (conditional on passing the method transfer) as

$$\Pr(S1|S1) = \frac{\int_{\Delta} \Pr(S2|\Delta)\Pr(S1|\Delta)\pi(\Delta)d\Delta}{\Pr(S1)}. \tag{4.8}$$

The above now only requires knowledge of $\Pr(S2|\Delta)$, i.e. the probability of a batch meeting the quality criteria given a shift of Δ in the measured results due to the measurement bias introduced during the transfer. This quantity is straightforward to compute. For example, we might know measured dosage units from the manufacturing process can be characterised as following a normal distribution with an overall process mean of μ, a between-batch variance component σ_b^2 and a within-batch variance component σ_w^2, so that if Y_{ij} is the measured value of dosage unit j from batch i then

$$Y_{ij} = \mu + b_i + \varepsilon_{ij} \tag{4.9}$$

where $b_i \sim N(0, \sigma_b^2)$ is a random batch effect and $\varepsilon_{ij} \sim N(0, \sigma_w^2)$ represents random variation of individual dosage units within each batch. In this case, the measurement bias of Δ introduced during the method transfer would have the effect of changing the process mean of the measured values from μ to $\mu + \Delta$.

Figure 4.3 presents this idea pictorially; the solid line represents $\Pr(S2|\Delta)$ the probability a batch meets the release criteria when the measured results are biased by an offset of Δ, whilst the dotted line and light gray area represents $\pi(\Delta|S1)$ assuming the power curve and prior based on Figure 4.2. The dashed line is the product $\Pr(S2|\Delta)\pi(\Delta|S1)$ whilst the conditional assurance is then the size of the dark gray area underneath. (The associated code will be given in Section 4.3, when we work through a practical example.)

4.3 A Practical Example

The practical example used throughout this section is for an assay analytical method used to determine the content of active pharmaceutical ingredient (API) in an oral solid dose product via high performance liquid chromatography (HPLC). An individual analytical measurement is obtained by taking 5 dosage units and dissolving them in solvent to create an analytical sample which is then then used in multiple injections into an HPLC instrument. The measurement result for the analytical sample is then the average content of the injections for that sample (divided by 5 to account for the use of 5 dosage units) and then expressed as a percentage of the label claim for the product.

In this example, the transfer study acceptance criteria are pre-defined as $\pm 2\%$, the analytical method standard deviation is 0.9%, and the sample size for the planned transfer study is 5 analytical samples per group. All analytical samples are to be obtained from the same product batch and a single analyst will perform the analytical method at both sites. Following discussion with an expert panel of analytical chemists, it has been agreed that a uniform distribution ranging from -2 to $+2$ adequately represent the experts prior belief about the likely site mean bias between the R&D and manufacturing sites.

In order to meet the batch release requirements for Assay, the results for two independent analytical samples created from the batch must both be within 95% to 105%. Data already collected on the performance of the manufacturing process assessed using the R&D analytical testing facilities indicate that individual analytical measurements can be adequately modeled using a one-way random effects model assuming normally distributed random components. The current estimates for the process mean, between-batch variability and within-batch variability are known to be 101%, 2%, and 2%, respectively.

4.3.1 PoS of Transfer Study

The assurance, $\Pr(S1)$, can be approximated in R using multiple approaches. We give three here.

Direct use of trapezoidal rule

1. Create a sufficiently large sequence of site differences that encompasses the range of the prior: $(\delta_1, ..., \delta_n)$.
2. Calculate the statistical power of passing the transfer for each value from the sequence of site differences in step 1: $(\Pr(S1|\delta_1), ..., \Pr(S1|\delta_n))$.
3. Based on the prior, calculate the probability density of each of the site differences from step 1: $(\pi(\delta_1), ..., \pi(\delta_n))$.
4. For each value from step 1, multiply the power (step 2) by the probability density (step 3): $(y_1, ..., y_n)$ where $y_i = \Pr(S1|\delta_i)\pi(\delta_i)$.

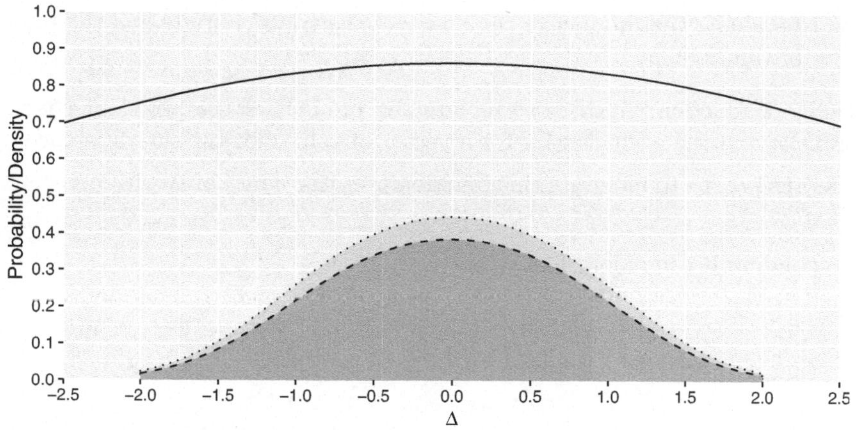

FIGURE 4.3
Illustration of conditional assurance. The solid line represents $\Pr(S2|\Delta)$ the probability of meeting the product quality criteria given a measurement bias of Δ. The dotted line and light gray shaded region represent $\pi(\Delta|S1)$. The dashed line is the product $\Pr(S2|\Delta)\pi(\Delta|S1)$ whilst the conditional assurance is then the size of the dark gray area underneath.

5. Use the trapezoidal rule to obtain the approximate value of the assurance based on the formula $0.5 \times \sum_{i=2}^{n}(\delta_i - \delta_{i-1})(y_{i-1} + y_i)$.

The corresponding R code looks like this:

```
data <- tibble(Delta=seq(-2.5, 2.5, length.out=101), #Step 1
               Power=power.TOST.equiv(Delta=Delta,    #Step 2
               Sigma=0.9,
               UpperLimit=2,
               SampleSizes=rep(5,2)))

data <- data %>%
        mutate(Prior=dunif(Delta, min=-2, max=2),     #Step 3
               Product=Power*Prior)                   #Step 4

AssuranceData <- filter(data, abs(Delta)<=2)
Assurance <- 0.5*sum(diff(AssuranceData$Delta)*       #Step 5
                  (AssuranceData$Product[-1] +
     AssuranceData$Product[-length(AssuranceData$Delta)]))

Assurance
## [1] 0.4805504
```

Use of R's adaptive integration functionality

Within R there is an `integrate` function which can be used to evaluate the integral of a function over a specified range. We can use this to calculate the assurance if we first define a function to evaluate the product of the power of the transfer study and the prior density for a vector of values of Δ.

1. Define a function which can evaluate the product of the power of passing the transfer and the prior density for a vector of values for the site difference.
2. Use `integrate` to integrate this function over the values of Δ with non-zero prior density.

The corresponding R code looks like:

```
fn1 <- function(x){                                        #Step 1
    Power <- power.TOST.equiv(Delta=x, Sigma=0.9,
                    UpperLimit=2, SampleSizes=rep(5,2))
    Prior <- dunif(x, min=-2, max=2)
    return(Power*Prior)
}

Assurance2 <- integrate(f=fn1, lower=-2, upper=2)    #Step 2
Assurance2

## 0.4805678 with absolute error < 3e-10
```

Use of Monte Carlo Simulation

Our final approach is to note that the integral calculation for assurance is actually the expected power, where the expectation is taken with respect to the prior distribution for Δ. This suggests the following Monte Carlo strategy:

1. Create an independent sample of values of $(\delta_1, ..., \delta_n)$ from the prior distribution for the site difference.
2. Calculate the corresponding value of the power of passing the transfer for each of these simulated values $(\Pr(S1|\delta_1), ..., \Pr(S1|\delta_n))$.
3. Estimate the assurance by taking the sample mean of the calculated power values $\sum_{i=1}^{n} \Pr(S1|\delta_i)/n$.

The corresponding R code looks like:

```
nSim <- 1e4
Sim.Delta <- runif(nSim, min=-2, max=2)             #Step 1

#Step 2
Sim.Power <- power.TOST.equiv(Delta=Sim.Delta, #Step 2
  Sigma=0.9, UpperLimit=2,
  SampleSizes=rep(5,2))


Assurance3 <- mean(Sim.Power)                        #Step 3
```

```
Assurance3
## [1] 0.4791226
```

For this example, we see close agreement between all three of the approaches. Based on our prior knowledge and the intended design of our method transfer, we conclude that there is slightly less than a 50% chance that this transfer will be successful.

4.3.2 PoS for Batch Release, Prior to Transfer

We now turn our attention to evaluation of what the potential impact of our transfer study design is on our ability to release batches. We want to reiterate that we are able to do this evaluation before we have even commenced the transfer study. In introducing this example we stated that in order to meet the batch release requirements for an assay, the results for two independent analytical samples created from the batch must both be within 95% to 105%. If Y_{ij} represents the measured result on analytical sample j from batch i in this example we believe we can adequately model this by assuming $Y_{ij} = \mu + b_i + \varepsilon_{ij}$, where $b_i \sim N(0, \sigma_b^2)$ and $\varepsilon_{ij} \sim N(0, \sigma_w^2)$ or equivalently $Y_{ij} = X_i + \varepsilon_{ij}$, where $X_i \sim N(\mu, \sigma_b^2)$ and $\varepsilon_{ij} \sim N(0, \sigma_w^2)$.

We previously defined $S2$ to denote the event that a future batch meets the required quality criteria for commercial release when tested using our analytical method of interest. For this example that means each analytical sample tested from the product batch must give a result which lies between set limits. One could use a simulation based approach to estimating $\Pr(S2)$ for known values of μ, σ_b^2, σ_w^2, but here we prefer to use the properties of the assumed model to reduce the calculation to a one-dimensional integral. Treating μ, σ_b^2 and σ_w^2 as known fixed quantities we can show that for a pair of limits (LSL, USL)

$$\Pr(S2) = \Pr(LSL \leq Y_{ij} \leq USL; \forall j = 1, ..., n) \tag{4.10}$$

$$= \int_x \left[\prod_{j=1}^{n} \Pr(LSL \leq Y_{ij} \leq USL | X_i = x) \right] f_{X_i}(x) dx \tag{4.11}$$

where f_{X_i} denotes the normal density function associated with X_i. Noting that

$$\Pr(LSL \leq Y_{ij} \leq USL | X_i = x) = \Phi\left(\frac{USL - x}{\sigma_w}\right) - \Phi\left(\frac{LSL - x}{\sigma_w}\right) \tag{4.12}$$

where Φ is the cumulative probability distribution function of the standard normal, it follows that

$$\Pr(S2) = \int_x \left[\Phi\left(\frac{USL - x}{\sigma_w}\right) - \Phi\left(\frac{LSL - x}{\sigma_w}\right) \right]^n \left[\frac{1}{\sqrt{2\pi\sigma_b^2}} \exp\left(-\frac{(x-\mu)^2}{2\sigma_b^2}\right) \right] dx. \tag{4.13}$$

We create an R function to calculate $\Pr(S2)$ using the following source code:

```
AssayBatchPassRate <- function(Mu, Sigmab, Sigmaw,
                               n, LSL, USL){
   f <- function(x, Sigmab=Sigmab, Sigmaw=Sigmaw,
```

```
                    n=n, LSL=LSL, USL=USL){
        (pnorm(USL, mean=x, sd=Sigmaw) -
         pnorm(LSL, mean=x, sd=Sigmaw))^n *
         dnorm(x, mean=Mu, sd=Sigmab)
    }
    integrate.out <- integrate(f, lower=Mu-10*Sigmab,
                               upper=Mu+10*Sigmab,
                               Sigmab=Sigmab,
                               Sigmaw=Sigmaw, n=n,
                               LSL=LSL, USL=USL)
    return(integrate.out$value)
}
```

To use this to calculate the probability of a product batch successfully meeting the criteria for our example, i.e. the 2 analytical sample measurements from the batch must lie within 95% and 105% of label claim, the process mean is 101%, the between-batch standard deviation is 2% and the within-batch standard deviation is 2%, we use the following

```
AssayBatchPassRate(Mu=101, Sigmab=2, Sigmaw=2,
                   n=2, LSL=95, USL=105)

## [1] 0.834605
```

We see that when the analytical measurements are generated by the R&D lab we would expect 83% of product batches to meet these release criteria.

4.3.3 PoS for Batch Release, Post to Transfer

To approximate the conditional assurance or $\Pr(S2|S1)$, the following approach is provided:

1. As before, create a sufficiently large sequence of site differences that encompasses the range of the prior: $(\delta_1, ..., \delta_n)$.
2. Calculate the statistical power of passing the transfer for each value from the sequence of site differences in step 1: $(\Pr(S1|\delta_1), ..., \Pr(S1|\delta_n))$.
3. Based on the prior, calculate the probability density of each of the site differences from step 1: $(\pi(\delta_1), ..., \pi(\delta_n))$.
4. For each value from step 1, multiply the power (step 2) by the probability density (step 3): $(y_1, ..., y_n)$ where $y_i = \Pr(S1|\delta_i)\pi(\delta_i)$.
5. Use the trapezoidal rule to obtain the value of the assurance $\Pr(S1)$ based on the formula $0.5 \times \sum_{i=2}^{n}(\delta_i - \delta_{i-1})(y_{i-1} + y_i)$.
6. For each value from step 1, divide each of the values obtained in step 4 by the assurance (step 5) to obtain the "conditional prior": $(\pi(\delta_1|S1), ..., \pi(\delta_n|S1))$.
7. Calculate the probability of meeting the batch release criteria based on the original process mean being offset by each of the site differences given in step 1.
8. For each value from step 1, multiply the conditional prior from step 6 by the batch release probability from step 6: $(z_1, ..., z_n)$ where $z_i = \Pr(S2|\delta_i)\pi(\delta_i|S1)$.

9. Use the trapezoidal rule to obtain the approximate value of the conditional assurance based on the formula $0.5 \times \sum_{i=2}^{n}(\delta_i - \delta_{i-1})(z_{i-1} + z_i)$.

```
data <- data %>%
    mutate(row=row(data)) %>%
    group_by(row) %>%
    mutate(ConditionalPrior=Product/Assurance,           #Step 6
             BatchPassRate=AssayBatchPassRate(101+Delta, 2,
                                  2, 2, 95, 105),        #Step 7
        Product2=BatchPassRate*ConditionalPrior) %>%     #Step 8
    ungroup()

AssuranceData <- filter(data, abs(Delta)<=2)
                                                         #Step 9
ConditionalAssurance <- 0.5*sum(diff(AssuranceData$Delta)*
                              (AssuranceData$Product2[-1] +
        AssuranceData$Product2[-length(AssuranceData$Delta)]))

ggplot() +
    xlab(expression(Delta)) +
    ylab("Probability/Density") +
    scale_y_continuous(expand=c(0,0), breaks=seq(0,1,by=0.1),
                       limits=c(0,1)) +
    scale_x_continuous(expand=c(0,0),
                       breaks=seq(-2.5,2.5,by=0.5),
                       limits=c(-2.5,2.5)) +
    geom_area(data=filter(data, abs(Delta)<=2),
            aes(x=Delta, y=ConditionalPrior), colour="black",
               fill="lightgrey",
               outline.type="full", lwd=.5, lty=3) +
    geom_path(data=data, aes(x=Delta, y=BatchPassRate),
              colour="black", lty=1, lwd=.5) +
    geom_area(data=filter(data, abs(Delta)<=2),
           aes(x=Delta, y=Product2), color="black",
              fill="darkgrey", outline.type="upper",
              lwd=.5, lty=2)

ConditionalAssurance
## [1] 0.8174857
```

4.3.4 Example Wrap Up

This example demonstrates how to calculate the assurance of an analytical method equivalence study from a transferring site to a receiving site. Based on the example as detailed in the opening of Section 4.3, it is estimated that the probability of successfully claiming equivalence and transferring the analytical method is 48%. Prior to transfer, the current product performance using the R&D based method is assessed against batch release specifications,

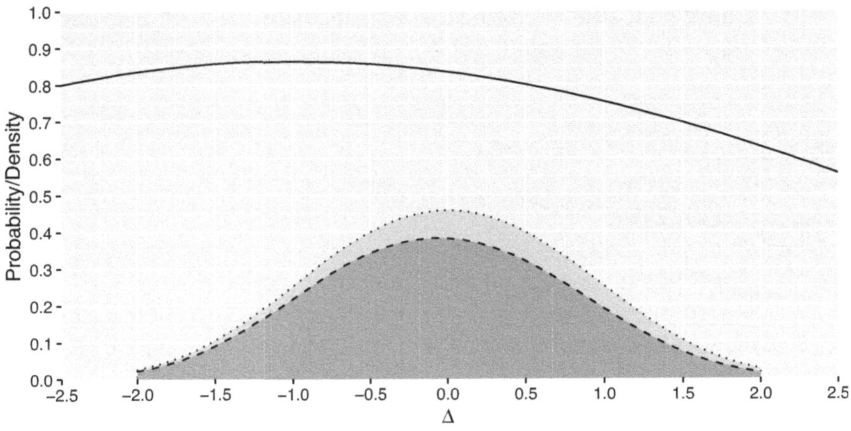

FIGURE 4.4
Probability of Successful Batch Release conditional on a successful method transfer (conditional assurance). The solid line represents $\Pr(S2|\Delta)$, the probability of meeting the batch release requirement that two independent analytical samples are both within 95% to 105% of the target given a measurement bias of Δ with an underlying process mean, between-batch variability and within-batch variability of 101%, 2%, and 2%, respectively. This line is asymmetric because the underlying process mean is offset from the target of 100%. The dotted line and light gray shaded region represent $\pi(\Delta|S1)$, the prior distribution of the measurement bias conditional on a successful method transfer. The dashed line is the product $\Pr(S2|\Delta)\pi(\Delta|S1)$ whilst the conditional assurance is then the size of the dark gray area underneath.

and is estimated to be approximately 83%. Finally the conditional assurance is calculated, which can be interpreted as the expected probability of meeting batch release specifications using the manufacturing site based method following a successful method transfer. This is estimated to be 82%.

4.4 Conclusions

The approach discussed in this chapter can help the business make good, smart choices at the design stage of an analytical method transfer study. Before conducting the transfer study the project teams can evaluate the assurance and conditional assurance and decide if (i) the transfer study design needs to be modified and (ii) the analytical method (prior to transfer) is sufficient; ultimately all parties are clear on the risks (in a quantitative form) going forward.

The example does not discuss the choice of prior. Within GSK the choice of prior (recommended by CMC Statistics) has been based on prior data and prior experience (especially in the absence of data). No priors are placed on the variability estimates to calculate the assurance and conditional assurance, nor is any prior placed on the underlying manufacturing process mean. The example shows a simple case of a parallel group design where the sets of measurement results at the transferring and receiving sites can be treated as two independent samples with no additional correlation structure. There are obvious extensions to what we have covered here to incorporate prior uncertainty on additional parameters and different transfer study designs as well as other product quality criteria. In order to embed assurance and conditional assurance into ways of working, the calculations now form part of a Shiny application routinely used for discussing method transfers. This application is fast and easy to use so that statisticians and scientists can have live discussions about risks, reducing any additional burden on statisticians and accelerating decisions for projects.

4.5 Acknowledgments

We would like to thank the CMC Statistics group for their on-going support in reviewing the methodology, developing a Shiny application, and advocating the use of assurance in projects. We would also like to thank the CMC Analytical group in R&D, in particular Adam Jones and Elizabeth Schmidt for their key contributions and collaboration in building acceptance of the approach within the analytical community.

5

Bayesian Dissolution Testing

Tony Pourmohamad

Genentech, Inc.

Robert Richardson

Brigham Young University

CONTENTS

5.1 Introduction

Changes in the formulation of a solid oral dosage form can have a major impact on both the safety and efficacy of the drug. Formulation changes are not limited solely to the formulated ingredients that make up the solid oral dosage form, but can also include changes to the manufacturing process, the manufacturing site, or other drug development factors. To ensure continuing drug product quality after changes in the drug formulation, dissolution studies are conducted to establish similarity between different solid oral dosage forms. At its simplest, a dissolution study seeks to show that a test product (solid oral dosage form after changes in the formulation) is deemed to be similar to a reference product (solid oral dosage form before changes in the formulation). Unfortunately, no universally accepted definition of similarity exists yet many definitions have been proposed (Podcseck, 1993; Moore and Flanner, 1996; Sathe et al., 1996; FDA, 1997a; Yuksel et al., 2000; Saranadasa and Krishnamoorthy, 2005; Mollenhoff et al., 2018, to name a few). And although the definition of similarity may vary from study-to-study, fundamentally all dissolution studies collect the same type of outcome data. For a predefined number of sample time points, a typical dissolution study proceeds by placing a fixed number of solid oral dosage forms (both from the reference and test products) one at a time into an agitated media where either chromatography or ultraviolet spectroscopy is used to calculate the percent dissolution of the solid oral dosage forms. These percent dissolution measurements of both the reference and

DOI: 10.1201/9781003255093-5

test products are then used, in conjunction with a given definition of similarity, to establish the similarity of the two drug products.

More specifically, suppose that a total of n_R and n_T solid oral dosage forms from the reference and test products, respectively, are to be tested in a dissolution study. For a given product group (i.e., reference or test group), the measurement $Y_{i,j,k}$ is defined to be the observed cumulative percentage dissolved for dosage unit j at sampling time t_k for product i, where $i = R$ or T denotes the reference and test products respectively, $j = 1, 2, ..., n_i$, and $k = 1, 2, ..., p$. The dissolution profile of a product can then be calculated as the curve of the mean dissolution rates over time, i.e.,

$$\bar{Y}_{i,t_k} = \frac{1}{n_i} \sum_{j=1}^{n_i} Y_{i,j,k}, \tag{5.1}$$

where $\bar{Y}_{R,t_k}$ and $\bar{Y}_{T,t_k}$ are the dissolution profiles at time point t_k for the reference and test products, respectively. Under these definitions and setup, Moore and Flanner (1996) introduced a similarity factor, known now as the f_2 statistic, which has become one of the most widely used criteria for assessing similarity of two solid oral dosage products. A simple model independent approach based on the observed dissolution data, the f_2 statistic is defined as

$$f_2 = 50 \log_{10} \left[100 \left(1 + \frac{1}{p} \sum_{k=1}^{p} w_k (\bar{Y}_{R,t_k} - \bar{Y}_{T,t_k})^2 \right)^{-1/2} \right] \tag{5.2}$$

where w_k are pre-specified weights that can be set to reflect possible heterogeneity across time for a given dissolution profile. The weights, however, are often viewed as optional and therefore are typically set to one.

The popularity of the f_2 statistic is due in part to its ease of calculation and interpretation. Furthermore, the f_2 statistic is perhaps one of the most widely used criterion for dissolution testing due to the numerous guidances issued by health authorities (FDA, 1995, 1997a,b,c, 2000, 2003; ICH Q8(R2), 2009; EMA, 2010b). A simple calculation, the US Food and Drug Administration (FDA) and European Medical Agencies (EMA) state that a reference and test product can be declared similar when the f_2 statistic is calculated to be at least 50, i.e., $f_2 \geq 50$. When the observed reference and test dissolution profiles are identical, the f_2 statistic is equal to $f_2 = 50 \log_{10}(100) = 100$, and $f_2 \geq 50$ implies that there is at most an average difference of about 10% across time points for the two dissolution profiles.

At face value, the notion that an average difference of about 10% across time points (i.e., $f_2 \geq 50$) would imply the similarity of dissolution profiles seems somewhat arbitrary. However, due to measurement noise, say, even when the dissolution profiles of the reference and test products are truly identical, the chance of observing $f_2 = 100$ is extremely unlikely, and so, some acceptable threshold for f_2 statistic must be specified. It turns out that the average difference of about 10% across time points is not actually so arbitrary. As pointed out in Shah et al. (1998), empirical evidence collected from dissolution studies suggests that an average difference in dissolution profiles of up to 10% at any sample time point can occur when two dissolution profiles generated from the same reference product are compared to each other. And so, this empirically derived average difference of up to 10% can be viewed as forming the basis for the criterion that $f_2 = 50 \log_{10}(10) = 50$ is the lowest necessary threshold for determining similarity of the reference and test products.

Despite the rise in popularity of the f_2 statistic, the f_2 statistic is not without its criticisms (LeBlond et al., 2015). Arguably the most problematic issue with the f_2 statistic (amongst potentially many) is that there is no uncertainty quantification associated with the statistic (e.g., it is not a point estimate with an associated margin of error), nor the decision criterion based upon it. The f_2 statistic is simply a calculated quantity of the data from which a binary (i.e., yes or no) decision will be made about the similarity of the dissolution profiles of the reference and test products. This lack of uncertainty quantification has not gone unnoticed by pharmaceutical companies nor health authorities. For example, the FDA has released regulatory guidance for industry (ICH Q8(R2), 2009) that acknowledges the uncertainty quantification issue and directly challenges the use of the f_2 statistic for decision making without some form of proper uncertainty quantification.

Uncertainty quantification for the f_2 statistic is not an insurmountable feat. Under reasonable assumptions, many authors have proposed ways for quantifying the uncertainty around the calculation of the f_2 statistic by means of, say, bootstrapped confidence intervals (Sathe et al., 1996; Shah et al., 1998; Ng et al., 2018) and probabilistic statements (Novick et al., 2015; Pourmohamad et al., 2022), for example. In fact, for the remainder of this chapter, we will explain and show how to use some of the Bayesian methods outlined in Novick et al. (2015) and Pourmohamad et al. (2022) for quantifying the uncertainty around the f_2 statistic, and then how to use that knowledge to make decisions about the similarity of the reference and test products.

Lastly, while not a concern for the case study shown in this chapter, it is worth noting that the use of the f_2 statistic is only deemed valid when the following criteria are met (EMA, 2010b):

1. A minimum of three time points must be tested (time zero excluded).
2. The time points should be the same for reference and test products.
3. Twelve individual dissolution measurements for every time point for each product.
4. No more than one mean value of greater than 85% dissolved for any of the two products.
5. The relative standard deviation, or coefficient of variation, of any dissolution profile should be less than 20% for the first time point, and less than 10% from the second to last time point.

In the event that any of the above criteria is violated, an alternative method for comparing the dissolution of the reference and test product must be developed. Some examples of such alternative methods include an inferential framework for testing comparability of dissolution curves based on the maximum deviation between curves (Mollenhoff et al., 2018), the T^2 test for equivalence (Hoffelder, 2018), and the recent work on Bayesian model selection for dissolution testing (Pourmohamad et al., 2022).

5.1.1 The F_2 Parameter

No implied probability distribution accompanies the use of the f_2 statistic without some sort of statistical assumptions. For clarity, let us define

$$D = \frac{1}{p}\sum_{k=1}^{p}(\bar{Y}_{R,t_k} - \bar{Y}_{T,t_k})^2 \tag{5.3}$$

so that we may re-express the f_2 statistic as the following

$$f_2 = 50\log_{10}\left(\frac{100}{\sqrt{1+D}}\right). \tag{5.4}$$

Given the form of D, it is easy to see that the f_2 statistic is a function of sample statistics for the mean dissolution profiles. Now consider replacing the sample statistics, $\bar{Y}_{R,t_k}$ and $\bar{Y}_{T,t_k}$, with the parameters μ_{R,t_k} and μ_{T,t_k} in (5.3), i.e., define the parameterized version of D to be Δ where

$$\Delta = \frac{1}{p}\sum_{k=1}^{p}(\mu_{R,t_k} - \mu_{T,t_k})^2. \tag{5.5}$$

Based on (5.5), the f_2 statistic can now be viewed as an estimator of the parameter F_2 where

$$F_2 = 50\log_{10}\left(\frac{100}{\sqrt{1+\Delta}}\right). \tag{5.6}$$

Now that we are dealing with a parameter rather than a statistic (i.e., the F_2 parameter vs the f_2 statistic), statistical inference can proceed for the F_2 parameter. For example, showing that two dissolution profiles are similar could correspond to testing the following pair of null and alternative hypotheses:

$$\begin{aligned} H_0 &: F_2 < 50 \\ H_a &: F_2 \geq 50. \end{aligned} \tag{5.7}$$

Note that it is by no means a simple task to perform inference under the frequentist paradigm for the F_2 parameter given the complex nonlinear form of the f_2 statistic. In fact, most all of the current frequentist literature relies upon use of bootstrapping procedures in order to obtain uncertainty quantification (via bootstrapped confidence intervals) for the f_2 statistic since deriving the distribution of the F_2 parameter is likely infeasible. However, this is not an issue from the Bayesian perspective (as will be shown in Section 5.2) since posterior samples of the distribution of the F_2 parameter can be obtained directly via the much easier to obtain samples of the posterior distributions for μ_{R,t_k} and μ_{T,t_k}. That is, posterior samples of μ_{R,t_k} and μ_{T,t_k} can be plugged in directly to equation (5.6) to obtain posterior samples of F_2. Probabilistic statements and credible intervals can then be computed for the F_2 parameter based on these posterior samples.

As pointed out in Novick et al. (2015), additional local equivalence testing criterion can be added to strengthen the dissolution profile similarity comparison. Based on the testing criteria in FDA (1997c), Novick et al. (2015) proposed testing the following set of hypotheses:

$$\begin{aligned} H_0 &: |\mu_{R,t_k} - \mu_{T,t_k}| > 15 \text{ for some } k = 1, ..., p \text{ or } F_2 < 50 \\ H_a &: |\mu_{R,t_k} - \mu_{T,t_k}| \leq 15 \text{ for all } k = 1, ..., p \text{ and } F_2 \geq 50. \end{aligned} \tag{5.8}$$

This new proposed set of hypotheses ensures that on average the difference across all of time for the dissolution profiles is no more than 10%, but also that at any given time point the average difference is no more than 15%. Although in practice one could test either set of hypotheses in (5.7) or (5.8), we prefer the latter set of hypotheses and will use that set for the remainder of the chapter.

So, from the Bayesian perspective, how do we actually go about testing the hypotheses in (5.8)? Let us first define the quantity δ such that

$$\delta = \max_{k=1,\ldots,p} |\mu_{R,t_k} - \mu_{T,t_k}|. \tag{5.9}$$

One way to test the hypotheses in (5.8) would be to calculate $100(1-\alpha)\%$ credible intervals for both δ and F_2, and to reject H_0 (i.e., conclude similarity of the reference and test product) if the $100(1-\alpha)\%$ credible interval for δ is entirely below 15, and if the $100(1-\alpha)\%$ credible interval for F_2 is entirely above 50. Here α would be prespecified and would be chosen to reflect the desired level of probabilistic certainty for the similarity conclusion to be true. An alternative approach would be to define the probability q such that

$$q = \Pr(\delta \leq 15 \text{ and } F_2 \geq 50|\mathcal{D}) \tag{5.10}$$

where $\mathcal{D}$ represents the collection of all of the dissolution data for the reference and test product. For a presepecified value of q_0, we would accept H_a if $q \geq q_0$.

Lastly, Pourmohamad et al. (2022) showed that, under the assumption that the dissolution profiles are continuous over time, the f_2 statistic is a biased time discretized estimator. The true underlying dissolution profiles for the reference and test products are continuous curves in time, however, in practice we only get to observe the dissolution curves at a discrete set of time points. Given the discreteness of the dissolution data collected, the f_2 statistic estimates a discrete similarity factor rather than a continuous one. However, a continuous similarity factor is the true quantity of interest for correct decision making. To rectify this issue, (Pourmohamad et al., 2022) suggests replacing the Δ in (5.5) with

$$\Delta = \frac{1}{t_p - t_1} \int_{t_1}^{t_p} \left[\mu_R(t) - \mu_T(t)\right]^2 dt \tag{5.11}$$

where $\mu_R(t)$ and $\mu_T(t)$ are the dissolution profiles for the reference and test products, respectively, for all time $t \in [t_1, t_p]$. Testing the hypotheses in (5.8) with the Δ in (5.11) proceeds analogously as before with the exception that now posterior samples of $\mu_R(t)$ and $\mu_T(t)$ must be obtained rather than μ_{R,t_k} and μ_{T,t_k}. Pourmohamad et al. (2022) showed that using the Δ in (5.11), rather than the Δ in (5.5), leads to an increase in correct similarity decisions, however, both definitions of Δ can be used in practice and so we illustrate the use of both in Sections 5.2 and 5.3.

5.2 The Statistical Models

Sections 5.2.2 and 5.2.3 describe some of the Bayesian models used in Novick et al. (2015) and Pourmohamad et al. (2022), respectively, for dissolution testing. Readers interested in the finer details of the models are advised to see those two papers. Section 5.2.2 provides the tools necessary to sample from the posterior distributions of μ_{R,t_k} and μ_{T,t_k}, while Section 5.2.3 will demonstrate how to obtain posterior samples of $\mu_R(t)$ and $\mu_T(t)$.

5.2.1 Basic Data Format and Requirements in R

Before launching into the descriptions of the two Bayesian models that will be used for dissolution testing, we first define the basic dissolution data structure that will be used in the R code explanantions for the remainder of the chapter. We assume that the data is stored in a $(n_R + n_T) \times (p+1)$ data frame (i.e., matrix) X that looks, in general, like the following

$$X = \begin{bmatrix} \text{Reference} & Y_{R,1,1} & Y_{R,1,2} & \cdots & Y_{R,1,p} \\ \text{Reference} & Y_{R,2,1} & Y_{R,2,2} & \cdots & Y_{R,2,p} \\ \vdots & \vdots & \vdots & \vdots & \vdots \\ \text{Reference} & Y_{R,n_R,1} & Y_{R,n_R,2} & \cdots & Y_{R,n_R,p} \\ \text{Test} & Y_{T,1,1} & Y_{T,1,2} & \cdots & Y_{T,1,p} \\ \text{Test} & Y_{T,2,1} & Y_{T,2,2} & \cdots & Y_{T,2,p} \\ \vdots & \vdots & \vdots & \vdots & \vdots \\ \text{Test} & Y_{T,n_T,1} & Y_{T,n_T,2} & \cdots & Y_{T,n_T,p} \end{bmatrix}. \quad (5.12)$$

Here the first column of X will always denote the group labels identifying whether a given dissolution run, i.e., $(Y_{i,j,1}, ..., Y_{i,j,p})$, belongs to the reference or test formulation group. For a given dissolution run, the remaining p columns of X contain the individual run's dissolution measurements sorted ascending in time.

In order to be able to use the code for the Bayesian models outlined in Sections 5.2.2 and 5.2.3, the following R packages must also be installed and loaded using the `library()` command

```
library(geoR)
library(ggplot2)
library(LaplacesDemon)
library(MCMCpack)
library(mnormt)
library(pscl)
```

5.2.2 Bayesian Multivariate Normal Model

Originally described in Novick et al. (2015), a very simple and straightforward approach to modeling the dissolution data is to assume a multivariate normal distribution for the data likelihood, i.e., if we let $\mathbf{Y}_{i,j} = (Y_{i,j,1}, ..., Y_{i,j,p})'$ for $i = R$ or T, then $\mathbf{Y}_{i,j} \sim \text{N}(\boldsymbol{\mu}_i, \boldsymbol{\Sigma}_i)$ for $j = 1, ..., n_i$ where $\boldsymbol{\mu}_i = (\mu_{i,t_1}, ..., \mu_{i,t_p})$. From there, priors are to be placed on the parameters $\boldsymbol{\mu}_i$ and $\boldsymbol{\Sigma}_i$ reflecting potential prior knowledge about the means and variances of the dissolution profiles. Luckily, in the absence of good prior knowledge, it turns out that noninformative priors tend to work well in practice. Here we recommend working with the multivariate Jeffrey's prior (Gelman et al., 2013, see chapter 3.6) for $\boldsymbol{\mu}_i$ and $\boldsymbol{\Sigma}_i$, i.e.,

$$p(\boldsymbol{\mu}_i, \boldsymbol{\Sigma}_i) \propto |\boldsymbol{\Sigma}_i|^{-(p+1)/2}. \quad (5.13)$$

Under this choice of prior, the posterior distribution can be written as follows:

$$\boldsymbol{\Sigma}_i | \mathbf{Y}_{i,1}, ..., \mathbf{Y}_{i,n_i} \sim \text{Inv-Wishart}(\mathbf{S}_i, n_i - 1) \quad (5.14)$$

$$\boldsymbol{\mu}_i | \mathbf{Y}_{i,1}, ..., \mathbf{Y}_{i,n_i}, \boldsymbol{\Sigma}_i \sim \text{N}(\bar{\mathbf{Y}}_i, \boldsymbol{\Sigma}_i / n_i) \quad (5.15)$$

where $\mathbf{S}_i = \sum_{j=1}^{n_i} (\mathbf{Y}_{i,j} - \bar{\mathbf{Y}}_i)(\mathbf{Y}_{i,j} - \bar{\mathbf{Y}}_i)'$ and $\bar{\mathbf{Y}}_i = \frac{1}{n_i} \sum_{j=1}^{n_i} \mathbf{Y}_{i,j}$ are the sample covariance matrix and sample mean, respectively. Working with the structure of the data frame X in (5.12), we can calculate the sample means and sample covariance matrices in R as follows:

```
names(X)[1] <- "Group"

dat_R <- X[X$Group == "Reference", -1] # Reference data
dat_T <- X[X$Group == "Test", -1]      # Test data
nlocs <- ncol(dat_R)                   # No. of time points
nreps <- nrow(dat_R)                   # No. of runs

Ybar_R <- apply(dat_R, 2, mean)        # Ref. sample mean
Ybar_T <- apply(dat_T, 2, mean)        # Test sample mean

# Calculation of ref. sample covariance matrix
anoms <- as.matrix(t(t(dat_R) - Ybar_R))
S2_R <- matrix(0, nlocs, nlocs)
for(i in 1:nreps){
  S2_R <- S2_R + (anoms[i,]) %*% t(anoms[i,])
}

# Calculation of test sample covariance matrix
anoms <- as.matrix(t(t(dat_T) - Ybar_T))
S2_T <- matrix(0, nlocs, nlocs)
for(i in 1:nreps){
  S2_T <- S2_T + (anoms[i,]) %*% t(anoms[i,])
 }
```

From here, posterior samples of $\boldsymbol{\mu}_R, \boldsymbol{\mu}_T, \boldsymbol{\Sigma}_R$, and $\boldsymbol{\Sigma}_T$ can be obtained, via Markov chain Monte Carlo (MCMC), by directly sampling from the distributions in (5.14) and (5.15) in an iterative fashion. That is, for a given number of posterior samples, say B, we start by sampling $\boldsymbol{\Sigma}_{\boldsymbol{R}}$, and $\boldsymbol{\Sigma}_T$ from the inverse Wishart distribution in (5.14), and then proceed to sample $\boldsymbol{\mu}_R$ and $\boldsymbol{\mu}_T$ from the multivariate normal distribution in (5.15) conditioned upon our previous samples of $\boldsymbol{\Sigma}_R$, and $\boldsymbol{\Sigma}_T$. This iterative process continues until B posterior samples have been drawn. Once obtained, the B posterior samples of $\boldsymbol{\mu}_R$ and $\boldsymbol{\mu}_T$ can be plugged directly into equations (5.6) and (5.9) in order to obtain B posterior samples of F_2 and δ. Implementing this rather straightforward sampling algorithm in R can be done as follows:

```
nrun <- B                  # No. of posterior samples
f2 <- rep(NA, nrun)
delta <- rep(NA, nrun)

for(i in 1:nrun){
  V_R <- riwish(nreps - 1, S2_R)
  mu_R <- rmnorm(1, Ybar_R, V_R)

  V_T <- riwish(nreps - 1, S2_T)
  mu_T <- rmnorm(1, Ybar_T, V_T)
```

```
    delta[i] <- max(abs(mu_R - mu_T))
    f2[i] <- 50 * log10(1 / sqrt(1 + (1 / length(mu_R)) *
              sum((mu_R - mu_T)^2)) * 100)
}
```

Lastly, the probability of interest, q in (5.10), can be calculated as the proportion of MCMC samples where both $\delta < 15$ and $f2 > 50$. Alternatively, $100(1-\alpha)\%$ credible intervals can be calculated for both F_2 and δ by computing the $100(\alpha/2)$ and $100(1-\alpha/2)$ percentiles from the B posterior samples of F_2 and δ. For a given value of α, these quantities can be calculated in R as follows:

```
q <- sum(delta < 15 & f2 > 50) / B
f2_credible <- c(quantile(f2, alpha / 2),
                 quantile(f2, 1 - alpha / 2))
delta_credible <- c(quantile(delta, alpha / 2),
                    quantile(delta, 1 - alpha / 2))
```

5.2.3 Hierarchical Gaussian Process Model

Pourmohamad et al. (2022) provide a good approximation to the integral in (5.11) by modeling the reference and test dissolution data using hierarchical Gaussian processes. A fully continuous Gaussian process model can be written as

$$\begin{aligned} Y_{i,j}(t) &\sim \mathrm{GP}(\mu_i(t), \sigma^2 k(t,t';\phi)), i = 1, ..., n, & (5.16)\\ \mu_i(t) &\sim \mathrm{GP}(m, \tau^2 h(t,t';\psi)), & (5.17)\end{aligned}$$

for i equal to R and T. For the upper level of the Gaussian process in (5.16), $\mu(t)$ is the mean function and $\sigma^2 k(t,t';\phi)$ is the covariance function with scale σ^2 and shape/range parameters denoted by ϕ. For the lower level in (5.17), the mean is a constant value m and the covariance is $\tau^2 h(t,t';\psi)$ where τ^2 is the scale and ϕ represents the shape and scale parameters.

When a Gaussian process is fit to data, a discrete version is used in which $\mathbf{Y}_{i,j} = (Y_{i,j}(t_1), ..., Y_{i,j}(t_p))$ and $\boldsymbol{\mu}_i = (\mu_i(t_1), ..., \mu_i(t_p))$. Covariance matrix $\sigma^2\mathbf{K}(\phi)$ is constructed where the (i,j)-th element of $\mathbf{K}(\phi)$ is $k(t_i, t_j; \phi)$, and $\tau^2\mathbf{H}(\psi)$ is built in a similar manner with respect to the covariance function h. The model for discretely observed data is then

$$\begin{aligned} \mathbf{Y}_{i,j} &\sim N(\boldsymbol{\mu}_i, \sigma^2\mathbf{K}(\phi)), i = 1, ..., n, & (5.18)\\ \boldsymbol{\mu}_i &\sim N(\boldsymbol{m}, \tau^2\mathbf{H}(\psi)). & (5.19)\end{aligned}$$

Gibbs sampling (Casella and George, 1992) will be used to sample from the posterior distributions of most all of the parameters. Draws can be taken from the posterior distributions of $\boldsymbol{\mu}_i$, τ^2, and σ^2 using closed form full conditionals when using inverse gamma priors for σ^2 and τ^2 with hyperparameters α_σ, β_σ, α_τ and β_τ. The covariance parameters ϕ and ψ must be estimated using Metropolis-Hastings methods (Hastings, 1970). We will assume gamma priors for ϕ and ψ with hyperparamaters α_ϕ, β_ϕ, α_ψ and β_ψ. For finer details about the model and mathematical derivations of the posterior distributions, please refer to Pourmohamad et al. (2022).

The following code we show here does not distinguish between the reference and test group, but rather a general Gaussian process that can be applied to either group. Draws from the posterior distributions for each of these parameters proceeds as follows:

```
# Draw mu
Xbar <- apply(X, 2, mean)
Vinv <- solve(tau2 * solve(H) + n * sigma2 * solve(K))
mstar <- n * sigma2 * Vinv %*% K %*% Ybar
mu <- rmnorm(1, mstar, Vinv)

# Draw sigma^2
Xcent <- as.matrix(t(t(X) - mu))
wsse <- sum(diag(Xcent %*% K %*% t(Xcent)))
sigma2 <- rigamma(1, alpha_v + nloc*n/2, beta_v + 1/2 * wsse)

# Draw tau^2
tau2 <- rigamma(1, alpha_v + nloc * 1 / 2,
        beta_v + 1 / 2 * mu %*% solve(H, mu))

# Draw phi
phi_new <- exp(rnorm(1, log(phi), prop_phi))
Knew <- exp(-D^2/phi_new)
alph <- dmnorm(X, mu, sigma2*Knew, log = TRUE) +
        dgamma(phi_new, alpha_r, beta_r, log = TRUE) -
        dmnorm(X,mu, sigma2*K, log = TRUE) -
        dgamma(phi, alpha_r, beta_r, log = TRUE)

if(log(runif(1)) < alph){
      phi <- phi_new
      K <- Knew
}


# Draw psi
psi_new <- exp(rnorm(1, log(psi), prop_psi))
Hnew <- exp(-D^2/psi_new)
alph <- dmnorm(mu, m, tau2*Hnew, log = TRUE) +
        dgamma(psi_new, alpha_v, beta_v, log = TRUE) -
        dmnorm(mu, m, tau2*H, log = TRUE) -
        dgamma(psi, alpha_r, beta_r, log = TRUE)

if(log(runif(1)) < alph){
      psi <- psi_new
      H <- Hnew
}
```

For the interpolation of the process to points between the observed data (i.e., predicting the dissolution values at unobserved time points), we work specifically with the Gaussian process of the mean function using (5.17). Let $\boldsymbol{t}^*$ be the set of r time points where the process will be estimated between time points, $\boldsymbol{t}^* = \{t_1^*, ..., t_r^*\}$, and $\boldsymbol{\mu}_{\boldsymbol{t}^*}$ be the vector of process values at those time points. The matrix $\mathbf{H}_{\boldsymbol{t}^*}$ is a covariance matrix of unobserved time points, meaning that the $(i,j)-$th element of $\mathbf{H}_{\boldsymbol{t}^*}$ is $h(t_i^*, t_j^*; \psi)$. The vector $\mathbf{h}_{\boldsymbol{t}^*}$ is the cross covariance between unobserved and observed time points, again using the covariance function h. Then the interpolated points can be drawn using the following code.

```
mnew <- m + t(hstar) %*% solve(H, mu-m)
signew <- Hstar - t(hstar) %*% solve(H, hstar)
mu_tstar <- rmnorm(1, mnew, signew)
```

The full estimating procedure involves sampling repeatedly, say B times, from each of the conditional posterior distributions, including performing the Metropolis-Hastings steps for the range parameters.

Now, let $\mu_R(t)$ and $\mu_T(t)$ be the mean functions for the reference and test sets respectively, meaning that they will take the place of $\mu(t)$ in the above formulas. Also let $\boldsymbol{\mu}_{R,\mathcal{A}} = (\boldsymbol{\mu}_R', \boldsymbol{\mu}_{R,\boldsymbol{t}^*}')'$ be the vector of observed and unobserved posterior draws for the mean function of the reference product, with a similar definition for $\boldsymbol{\mu}_{T,\mathcal{A}}$ and the test product. To calculate an estimate of the F_2 parameter under the hierarchical Gaussian process model, we can use

$$F_2 = 50 \log_{10} \left[100 \left(1 + \frac{1}{p+r} ||\boldsymbol{\mu}_{R,\mathcal{A}} - \boldsymbol{\mu}_{T,\mathcal{A}}||^2 \right)^{-1/2} \right]. \tag{5.20}$$

Posterior samples of F_2 can be obtained be making draws of $\boldsymbol{\mu}_{R,\mathcal{A}}$ and $\boldsymbol{\mu}_{T,\mathcal{A}}$ over the course of the MCMC sampling algorithm to generate a full posterior distribution for F_2. Likewise, the δ parameter introduced in Novick et al. (2015) can also be calculated via posterior draws of $\boldsymbol{\mu}_{R,\mathcal{A}}$ and $\boldsymbol{\mu}_{T,\mathcal{A}}$ using the following formula,

$$\delta = \max\left(|\boldsymbol{\mu}_{R,\mathcal{A}} - \boldsymbol{\mu}_{T,\mathcal{A}}|\right). \tag{5.21}$$

Posterior samples of F_2 and δ can be obtained as follows

```
f2 <- 50 * log10(1 / sqrt(1 + (1 / (nlocs + ninterp)) *
    sum((mustar_R - mustar_T)^2)) * 100)
delta <- max(abs(mustar_R - mustar_T))
```

5.2.4 R Function Wrappers

For ease of use, we took the methodology and code from Sections 5.2.2 and 5.2.3 and wrapped them as R functions. The functions can be downloaded for use at the following location: `https://github.com/BayesCMC/Book`.

The function `bmn()` implements the Bayesian multivariate normal model and takes two arguments as inputs. The first input to the function is the data frame `dis_data` containing the dissolution data set. `dis_data` should be formatted in the same orientation as X in (5.12). The second input is an integer value `B` which specifies the number of posterior draws to make. The function then returns the B posterior draws of δ and F_2 as a list that can be used to calculate further quantities of interest such as credible intervals, or the probability q. Likewise, the function also returns the posterior draws of μ_{R,t_k} and μ_{T,t_k}.

The function `hgp()` implements the hierarchical Gaussian process model and takes several arguments as inputs. The first input to the function is again the data frame `dis_data` containing the dissolution data set. The second input, `locs`, is an ordered vector of length p that corresponds to the time points at which the dissolution data was measured at. The input `n_interp` is an integer value specifying the number of time points to interpolate at. The interpolated time points are taken on an equally spaced grid starting at the first observed time point and ending at the last observed time point. The input `control` is a list of potential priors and initial values. More specifically, `control` can be used to define the following settings:

- `sigma2_starting` – starting value for σ^2
- `tau2_starting` – starting value for τ^2
- `phi_starting` – starting value for ϕ
- `psi_starting` – starting value for ψ
- `sigma2_alpha` and `sigma2_beta` are the parameters for the inverse gamma prior for σ^2
- `tau2_alpha` and `tau2_beta` are the parameters for the inverse gamma prior for τ^2
- `phi_alpha` and `phi_beta` are the parameters for the gamma prior for ϕ
- `psi_alpha` and `psi_beta` are the parameters for the gamma prior for ψ
- `prop_phi` – proposal variance for the parameters ϕ
- `prop_psi` – proposal variance for the parameters ψ

These values can be adjusted using input arguments such as `control = list(sigma2_starting = 1)`, for example. However, the `control` parameter does not need to be specified by the user as the default values for each of the settings tend to work well based on empirical evidence in a number of examples. The last parameter to the `hgp()` function is for the option of using a form of adaptive MCMC. If `adaptive = TRUE`, this would replace both `prop_phi` and `prop_psi` by using past MCMC draws to inform the proposal variance.

5.3 Case Study

We will apply the Bayesian methods described in Sections 5.2.2 and 5.2.3 to a real dissolution data set taken from Ocaña et al. (2009). The data consists of dissolution measurements taken on oral tablets made with metoclopramide hydrochloride. Of interest is to test the similarity of metoclopramide hydrochloride tablets made with and without the ingredient tensioactive. Here there are $n_T = 12$ tablets with tensioactive (test product) and $n_R = 12$

TABLE 5.1
Dissolution data (in %) for the reference and test products presented in Ocaña et al. (2009).

		Time Points							
	Tablet	1	2	3	4	5	6	7	8
Reference	1	19.78	37.61	48.53	60.62	63.34	68.72	75.76	83.42
	2	22.05	36.74	46.12	53.90	61.35	67.35	72.85	77.88
	3	21.50	34.58	44.88	53.46	61.09	66.83	73.11	77.28
	4	20.24	35.23	50.27	66.49	75.87	79.84	83.33	87.57
	5	17.66	33.51	47.97	59.29	67.52	70.05	77.04	80.88
	6	18.16	33.75	49.02	58.26	71.63	74.98	80.38	84.33
	7	20.94	33.31	47.40	59.26	68.65	75.82	79.98	82.96
	8	19.43	31.40	44.18	56.20	67.36	75.03	79.70	83.98
	9	19.12	32.93	47.79	60.19	69.71	76.26	80.84	83.95
	10	19.76	31.67	44.92	56.79	66.83	74.41	78.77	82.30
	11	20.64	32.42	45.80	58.11	69.46	76.81	81.57	85.83
	12	19.22	32.14	46.60	58.16	64.18	75.79	81.49	83.94

		Time Points							
	Tablet	1	2	3	4	5	6	7	8
Test	1	35.70	48.81	57.05	65.01	71.92	75.32	80.64	83.52
	2	36.10	52.88	61.79	67.54	74.47	78.71	80.71	83.23
	3	41.66	52.52	63.22	70.21	76.71	80.00	83.25	85.61
	4	35.49	50.39	58.99	65.68	72.59	76.58	80.52	83.00
	5	36.06	52.09	63.46	69.84	75.23	78.57	81.53	84.37
	6	35.53	51.63	62.59	68.68	75.64	79.43	82.99	85.81
	7	32.70	46.85	57.51	65.00	71.26	75.24	79.18	81.21
	8	33.85	44.89	53.64	60.87	67.34	71.18	73.51	76.42
	9	32.33	46.58	56.46	64.38	70.30	75.17	77.83	79.86
	10	32.80	46.37	56.66	65.37	70.04	75.33	77.11	80.45
	11	33.86	46.72	57.45	65.40	71.05	75.78	76.22	79.38
	12	32.46	45.60	55.04	62.78	68.54	73.06	75.73	77.68

tablets without tensioactive (reference product) at $p = 8$ time points. The dissolution data from Ocaña et al. (2009) is given in Table 5.1.

The data can be downloaded from `https://github.com/BayesCMC/Book`, or loaded into R as follows:

```
X <- matrix(c(
19.78, 37.61, 48.53, 60.62, 63.34, 68.72, 75.76, 83.42,
22.05, 36.74, 46.12, 53.90, 61.35, 67.35, 72.85, 77.88,
21.50, 34.58, 44.88, 53.46, 61.09, 66.83, 73.11, 77.28,
20.24, 35.23, 50.27, 66.49, 75.87, 79.84, 83.33, 87.57,
17.66, 33.51, 47.97, 59.29, 67.52, 70.05, 77.04, 80.88,
18.16, 33.75, 49.02, 58.26, 71.63, 74.98, 80.38, 84.33,
20.94, 33.31, 47.40, 59.26, 68.65, 75.82, 79.98, 82.96,
19.43, 31.40, 44.18, 56.20, 67.36, 75.03, 79.70, 83.98,
19.12, 32.93, 47.79, 60.19, 69.71, 76.26, 80.84, 83.95,
19.76, 31.67, 44.92, 56.79, 66.83, 74.41, 78.77, 82.30,
20.64, 32.42, 45.80, 58.11, 69.46, 76.81, 81.57, 85.83,
19.22, 32.14, 46.60, 58.16, 64.18, 75.79, 81.49, 83.94,
```

```
35.70, 48.81, 57.05, 65.01, 71.92, 75.32, 80.64, 83.52,
36.10, 52.88, 61.79, 67.54, 74.47, 78.71, 80.71, 83.23,
41.66, 52.52, 63.22, 70.21, 76.71, 80.00, 83.25, 85.61,
35.49, 50.39, 58.99, 65.68, 72.59, 76.58, 80.52, 83.00,
36.06, 52.09, 63.46, 69.84, 75.23, 78.57, 81.53, 84.37,
35.53, 51.63, 62.59, 68.68, 75.64, 79.43, 82.99, 85.81,
32.70, 46.85, 57.51, 65.00, 71.26, 75.24, 79.18, 81.21,
33.85, 44.89, 53.64, 60.87, 67.34, 71.18, 73.51, 76.42,
32.33, 46.58, 56.46, 64.38, 70.30, 75.17, 77.83, 79.86,
32.80, 46.37, 56.66, 65.37, 70.04, 75.33, 77.11, 80.45,
33.86, 46.72, 57.45, 65.40, 71.05, 75.78, 76.22, 79.38,
32.46, 45.60, 55.04, 62.78, 68.54, 73.06, 75.73, 77.68),
nrow = 24, byrow = TRUE)

X <- data.frame(group = rep(c("Reference", "Test"),
                             each = 12), X)
```

Before any Bayesian modeling approach is taken, we recommend a visual inspection of the dissolution data to get an informal sense of how similar the two products may be. Additionally, one may want to check such things as whether or not there is a substantial amount of within time point variability for a given product, or if there are any "odd" or "extreme" dissolution curves that might affect the Bayesian model fitting process. A useful plot for this sort of assessment can be seen in Figure 5.1 and can be generated with the following code:

```
matplot(t(X[,-1]), pch = rep(c(19, 17), each = 12),
        col = rep(c("gray65","black"), each = 12),
        xlab = "Time Points",
        ylab = "Percentage Dissolved")
legend("bottomright", c("Reference", "Test"), pch = c(19, 17),
       col = c("gray65", "black"), bty = "n")
```

The addition of line segments connecting points on the same dissolution curve can be useful as well for further determining any odd curves in the data (for example, highly non-monotonic data). However, it was not necessary in our case. Based on our data, the sets of dissolution curves look rather well behaved, with the reference and test product looking slightly dissimilar at earlier time points, but becoming increasingly more similar at later time points. Again, this is not a formal assessment, but rather a first pass approach to get a feeling for the data, and whether or not it seems appropriate to apply 1) the f_2 statistic criteria, and 2) the Bayesian modeling approaches. Here, both assumptions seem reasonably satisfied based on the data.

Based on the dissolution data set, the calculated value of the f_2 statistic is $f_2 = 51.71$, i.e.,

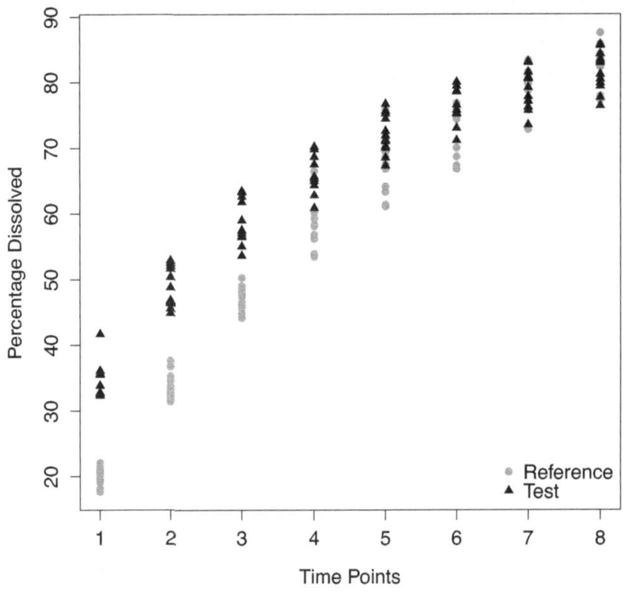

FIGURE 5.1
The dissolution data for the reference and test products presented in Ocaña et al. (2009).

```
ybar_R <- apply(X[X$group == "Reference", -1], 2, mean)
ybar_T <- apply(X[X$group == "Test", -1], 2, mean)
f2 <- 50 * log10(1 / sqrt(1 + (1 / length(ybar_R)) *
      sum((ybar_R - ybar_T)^2)) * 100)
> f2
[1] 51.70784
```

which would indicate that the reference and test products would be deemed similar based on health authority guidelines. Clearly in this instance though, the use of the F_2 parameter and its associated uncertainty quantification is extremely important since the value of the f_2 statistic is very close to the decision threshold of 50.

Now, we chose the Ocaña et al. (2009) data set as our case study example due to a particular issue with the data that highlights a very important point between the Bayesian multivariate normal (BMN) model (Section 5.2.2) and the hierarchical Gaussian process (HGP) model (Section 5.2.3). The BMN model, as well as the original f_2 statistic calculation, can be used without having knowledge about the actual values of the time points in which the dissolution curves are measured at. The same cannot be said for the HGP model. The HGP model cannot be run without specifying the values of the time points at which data collection is being made at. This critical dependence on the time point values stems from the fact that estimation of the HGP model's covariance parameters is highly dependent on the distance between time points (see, for example, Rasmussen and Williams (2006) for more details on Gaussian process parameter estimation). Now, the details of the dissolution data in Ocaña et al. (2009) did not include the actual values of the time points at which measurements of dissolution were taken at. Furthermore, upon requesting this information it was made apparent that this information would not be available due to unforeseen circumstances. In practice, when collecting one's own data this might not seem like an issue, but perhaps looking back at one's own data, for the sake of retrospective analyses, it seems entirely plausible that this issue may arise (say based on poor documentation of the data, for example). This certainly highlights a clear benefit for the BMN model. However, as shown in (Pourmohamad et al., 2022), the process of estimating and quantifying the uncertainty of the F_2 parameter and δ can be significantly improved by the extra information gain from the time point values when using the HGP model over the BMN model.

Under the assumption of equally spaced time points, the HGP model can still be used without the specification of time point values since parameter estimation under a Gaussian process is still valid based on a rescaling of the original input data. However, in the sections that follow, we will assume that we know the values of the time points at which dissolution measurements are taken in order to show how dissolution testing proceeds under both the BMN and HGP models.

5.3.1 Equally Spaced Time Points

We assume that the time points for the dissolution data from Ocaña et al. (2009) are equally spaced at ten minute increments starting at 10 minutes and ending at 80 minutes. We first proceed with dissolution testing of the reference and test product using the Bayesian multivariate normal model. In order to use the `bmn()` function, we specify the number of posterior samples, B, we wish to obtain as well as the number of samples we plan to burn-in.

```
tp <- seq(10, 80, 10)  # Time points
B <- 10000             # Number of posterior samples
burnin <- 0.1 * B      # Amount of samples to burn-in

method1 <- bmn(X, B)   # Bayesian multivariate normal model
```

The posterior samples of $\boldsymbol{\mu}_R, \boldsymbol{\mu}_T, \delta$, and F_2 are stored in an object called `method1`. Next, we must remove the burn-in samples. As a rule of thumb, we recommend removing 10% of the posterior samples for burn-in. In the BMN model, posterior samples are drawn using only a Gibbs sampler and so we do not recommend thinning the samples as the level of autocorrelation will tend to be extremely low.

```
# Removing samples for burn-in
method1$delta <- method1$delta[-(1:burnin)]
method1$f2 <- method1$f2[-(1:burnin)]
method1$mu_R <- method1$muR[,-(1:burnin)]
method1$mu_T <- method1$muT[,-(1:burnin)]
```

Checking the effective sample sizes (ESS) further validates our recommendations as the smallest ESS is 9000 (i.e., we achieved the maximum effective sample size possible). Here, the effective sample sizes of $\boldsymbol{\mu}_R$ and $\boldsymbol{\mu}_T$ can be calculated using the `ESS()` function.

```
> min(apply(method1$mu_R, 1, ESS))    # Effective sample size
[1] 9000
> min(apply(method1$mu_T, 1, ESS))
[1] 9000
```

Other qualitative checks (for example, see Chapter 3 of this book) of the posterior samples should be taken to ensure that the samples can be used for inference and dissolution testing. Trace plots of the posterior samples (Figure 5.2) and posterior density plots (Figure 5.3) can be used to check the adequacy of the posterior samples obtained. Here we obtain trace plots of the posterior samples of $\boldsymbol{\mu}_R$ and $\boldsymbol{\mu}_T$ as follows:

```
N <- B - burnin          # Number of samples after burn-in
chains <- data.frame( # Data frame holding posterior samples
          samples = rep(c(1:N, 1:N), each = ncol(X) - 1),
          group = rep(c("muR","muT"), each = (ncol(X) - 1)*N),
          timepoint = paste("Time Point",
                            rep(1:(ncol(X) - 1), 2 * N)),
          values = c(c(method1$mu_R), c(method1$mu_T)))

# Trace plots
ggplot(chains, aes(samples, values)) +
  geom_line() +
  labs(x = "Iterations", y = "Posterior Sample Values") +
  facet_wrap(group~timepoint) +
  theme(text = element_text(size = 16))
```

The trace plots in Figure 5.2 show good mixing of the chains of the posterior samples of μ_{R,t_k} and μ_{T,t_k} at all eight time points. Although we do not show it here, multiple restarts of the chains with different initial values did not have an impact on the convergence (or mixing) of the chains.

Posterior density plots of μ_{R,t_k} and μ_{T,t_k} (Figure 5.3) showed nice symmetric unimodal distributions at each of the eight time points. Posterior density plots can be obtained via the following code:

```
# Posterior density plots
ggplot(chains, aes(values)) +
  geom_density() +
  labs(y = "Posterior Density") +
  facet_wrap(group~timepoint, scales = "free") +
  theme(text = element_text(size = 16))
```

Once all of these posterior sample checks have been completed, dissolution testing of the reference and test product can be carried out. Here we illustrate the use of the probability

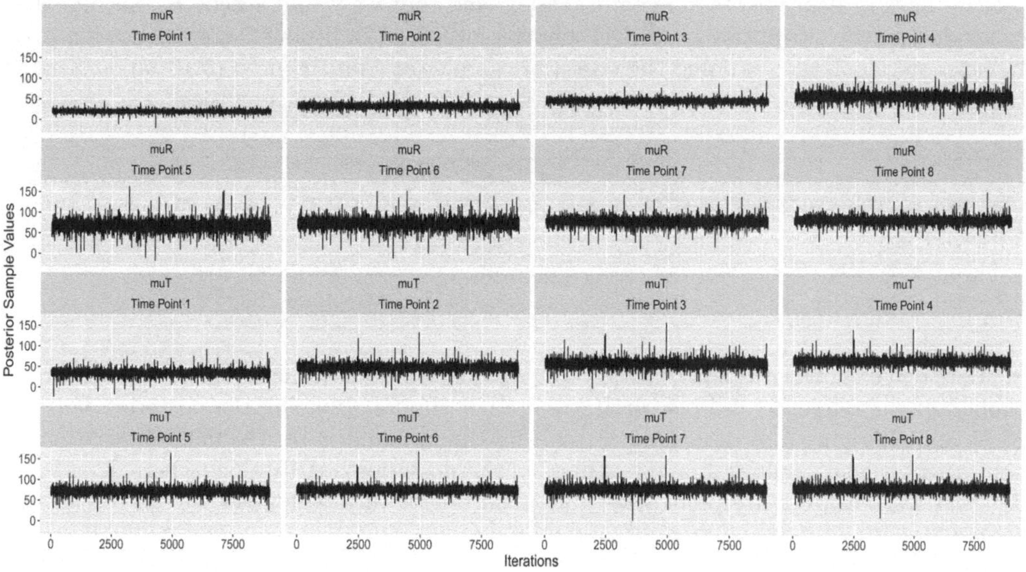

FIGURE 5.2
Trace plots of the posterior samples of μ_{R,t_k} and μ_{T,t_k} for the reference and test products (denoted `muR` and `muT`, respectively) at the 8 observed time points.

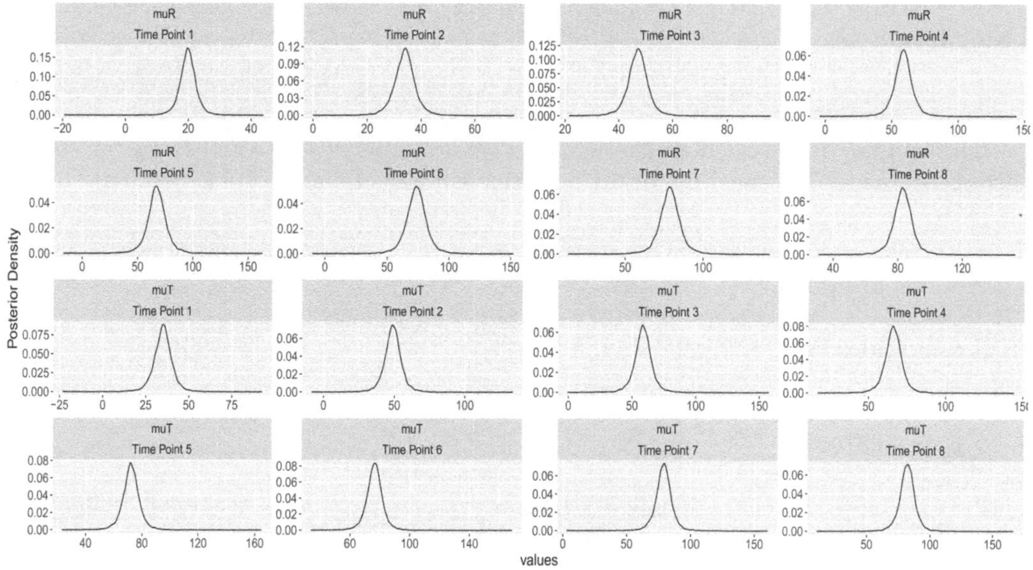

FIGURE 5.3
Posterior density plots of μ_{R,t_k} and μ_{T,t_k} for the reference and test products (denoted `muR` and `muT`, respectively) at the 8 observed time points.

q, as well as Bayesian credible intervals for δ and F_2, for dissolution testing. Let us assume that we have presepecified a value of $q_0 = 0.95$ and that we would accept H_a in (5.8) (i.e., conclude that the dissolution profiles of the reference and test products are similar) if $q \geq q_0$. In order to calculate q, we plug the posterior samples of δ and F_2 into (5.10) and calculate the proportion of times the posterior samples satisfy the set of inequalities, i.e.,

```
q <- sum(method1$delta < 15 & method1$f2 > 50) / (B - burnin)
> q
[1] 0.2383333
```

Here $q = 0.24$ which is less than $q_0 = 0.95$ and so we would conclude that the dissolution profiles of the reference and test products are not similar. Plotting the posterior densities of F_2 and δ (Figure 5.4), it is easy to see why the probability q is so much lower than q_0 since there is a substantial amount of mass of the posterior distributions where $\delta > 15$ and $F_2 < 50$. Posterior density plots of F_2 and δ can be obtained as follows:

```
plot(density(method1$f2), xlab = expression(F[2]),
      ylab = "Posterior Density",
      main = expression("Posterior Density of "*F[2]))
abline(v = 50, lty = 2)

plot(density(method1$delta), xlab = expression(delta),
      ylab = "Posterior Density",
      main = expression("Posterior Density of "*delta))
abline(v = 15, lty = 2)
```

If instead we wish to calculate the, say, 95% credible intervals for δ and F_2 we can simply take the 2.5 and 97.5 percentiles of the posterior samples of δ and F_2, i.e.,

```
alpha <- 0.05
f2_cred <- c(quantile(method1$f2, alpha / 2),
  quantile(method1$f2, 1 - alpha / 2))
> f2_cred
    2.5%    97.5%
29.52491 63.02059

delta_cred <- c(quantile(method1$delta, alpha / 2),
  quantile(method1$delta, 1 - alpha / 2))
> delta_cred
     2.5%     97.5%
 9.068288 37.995474
```

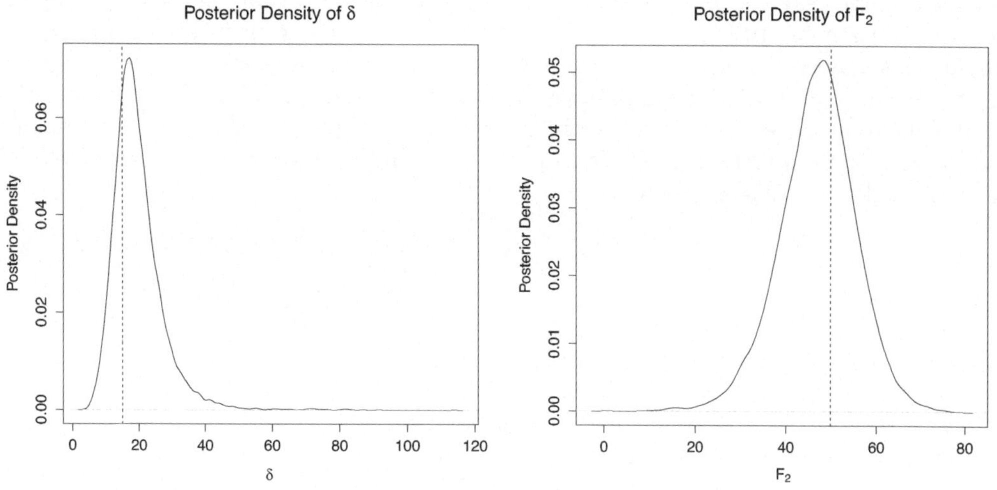

FIGURE 5.4
The posterior distribution of δ and F_2 based on the Bayesian multivariate normal model. Vertical dashed lines are placed at $\delta = 15$ and $F_2 = 50$.

The 95% credible interval for F_2 (i.e., (29.5, 63.0)) is not completely above 50, and the 95% credible interval for δ (i.e., (9.1, 40.0)) is not completely below 15, and so again we would conclude that the dissolution profiles of the reference and test products are not similar.

Using the hierarchical Gaussian process model (Section 5.2.3) proceeds analogously to the BMN model. To use the `hgp()` function we need to specify the number of posterior samples, B, and the number of samples to use for burn-in. Additionally, we must also specify the number of points to interpolate the HGP model at. As shown in Pourmohamad et al. (2022), the bias in the estimate of F_2 decreases as the number of interpolated points increases. However, it is best not to set the number of interpolated points too high as computations can be very slow for very fine grids of interpolated points. In general, we suggest using at least 30 interpolated points as a rule of thumb based off of our own experiences with using the method. For the Ocaña et al. (2009) dissolution data, we chose to use 100 interpolated points as the code still ran reasonably fast. If no lists of prior values are passed to the function, via the `control` parameter, then the default priors highlighted in Section 5.2.3 are used. Section 5.3.2 will give an example of when different priors may want to be specified. Running the `hgp()` command proceeds as follows:

```
B <- 100000
burnin <- 0.1 * B
thin <- 10

method2 <- hgp(X, locs = tp, B = B, n_interp = 100)
```

The posterior samples of all of the parameters are stored in an object called `method2`. Note now that we have specified an addiotional variable called `thin` that can be used to thin our posterior samples in case there is any autocorrelation within our MCMC sampler. Here setting `thin <- 10` is due to the fact that we plan to only keep every tenth posterior sample. This may seem a little high but we choose it this way since we are also sampling a very high number of posterior samples, i.e., $B = 100{,}000$, and again burning-in 10% of the samples. Thus, at the end we are left with 9,000 posterior samples to use (the same amount as the example of the BMN model). Burn-in and thinning for the covariance parameters of the HGP model proceeds as follows:

```
phi <- method2$mcmc_chains$cov_pars$phi[-c(1:burnin)]
phi <- phi[seq(1, (B-burnin), thin)]
psi <- method2$mcmc_chains$cov_pars$psi[-c(1:burnin)]
psi <- psi[seq(1, (B-burnin), thin)]
sigma_R <- method2$mcmc_chains$cov_pars$sigma_R[-c(1:burnin)]
sigma_R <- sigma_R[seq(1, (B-burnin), thin)]
sigma_T <- method2$mcmc_chains$cov_pars$sigma_T[-c(1:burnin)]
sigma_T <- sigma_T[seq(1, (B-burnin), thin)]
tau <- method2$mcmc_chains$cov_pars$tau[-c(1:burnin)]
tau <- tau[seq(1, (B-burnin), thin)]
```

Recall that the samples of $\mu_R(t)$ and $\mu_T(t)$ are actually taken from the posterior predictive distribution, and not the posterior distribution, which is why we do not necessarily need to concern ourselves with burn-in and thinning of these samples when checking the quality of our posterior samples taken from our MCMC sampler. Checking the minimum effective sample size of our posterior samples yields a large ESS of 2926, i.e.,

```
> min(ESS(phi), ESS(psi), ESS(sigma_R),
                          ESS(sigma_T), ESS(tau))
[1] 2926
```

Next we can check for convergence of the trace plots of the posterior samples. Here we plot the posterior samples over time for each parameter (Figure 5.5) with the following code:

```
chains <- data.frame( # Data frame holding posterior samples
           samples = rep(1:((B-burnin)/thin), times = 5),
           parameter = rep(c("phi", "psi", "sigma_R",
                             "sigma_T", "tau"),
                             each = (B-burnin)/thin),
          values = c(phi, psi, sigma_R, sigma_T, tau))

chains$parameter <- factor(chains$parameter,
                           labels = c(expression(phi),
                                      expression(psi),
                                      expression(sigma[R]),
```

```
                                    expression(sigma[T]),
                                    expression(tau)))

ggplot(chains, aes(samples, values)) +
  geom_line() +
  labs(x = "Iterations", y = "Posterior Sample Values") +
  facet_wrap(~parameter, scales = "free",
             labeller = label_parsed) +
  theme(text = element_text(size = 22))
```

All of the chains in Figure 5.5 appear to be well mixed with no convergence concerns. Similarly, starting the chains at different initial values would yield similar results (not shown).

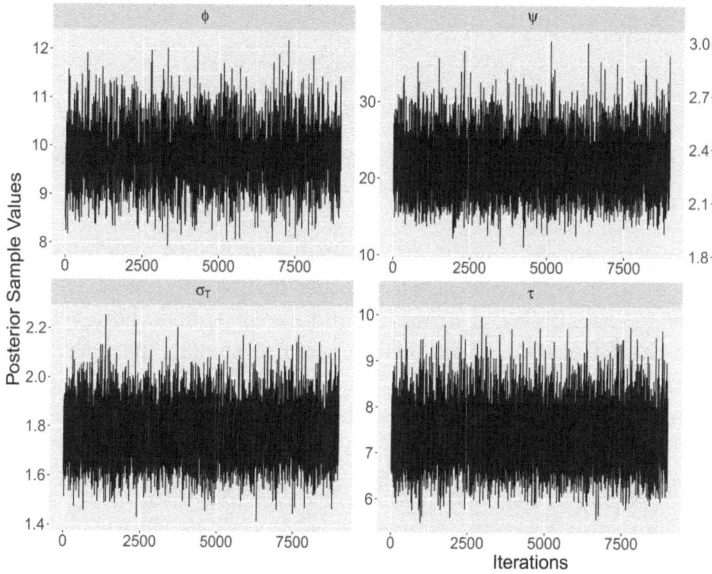

FIGURE 5.5
Trace plots of the posterior samples for the parameters of the covariance matrix of the hierarchical Gaussian process model.

Posterior density plots of the covariance parameters $\phi, \psi, \sigma_R, \sigma_T$, and τ (Figure 5.6) displayed nice symmetric unimodal distributions. Posterior density plots can be obtained via the following code:

```
ggplot(chains, aes(values)) +
  geom_density() +
  labs(x = "Values", y = "Posterior Density") +
  facet_wrap(~parameter, scales = "free",
             labeller = label_parsed) +
  theme(text = element_text(size = 22))
```

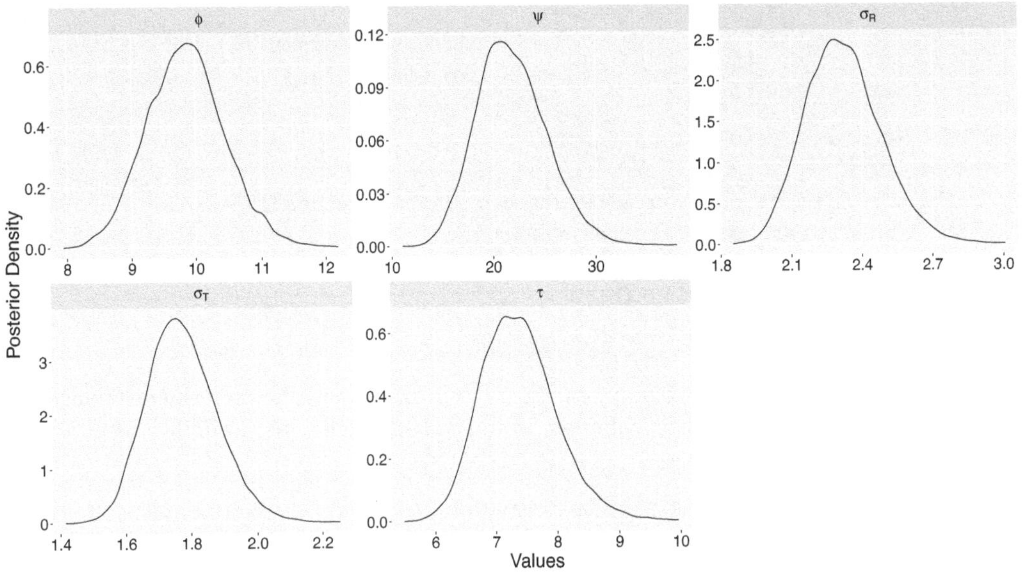

FIGURE 5.6
Posterior density plots for the parameters of the covariance matrix of the hierarchical Gaussian process model.

Once all posterior sample quality checks have been satisfied, one should next plot the prediction under the HGP model to qualitatively check whether or not the predictive distribution seems reasonable. Here, reasonable can mean many different things, however, we prefer to think of it as 1) does the HGP model's prediction seem to roughly pass through the center (or mean) of the observed data, and 2) does the prediction seem to be roughly monotone? If both seem satisfied, then the HGP model is likely producing a good fit to the data. A plot of the predicted dissolution curves and uncertainty bands (Figure 5.7) for the reference and test products under the hierarchical Gaussian process model can be achieved as follows:

```
matplot(tp, t(X[,-1]), pch = rep(c(19, 17), each = 12),
        col = rep(c("gray65","black"), each = 12),
        xlab = "Time (Minutes)",
        ylab = "Percentage Dissolved")
legend("bottomright", c("Reference", "Test"), pch = c(19, 17),
       col = c("gray65", "black"), bty = "n")

grid1 <- (1:B)[-(1:burnin)][seq(1, (B-burnin), thin)]
grid2 <- ((B+1):(2*B))[-(1:burnin)][seq(1, (B-burnin), thin)]
lines(grid, apply(method2$mcmc_chains$mu_pars[,grid1], 1,
                  mean), col = "gray65", lwd = 2)
lines(grid, apply(method2$mcmc_chains$mu_pars[,grid2], 1,
                  mean), col = "black", lwd = 2)

lower <- apply(method2$mcmc_chains$mu_pars[,grid1], 1,
               quantile, prob = 0.025)
```

```
upper <- apply(method2$mcmc_chains$mu_pars[,grid1], 1,
               quantile, prob = 0.975)
polygon(c(grid, rev(grid)), c(lower, rev(upper)),
        col = alpha("gray65",.2), border = NA)

lower <- apply(method2$mcmc_chains$mu_pars[,grid2], 1,
               quantile, prob = 0.025)
upper <- apply(method2$mcmc_chains$mu_pars[,grid2], 1,
               quantile, prob = 0.975)
polygon(c(grid, rev(grid)), c(lower, rev(upper)),
        col = alpha("black",.2), border = NA)
```

From Figure 5.7 we see that the HGP model prediction of the reference and test dissolution curves appears to pass roughly through the center of the data and is fairly monotone. A common feature of Gaussian processes is that predictive uncertainty at a given predicted point grows larger the farther away the predicted point is from observed data (and thus shrinking the closer it is to observed data). Given the spacing of the observed time points, the HGP model's uncertainty bands also seem to make sense. Overall, the HGP model seems like a reasonable fit to the data. Moreover, Figure 5.7 gives us an intuition into the similarity of the dissolution profiles of the reference and test products. Here, there is little overlap of the uncertainty bands for the reference and test products at early time points suggesting that the dissolution of the products is fairly dissimilar early on, but grows more similar as time increases.

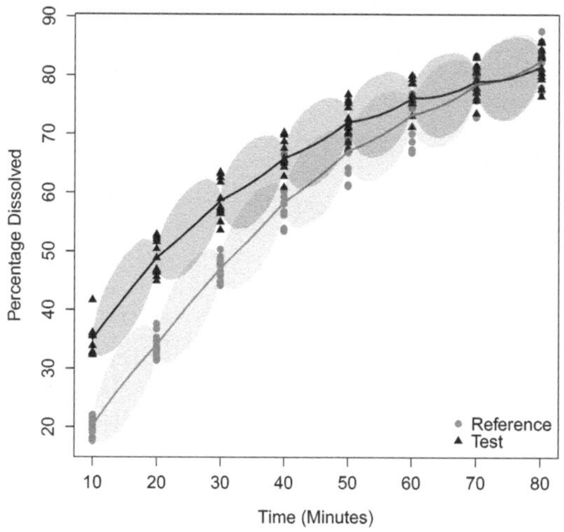

FIGURE 5.7
The predicted dissolution curves and uncertainty bands for the reference and test products under the hierarchical Gaussian process model.

A more formal assessment of the similarity of the reference and test products dissolution profiles can again be assessed via the probability q, and by calculating the credible intervals for F_2 and δ. Let us again assume that we have presepecified a value of $q_0 = 0.95$ and that

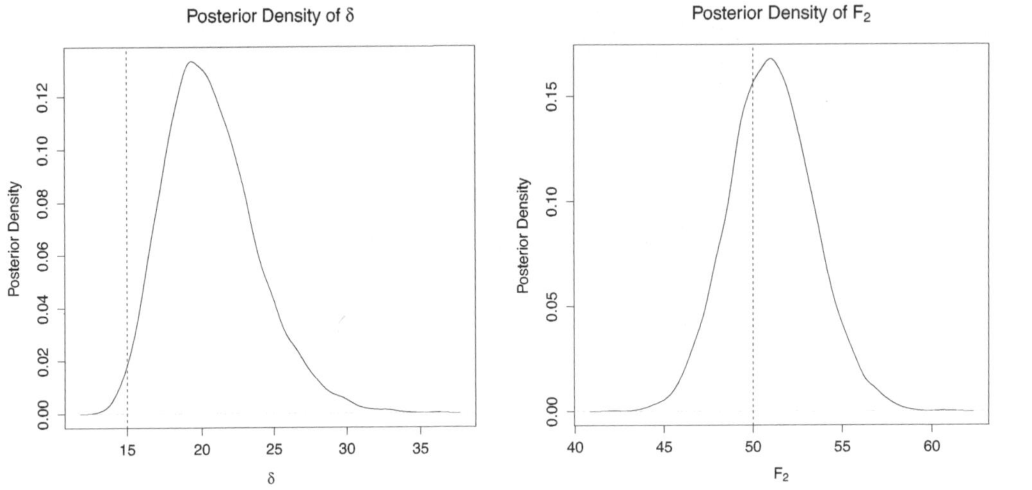

FIGURE 5.8
The posterior distribution of δ and F_2 based on the hierarchical Gaussian process model. Vertical dashed lines are placed at $\delta = 15$ and $F_2 = 50$.

we would conclude that the dissolution profiles of the reference and test products are similar if $q \geq q_0$. In order to calculate q, we plug the posterior samples of δ and F_2 into (5.10) and calculate the proportion of times the posterior samples satisfy the set of inequalities, i.e.,

```
q <- sum(method2$mcmc_chains$delta[grid1] < 15 &
     method2$mcmc_chains$f2[grid1] > 50) /
     ((B - burnin)/thin)
> q
[1] 0.01010101
```

We have $q = 0.01$ which is far less than $q_0 = 0.95$ and so we would conclude that the dissolution profiles of the reference and test products are not similar. Using Figure 5.8, it is easy to see why the probability q is so small given the posterior densities of F_2 and δ. There, we see that a significant proportion of the posterior density of F_2 is above 50, while almost all of the posterior density for δ is larger than 15. Plots of the posterior distributions of F_2 and δ can be obtained as follows:

```
plot(density(method2$mcmc_chains$f2[grid1]),
     xlab = expression(F[2]), ylab = "Posterior Density",
     main = expression("Posterior Density of "*F[2]))
abline(v = 50, lty = 2)

plot(density(method2$mcmc_chains$delta[grid1]),
     xlab = expression(delta), ylab = "Posterior Density",
```

```
      main = expression("Posterior Density of "*delta))
abline(v = 15, lty = 2)
```

Lastly, calculating 95% credible intervals for F_2 and δ yields an interval for F_2 that overlaps with 50, i.e., (46.5, 55.9), and an interval for δ that is completely above 15, i.e., (15.7, 27.6). In this case, using either the probability q or the credible intervals would lead to the same similarity conclusion. The following code calculates the 95% credible intervals for F_2 and δ:

```
alpha <- 0.05
f2_cred <- c(quantile(method2$mcmc_chains$f2[grid1],alpha/2),
      quantile(method2$mcmc_chains$f2[grid1], 1 - alpha / 2))
> f2_cred
    2.5%     97.5%
46.51777 55.85440

delta_cred <- c(quantile(method2$mcmc_chains$delta[grid1],
                alpha / 2),
                quantile(method2$mcmc_chains$delta[grid1],
                1 - alpha / 2))
> delta_cred
    2.5%     97.5%
15.65330 27.64504
```

5.3.2 Unequally Spaced Time Points

In Section 5.3.1, we made the assumption that all of the observed time points were equally spaced. Now, let us assume that the observed time points for the dissolution data in Ocaña et al. (2009) are unequally spaced at 5, 15, 30, 45, 60, 90, 120, and 180 minutes. The change in the configuration of the observed time points has absolutely no impact on the BMN model and so the results from Section 5.3.1 would remain exactly the same. This highlights the fact that the BMN model, while convenient to use, completely ignores the underlying shape of the dissolution curves. On the other hand, the results of the HGP model are highly dependent upon the spacing of the observed time points and so we shall examine how the results might change under a different time point configurations, as well as how to handle any necessary tweaks to the HGP model.

Conveniently, all of the code for the HGP model from Section 5.3.1 does not change at all and so we can simply reuse it. The only part of the code that will need to be tweaked is the specification of the location of the time points, and changing one of the prior distributions for a parameter of the covariance function. The code from Section 5.3.1 is updated as follows:

```
# Unequally spaced time points
tp <- c(5, 15, 30, 45, 60, 90, 120, 180)
```

```
method2 <- hgp(X, locs = tp, B = B, n_interp = 100,
               control = list(psi_alpha = 100,
                              psi_beta = 0.1))
```

Note that we are now using the `control` parameter of the `hgp()` function to change the prior distribution for the covariance parameter ψ. The reason we need to change the prior for ψ is perhaps best illustrated with an example of what happens if we instead use the default priors in the `hgp()` function. Fitting the HGP model with the default priors lead to the following non-monotonic dissolution curve predictions in Figure 5.9.

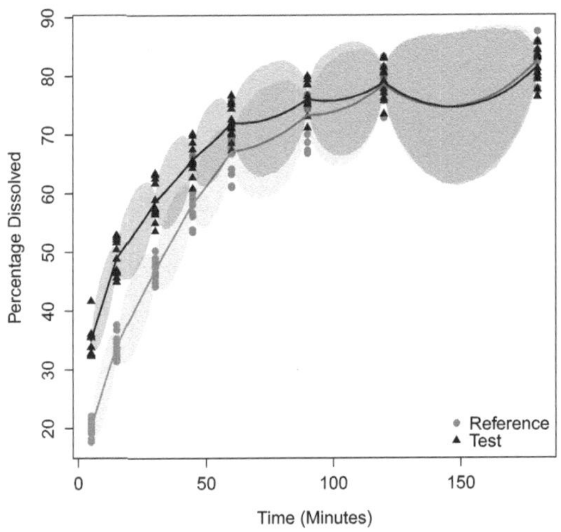

FIGURE 5.9
The predicted dissolution curves and uncertainty bands for the reference and test products under the hierarchical Gaussian process model using the default priors in the `hgp()` function.

As we can see from Figure 5.9, the dissolution curves become highly non-monotone after 60 minutes as the unequal spacing between time points greatly increases. Known as the shape/scale parameter in the Gaussian process literature, the parameter ϕ controls how fast the Gaussian process can wiggle or decay across time points. When the parameter ψ is not set to be large enough, the HGP prediction of the dissolution curves will tend toward the constant mean m in the lower level specification of the HGP model in (5.17). Here, in the `hgp()` function m is set to 50. To overcome the non-monotone behavior in Figure 5.9, a more informative prior must be specified. In this example, we let $\psi \sim \text{Gamma}(100, 0.1)$ which ensures a large prior expected value for the for the shape/scale parameter, and consequently for the posterior expected value as well. Under the newly suggested prior, the predicted dissolution curves for the reference and test products seem much more reasonable, and are indeed monotone (Figure 5.10).

Checking the quality of the posterior samples proceeds as before, and (although not shown) the trace plots show good mixing of all of the chains, as well the posterior densities look nicely unimodal and fairly symmetric. Moreover, the minimum effective sample size

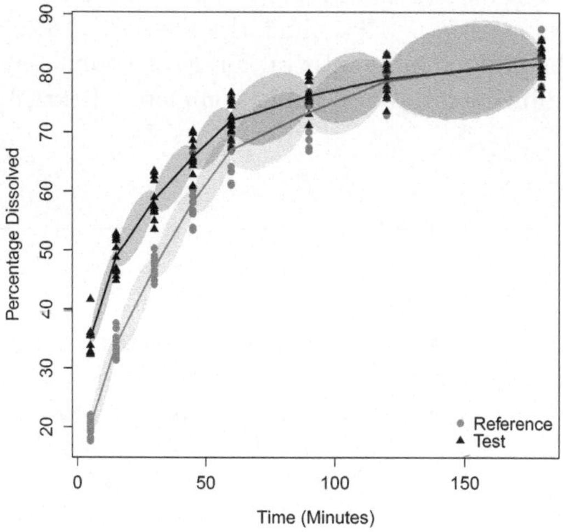

FIGURE 5.10
The predicted dissolution curves and uncertainty bands for the reference and test products under the hierarchical Gaussian process model with an adjusted prior for ϕ.

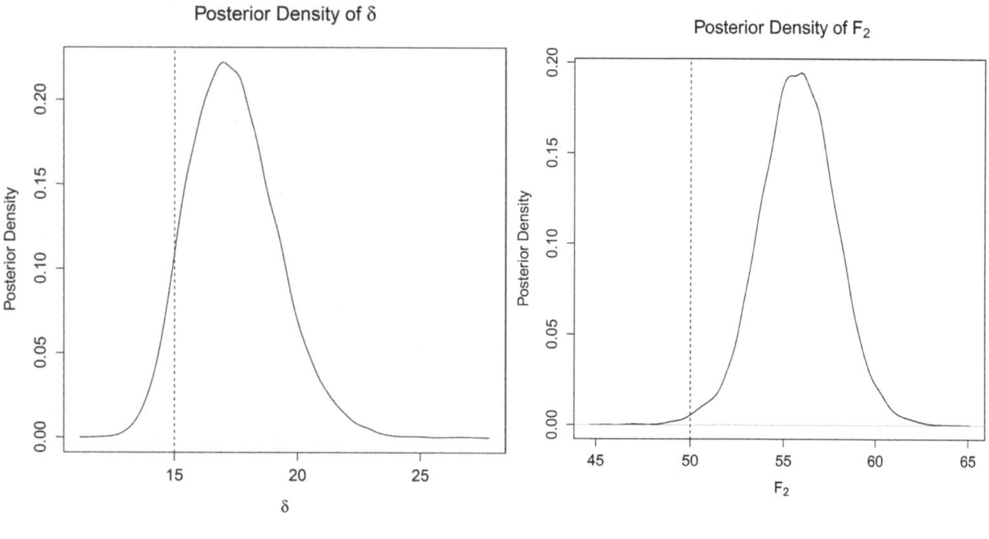

FIGURE 5.11
The posterior distribution of δ and F_2 based on the hierarchical Gaussian process model. Vertical dashed lines are placed at $\delta = 15$ and $F_2 = 50$.

is 2787 which is adequately large. Thus, dissolution testing can proceed via the use of the posterior samples of F_2 and δ.

Assume that we have prespecified a value of $q_0 = 0.95$. Plugging the posterior samples of F_2 and δ into (5.10) results in a value of $q = 0.076$. Thus, we would conclude that, since $q < q_0$, the dissolution profiles of the reference and test products are not similar. Interestingly, checking the posterior densities of F_2 and δ (Figure 5.11) actually shows that the reason the two products are not deemed similar has more to do with our δ criterion rather than the F_2 criterion. In fact, the $\Pr(F_2 \geq 50|\mathcal{D}) = 0.9959$ which is higher than our benchmark probability value of $q_0 = 0.95$. Similarly, the 95% credible intervals for F_2 and δ tell the same story. The 95% credible interval for F_2 is completely above 50, i.e., (51.7, 59.8), while the 95% credible interval for δ is not completely below 15, i.e., (14.3, 21.3).

5.4 Discussion

There are several health authority guidances on the topic of dissolution testing, but no particular guidance addressing the topic from the Bayesian point-of-view. We believe that this absence of guidances likely stems from a lack of available tools and resources for implementing dissolution testing from the Bayesian point-of-view. The recent papers by Novick et al. (2015) and Pourmohamad et al. (2022) provide a concrete framework for Bayesian dissolution testing. However, for those not used to the Bayesian paradigm, the task of practically implementing those methods may seem like a daunting proposition. It is our hope that by taking the methodology described in Novick et al. (2015) and Pourmohamad et al. (2022), and by condensing it into easy to use and understand R functions, that the use of Bayesian dissolution testing will become more commonly applied and accepted. As Bayesian methods for dissolution testing become more commonly used, we hope that such method will be acknowledged and addressed in health authority guidance documents.

6

A Non-Normal Bayesian Model for the Estimation and Comparison of Immunogenicity Screening Assay Cut-Points

David LeBlond

Robert Singer Consulting

Robert Singer

Robert Singer Consulting

Lu Xu

PRAV Biosciences

Rong Zeng

Amador Bioscience

CONTENTS

DOI: 10.1201/9781003255093-6

6.1 Introduction

6.1.1 Screening Clinical Subjects for Immunogenicity and Anti-Drug Antibodies

Immunogenicity, the capacity of a biological therapeutic drug to induce an immune response, may result in the production of anti-drug antibodies (ADA). The consequences of immunogenicity can range from no effect to life-threatening events (Civoli et al., 2019). Regulatory agencies mandate immunogenicity evaluation in clinical settings (FDA, 2019b; EMA, 2010a). Immunogenicity assessment strategies include a widely adopted multi-tiered testing and decision-tree (Shankar et al., 2008). The initial stage of this decision-tree includes screening of clinical samples for the presence of ADA.

The reportable value from such screening assays is usually $y = \pm\log(S/N)$ where S and N are assay signals from a test sample and from a pool negative control sera, respectively. The sign of the reportable value may be chosen to assure a positive correlation with ADA positivity.

ADA screening assays classify clinical samples as ADA positive or negative by comparing the assay reportable value to a decision cut-point (CP). FDA (2019) recommends that the screening assay CP be set to assure a false positive rate (FPR) of 5%.

6.1.2 Estimation of ADA Screening Assay CPs

Two different kinds of studies are described here. Following Shankar et al. (2008), we refer to these as either *pre-studies* or subsequent clinical *in-studies*. Sponsors conduct pre-studies to estimate the screening assay CP prior to the one or more clincial in-studies in which this screening assay will be used to screen subjects for ADA.

Pre-studies are typically conducted as part of ADA screening assay validation. Pre-studies sample a population of supposedly naïve normal human sera (often 30 – 50 depending on stage of assay development) which ideally represent the population of pre-dose subjects ultimately sampled in the clinical in-study. While pre-study protocols produce 3 or more independent reportable test results on each subject, which permits estimation of analytical variability, in-study protocols typically rely on a single pre-treatment screening assay result.

6.1.3 Traditional Statistical Methods for Pre-Study CP Assignments

According to Shankar et al. (2008), the process of assigning a screening CP consists of the following steps: 1) Investigate the distribution of reportable values and exclude outliers; 2) compare assay run means and variances to determine the type of CP strategy that is appropriate; and 3) calculate the screening CP. Traditionally these steps are implemented using an ad hoc collection of common statistical procedures that presume or approximate normality (e.g., outlier tests, normality or skewness tests, transformations, analysis of variance (ANOVA), hypothesis tests for means and variance), or robust or non-parametric methods when normality cannot be justified. These ad hoc procedures have been organized into flow charts for decision making (see for example Devanarayan (2017)). Such flow charts have been programmed into commonly available software platforms for general use.

Devanarayan (2017) recommends that statistical procedures for setting a preliminary screening CP to achieve a 5% FPR include properly powered "pre-studies," replicate testing of at least 50 naive human sera, ANOVA to identify an optimal control strategy, use of mixed effects modeling and box plots to distinguish analytical and biological effects, and normality tests of $\log(S/N)$ to decide between "parametric" (reportable result normality accepted) or nonparametric (normality rejected) CP estimation.

Analytical variation refers to intra-subject differences in observed reported values and includes intra-laboratory (i.e., "intermediate precision") sources such as operator, day, and plate. Analytical outliers are sometimes identified by applying the Grubbs test (Grubbs, 1950) to each pre-study subject replicate set.

A persistent challenge in estimating the reportable value is the fact that the distribution of the mean $\log(S/N)$ screening assay response from supposedly naïve donors often appears right skewed and normality tests frequently fail. These distributions often contain samples with remarkably elevated responses. This should not be surprising as the assay response may be impacted by unidentified prior subject-exposures, cross-reactivities, or other latent biological processes resulting in responses that may or may not be representative of a truly naive population. Samples with such elevated response are often referred to as "biological outliers".

Biological variation may arise from minor differences in serum components that interfere with the screening assay mechanism or from more significant effects such as the presence of pre-existing anti-drug antibodies. Biological outliers are sometimes identified by applying Tukey's exploratory visual box-plot (Wickham et al., 2019) to subject mean responses.

Assuming that analytical and biological outliers have been identified and removed, we can now move to CP assignment. Yang et al. (2015), section 3.3, provides an excellent description of the traditional state-of-the-art of screening CP assignment. We will not review all these details, but instead will focus in this chapter on the so called "floating CP" strategy. A floating CP is recommended when within-run variance can be assumed constant across analytical runs. It represents the most commonly applied strategy and involves adjusting each assay response (S) obtained in a given run for the mean response of negative controls in that same run (N). When the assay response is an increasing function of immunogenicity and is log transformed (in an effort to achieve normality), this amounts to expressing the reportable result of the screening assay as $\log(S/N)$. The screening CP is traditionally defined as the 95th percentile of reportable results. When normality is accepted (e.g., based on a Shapiro-Wilk test with a Type I error of 0.05), the CP is taken as $\text{mean}(\log(S/N)) + 1.645 \times \text{sd}(\log(S/N))$, where the mean() and sd() are taken over the observed pre-study reportable results. If normality is rejected, the CP is approximated nonparametrically as the 95th percentile of the observed pre-study reportable results.

6.1.4 Importance of an In-Study Specific CP (SSCP) Comparison

A fundamental assumption is that the 50 naïve sera and negative control pool used in the pre-study are representative of naive (pre-dose) portion of the target clinical in-study population(s). In-study FPRs must be monitored because unanticipated differences between the pre- and in-study populations, reagents, or sample handling procedures may result in different background activity in ADA assays which could render the pre-study CP inappropriate for screening in-study samples. FDA (2019b) therefore recommends that pre-study CPs be confirmed relative to the in-study target population.

Such SSCP comparisons are conducted using in-study pre-treatment screening results to re-estimate the CP. A comparison is then made with the CP estimated from the respective pre-study. The need to revise the provisional pre-study CP estimate is assessed in order to assure a 5% FPR when screening in-study subjects.

6.1.5 Traditional SSCP Comparison Methods

SSCP evaluations seem called for if the observed FPR in the in-study target population deviates greatly from the nominal 5%. To decide whether an in-study specific CP (SSCP) is needed, Devanarayan et al. (2017) and Devanarayan (2017) recommend a decision tree (a different decision tree than that used for CP assignment mentioned above) that includes ANOVA and Levene's tests comparing population means and variances, respectively. The properties of such tests of course depend on the assumption of normal error distribution. To avoid reacting to expected variability, Devanarayan et al. (2017) recommends that an in-study FPR outside the range of 2 to 11% trigger an SSCP comparison.

6.1.6 Challenges with Traditional Methods

Decision trees, such as those for CP and SSCP determination noted above, provide a practical, objective, and consistent basis for ADA screening CP determination. However, the specific statistical approaches to be employed remain controversial. The underlying biological mechanisms that govern the distributions of the $\log(S/N)$ responses in ADA screening assays are complex, vary with application, and are rarely well understood. This calls into question whether the various statistical test sizes and ultimate assay FPR levels will be nominal using methods dependent on a questionable assumption of normality.

Within-donor analytical error in these assays is generally normally distributed and "analytical outliers" can be properly identified by a preliminary analysis of ANOVA Studentized residuals. However, conducting separate outlier tests on each replicate set leads to an elevated family-wise type I error rate due to multiplicity. Also, the power of the Grubbs test to detect sizable deviations in small samples is remarkably low (Hawkins, 1980).

Dawson (2011) has shown that, for a normal distribution, the type I error of a box plot outlier procedure is never below 30%. Kubiak et al. (2018) have also commented on the negative impacts of excessive outlier removal in immunogenicity testing. Boxplots (Tukey, 1977) provide no information on the underlying data distribution and provide a somewhat arbitrary detection of extreme values especially for non-normal data distributions (Kampstra, 2008; Kryzwinski and Altman, 2014). In our work, non-normality often stubbornly persists even after removal of biological outliers by such approximate or ad hoc outlier procedures. Recently, Shen et al. (2015) and Shen et al. (2021) have argued that while basing a screening CP on a 95% sample percentile results in a 5% FPR on average, it does not provide sufficient statistical confidence that the FPR will be at least 5% in any particular case. These researchers compare various approaches under the assumption of normality and absence of outliers and recommend that a screening CP be determined as the estimated 95% lower confidence bound of the one-sided 95% percentile based on an exact t method. This philosophy is reflected in a more recent FDA (2019b) regulatory guidance which suggests a 90% confidence level.

The above traditional methods are conveniently available in simple statistical platforms and spreadsheets. Such tools can be linked together to form ad hoc algorithms for consistent and robust CP decision making. However, unless normality is confirmed, such algorithms lack an assumed underlying distributional model for biological variation that can motivate an understanding of the uncertainties in CP estimation and comparison. Without a distribution model of the underlying biological skewness, approximate methods that assume normality or less powerful robust or nonparametric approaches are traditionally employed.

The absence of a parametric working model calls into question the accuracy of FPR estimation, as well as the reliability of estimates and decisions made using mixed modeling that also depends on the assumption of normal error distributions. For instance, it is not clear how to identify unrepresentative responses or estimate the CP lower bound as advocated by Shen et al. (2015) and Shen et al. (2021) in order to assure a 5% FPR with high confidence in the non-normal case. Such challenges have been pointed out by Yang et al. (2015), JHoffelder (2016), Kubiak et al. (2018), and Tan (2019).

6.1.7 Benefits of a Bayesian Approach

This chapter is built on the earlier work of others. We describe a comprehensive approach to screening assay CP determination and SSCP comparisons based on 1) Rosner's test for analytical outliers, 2) distributional modeling for biological outlier identification, 3) Bayesian non-normal hierarchical modeling, 4) CP estimation and SSCP comparisons based on posterior distributions. We show that this choice of full probability modeling and comparison based on posterior probabilities better supports coherent risk-based decision making and the recommendations of Shen et al. (2015) and Shen et al. (2021). Such modeling may play an informative role in critical applications. We contrast this Bayesian approach with traditional methods such as those described in Sections 6.1.3 and 6.1.5.

The rest of this chapter is organized as follows: In Section 6.2, we motivate the use of an exponential Gaussian model for biological variability and describe its useful properties. In Section 6.3, we describe a Bayesian hierarchical model and give R and Stan code for analysis of pre- and in-study screening assay reportable results. In Section 6.4, we introduce a pre-study and two corresponding in-studies. We use Rosner's test to identify analytical outliers in the pre-study and a model based procedure ("INRQP") to identify biological outliers in all 3 studies. We use the Bayesian hierarchical model for pre-study CP determination and perform SSCP comparisons with two corresponding in-studies. Finally in Section 6.5, we describe some challenges in implementing these Bayesian procedures and offer arguments that the value gained is worth the extra effort.

6.2 Exponential Gaussian Model of Biological Effects

FDA (2019b) recommends that "The statistical method used to determine the cut-point should be based on the statistical distribution of the data." Schlain et al. (2010) pioneered the use of a 3-parameter gamma distribution and Zhang et al. (2015) examined both skew-t and log-gamma distribution random effects Bayesian models for ADA screening assay CP determination.

Recognizing that the traditional normal distribution does not always offer an ideal approximation for CP determination, we investigated a variety of distributional models that accommodate positive skewness and the presence of elevated results commonly encountered when screening in-study populations for ADA. The R package `gamlss` provides a number of distribution and other utility functions for a wide range of non-normal distributions. The `gamlss` package and available distributions are well documented in Rigby et al. (2020) (see especially Section 4.6.1, Table 4.1, and Chapter 18). The `fitDist()` function was used to fit, by maximum likelihood, 29 2-, 3-, or 4-parameter common distributional models of location, spread, and shape (including the normal) with support on the real line to the $\log(S/N)$ responses from 14 pre- and in-studies.

Out of the 29 possible distributions considered, the exponential Gaussian appeared to be a parsimonious choice to model biological variation based on the Akaiki information criterion (AIC). Four parameter choices (which separately model both skewness and kurtosis) seemed over-parameterized to support studies that include only 50 or fewer subject means. Further, many distributions model both left and right skewness. In our experience with CP estimation, left skewness is rarely observed. The exponential Gaussian distribution was the best choice among all tested 3-parameter distributions with respect to AIC.

There is no assurance that this choice is universally optimal. However, the exponential Gaussian provides a somewhat compelling, if empirical, model of biological effects. As described in the next Section, Its 3 parameters offer an intuitive description and some insight by separately quantifying normal and non-normal biological effects.

6.2.1 Structure, Properties, and Motivation for the Exponential Gaussian Distribution

In this section, we provide some motivation for this distribution which is a generalization of the normal distribution,

$$N(y|\mu,\sigma^2) = \frac{1}{\sigma\sqrt{2\pi}} \exp\left(-\frac{(y-\mu)^2}{2\sigma^2}\right) \tag{6.1}$$

with $N(y|0,1) = \phi(y)$, results from the sum of many small effects and is a maximum entropy (minimal assumptions, see McElreath (2020)) choice among all distributions defined by a fixed mean and variance.

The exponential Gaussian (Rigby et al., 2020) having pdf

$$\text{exGAUS}(y|\mu,\sigma,\nu) = \frac{1}{\nu} \exp\left[\frac{\mu-y}{\nu} + \frac{\sigma^2}{2\nu^2}\right] \Phi\left(\frac{y-\mu}{\sigma} + \frac{\sigma}{\nu}\right), \tag{6.2}$$

with $\Phi(\cdot)$ the cumulative density function of the normal distribution, and has a mean of $\mu+\nu$, a variance of $\sigma^2+\nu^2$, and a moment skewness of $2\times(1+\sigma^2/\nu^2)^{-3/2}$. The exponential Gaussian distribution introduces positive skewness by assuming that one of those many effects may be large and follows an exponential distribution, having pdf

$$\text{Exp}(y|\nu) = \frac{1}{\nu} \exp\left(-\frac{y}{\nu}\right). \tag{6.3}$$

While the exponential distribution is often associated with time-to-event models, it has many other applications such as wealth distribution (Lopez-Ruiz et al., 2012). Further, the exponential distribution is the maximum entropy distribution among all distributions defined on a non-negative support by a fixed mean ν (see page 314 of McElreath (2020)). As the mean ν of the exponential component tends toward zero, the exponential Gaussian distribution tends toward the normal and its moment skewness tends toward zero. Below we symbolize cumulative distribution functions (cdfs) of the normal and exponential Gaussian distributions as: $T_y = \Phi(y|\mu,\sigma) = \mu+\sigma\Phi(y)$ with $\Phi(y) = \Phi(y|0,1)$, and $\text{pexGAUS}(y|\mu,\sigma,\nu)$, respectively. The pth quantiles (inverse cdf function) are symbolized as: $\Phi^{-1}(p|\mu,\sigma)$ with $\Phi^{-1}(p) = \Phi^{-1}(p|0,1)$, or $\text{qexGAUS}(p|\mu,\sigma,\nu)$, respectively. A random variable having a normal, exponential, or exponential Gaussian distributions is indicated as: $y \sim N(\mu,\sigma^2)$, $y \sim \text{Exp}(\nu)$, or $y \sim \text{exGAUS}(\mu,\sigma,\nu)$, respectively.

6.3 Bayesian Hierarchical Pre-Study and SSCP Model

In both pre- and in-studies, many sources of variation in y can be identified. We focus here on two sources: biological and analytical. Biological variation refers to inter-subject differences in mean reported values. Biological and analytical sources can be identified and quantified only in pre-studies which include intra-subject replication. With in-studies, these two sources are confounded. However, in-study biological variation can be inferred from a prior pre-study estimate when the pre- and in-study are performed in the same laboratory using a screening assay that is under statistical control.

We incorporate Bayesian hierarchical modeling (as advocated by Shen et al. (2021)) to better inform risk with probabilities associated with the events of interest (e.g., values of the true CP or differences between two CPs).

6.3.1 Mathematical Description of the Model

Consider a pre-study in which n results are obtained from S subjects. The ith observed $\log(S/N)$ result from the s_i^{th} subject, y_i, is modeled as the sum of 3 independent random components $y_i = G_{s_i} + E_{s_i} + A_i$. Components $G_{s_i} \sim N(\mu, \sigma^2)$ and $E_{s_i} \sim \text{Exp}(\nu)$ are subject specific and together represent biological variation with $G_{s_i} + E_{s_i} \sim \text{exGAUS}(\mu, \sigma, \nu)$. Component $A_i \sim N(0, \sigma_e^2)$ accounts for analytical variation. Thus, pre-study results, where a given subject is tested multiple times, arise from a hierarchical structure (an intra-subject level within an inter-subject level). Ultimately however, the intention is to use this model for determination and decision making regarding a screening assay CP.

Model parameter estimates are available using traditional statistical methods. An estimate for analytical standard deviation, $\hat{\sigma}_e$, is available by pooling within subject variances. This estimate will have an associated pooled degrees of freedom, df. Approximate maximum likelihood estimates $\hat{\mu}_{\text{MLE}}$, $\hat{\sigma}_{\text{MLE}}$, and $\hat{\nu}_{\text{MLE}}$, and their respective standard errors $se(\hat{\mu}_{\text{MLE}})$, $se(\hat{\sigma}_{\text{MLE}})$, and $se(\hat{\nu}_{\text{MLE}})$, are readily obtained by analysis of pre-study subject means using the R package `gamlss` (Rigby et al., 2020), as illustrated in the case study below.

Posterior distributional estimates of these parameters are useful as they provide insight into CP estimation uncertainty for risk based decision making. However, posterior estimation requires prior distributional assumptions of model parameters, i.e.,

$$\mu \sim N(0, k^2) \tag{6.4}$$

$$\sigma, \nu, \sigma_e \sim \text{Half-}N(0, k^2) \tag{6.5}$$

where the Half-$N()$ indicates a normal distribution truncated below zero.

In the case study below, we found no discernible impact of k on posterior estimates when $k \geq 3$. Of course applications that result in other response ranges may require other prior distributions.

Because the CP is meant to apply to an in-study in which each subject is tested only once (i.e., there is no intra-subject level), it is necessary to use the pre-study estimate of σ_e to anticipate the expected distribution of individual results

$$y_i = G_i + E_i + A_i = (G_i + A_i) + E_i \tag{6.6}$$

where, by definition of the exponential Gaussian distribution,

$$y_i \sim \text{exGAUS}\left(\hat{\mu}, \sqrt{\hat{\sigma}^2 + \hat{\sigma}_e^2}, \hat{\nu}\right). \tag{6.7}$$

The CP is defined here as the 0.95^{th} quantile of this distribution, i.e., CP = qexGAUS$\left(0.95, \hat{\mu}, \sqrt{\hat{\sigma}^2 + \hat{\sigma}_e^2}, \hat{\nu}\right)$, where the qexGAUS() function is supplied by the `gamlss` R package. When these fixed formulae are applied to each draw from the joint posterior sample of model parameters, the result is a sample from the posterior distribution of either expected in-study result y_i or the CP distribution, respectively.

6.3.2 Computing Methods

All analyses were performed using R Studio, under MSWindows version 10. The following R packages were used: `tidyverse` (Wickham et al., 2019) for data formatting and graphics, `gamlss` (Rigby and Stasinopoulos, 2005) for non-normal distributional functions and regression, `EnvStats` (Millard, 2013) for Rosner's outlier test, `outliers` (Komsta, 2022) for the Grubb's outlier test, `qqplotr` (Almeida et al., 2018) for normalized residual quantile plot confidence bands, `rstan` and Stan (Stan Development Team, 2021a,b) for posterior estimation, and `gridExtra` (Auguie, 2017) for graphical layout. Code snippets E, G, and K were borrowed from the freely available CP tool (Zhang et al., 2013). The R code used for all analyses presented here is available from `https://github.com/BayesCMC/Book`.

6.3.3 Stan Code for a Pre-Study Model

The model consisting of analytical and biological hierarchical levels described above is used for analysis. The analytical level identifies analytical effect, A_i for the ith observation y_i, conditional on the biological effect $G_{s[i]} + E_{s[i]}$ from the sth subject associated with the ith observation. These analytical effects are assumed to be normally distributed with mean zero and standard deviation σ_e. Thus the conditional observed result at the analytical level is

$$y_i|G_{s[i]}, E_{s[i]} \sim N\left(G_{s[i]} + E_{s[i]}, \sigma_e^2\right). \tag{6.8}$$

The biological level identifies the biological effect, $G_s + E_s$, for the sth subject. At this level, non-centered parameterizations were found to speed convergence and improve mixing. This was implemented by introducing intermediate variables G_s^{raw} and E_s^{raw} whose distributions were independent of model parameters, resulting in a more homogeneous parameter space for executing Stan's Hamiltonian Monte-carlo, i.e.,

$$G_s^{\text{raw}} \sim N(0, 1) \tag{6.9}$$
$$E_s^{\text{raw}} \sim \text{Uniform(0,1)}. \tag{6.10}$$

The Gaussian component G_s of biological effects is assumed normally distributed with mean μ and standard deviation σ. G_s is recovered by re-parameterization of G_s^{raw} as follows

$$G_S = \mu + G_s^{\text{raw}} \times \sigma. \tag{6.11}$$

Similarly, the exponential component E_s, assumed exponentially distributed with mean ν, is recovered from E_s^{raw} by the well-known transformation

$$E_s = -\nu \log(1 - E_s^{\text{raw}}). \tag{6.12}$$

This hierarchical model is implemented in Stan using the following model text file that is created and given a suitable file name such as `prestudy model.stan`.

```
// A. Stan model for a pre-study
data {
int<lower=0> nsubjects;
int<lower=0> nobs;
int<lower=0> Subject[nobs];
vector[nobs] y;
real k;
}
parameters {
real mu;
real<lower=0> sigma; // implies prior truncated below zero
real<lower=0> nu; // implies prior truncated below zero
real<lower=0> sigma_e; // implies prior truncated below zero
vector[nsubjects] G_raw;
vector<lower=0,upper=1>[nsubjects] E_raw; // implies
                                           //uniform(0,1) prior
}
transformed parameters{
real lsigma;
real lnu;
vector[nsubjects] G;
vector[nsubjects] E;
lsigma = log(sigma);
lnu = log(nu);
G = mu + G_raw*sigma;
E = -nu*log( 1 - E_raw);
}
model {
// Priors (k is the prior discount factor)
mu ~normal(0, k);
sigma ~normal(0, k);
nu ~normal 0, k);
sigma_e ~normal(0, k);
// Likelihood exponential Gaussian likelihood on biological
//effects
for(i in 1:nsubjects){
G_raw[i] ~ std_normal();
}// Normal likelihood on analytical effects
for(i in 1:nobs){
y[i] ~ normal(G[Subject[i]] + E[Subject[i]] ,sigma_e);
}
}
```

Note in the above Stan model that while prior distributions are specified for σ and ν, log transformations of these parameters (`lnu` and `lsigma`, respectively) are ultimately saved in the R code described below. This is an arbitrary choice. In any case, posterior samples of the untransformed parameters can always be recovered by exponentiation.

6.3.4 Fitting the Stan Model to Pre-Study Results in R

Let y denote a vector of nobs $\log(S/N)$ values and Subject a corresponding vector of subject indices from 1 to nsubjects. Code snippet B will estimate the joint posterior distribution of model parameters.

```
# B. Fit Stan model to pre-study results
# Define data for Stan
dataList = list(
nobs = length(y),
nsubjects = length(unique(Subject)),
y = y,
Subject=Subject,
k=5 # prior discount factor
)
# Define the parameters for Stan
parameters = c("mu","lsigma","lnu","sigma_e")
# Translate model to C++ and compile to DSO
StabDSO <- stan_model( 'prestudy model.stan' )
# Obtain sample of n.chains*(iter - warmup)/thin
# posterior draws
n.chains <- 4

options (mc.cores = n.chains)
stanFit <- sampling( object=StabDSO ,
pars=parameters,
data = dataList ,
chains = n.chains ,
iter = 8000 ,
warmup = 4000 ,
thin = 1,verbose=TRUE , control=list(
adapt_delta=0.995, max_treedepth=15))
# Examine the quality of the fit
stan.sum<-summary(stanFit)
stan.sum$summary
```

6.3.5 Stan Code for SSCP Model

The Stan model for an SSCP comparison is identical to that for a pre-study except additional parameters are included to describe the in-study data generation. The respective parameters are identified in code snippet C below using _pre or _in suffixes. This is created as a text file and given a suitable file name such as SSCP model.stan.

```
// C. Stan model for SSCP comparison
data {
int<lower=0> nsubjects_pre;
```

```
int<lower=0> nsubjects_in;
int<lower=0> nobs_pre;
int<lower=0> nobs_in;
int<lower=0> Subject_pre[nobs_pre];
int<lower=0> Subject_in[nobs_in];
vector[nobs_pre] y_pre;
vector[nobs_in] y_in;
real k;
}
parameters {
real mu_pre;
real mu_in;
real<lower=0> sigma_pre; // implies prior truncated below zero
real<lower=0> sigma_in; // implies prior truncated below zero
real<lower=0> nu_pre; // implies prior truncated below zero
real<lower=0> nu_in; // implies prior truncated below zero
real<lower=0> sigma_e; // implies prior truncated below zero
vector[nsubjects_pre] G_pre_raw;
vector[nsubjects_in] G_in_raw;
vector<lower=0,upper=1>[nsubjects_pre] E_pre_raw;//implies uniform(0,1) prior
vector<lower=0,upper=1>[nsubjects_in] E_in_raw;// implies uniform(0,1) prior
}
transformed parameters{
real lsigma_pre;
real lsigma_in;
real lnu_pre;
real lnu_in;
vector[nsubjects_pre] G_pre;
vector[nsubjects_in] G_in;
vector<lower=0>[nsubjects_pre] E_pre;
vector<lower=0>[nsubjects_in] E_in;
lsigma_pre = log(sigma_pre);
lsigma_in = log(sigma_in);
lnu_pre = log(nu_pre);
lnu_in = log(nu_in);
G_pre = mu_pre + G_pre_raw*sigma_pre;
G_in = mu_in + G_in_raw*sigma_in;
E_pre = -nu_pre*log( 1 - E_pre_raw);
E_in = -nu_in*log( 1 - E_in_raw);
}
model {
// Priors
mu_pre ~ normal(0,k);
mu_in ~ normal(0,k);
sigma_pre ~ normal(0,k);
sigma_in ~ normal(0,k);
nu_pre ~ normal(0,k);
nu_in ~ normal(0,k);
sigma_e ~ normal(0,k);
// Likelihood for pre-study
// exponential Gaussian likelihood on biological effects
for(i in 1:nsubjects_pre){
G_pre_raw[i] ~ std_normal();
}// Normal likelihood on analytical effects
for(i in 1:nobs_pre){
y_pre[i] ~ normal(G_pre[Subject_pre[i]] + E_pre[Subject_pre[i]] ,sigma_e);
}
// Likelihood for in-study
// exponential Gaussian likelihood on biological effects
for(i in 1:nsubjects_in){
G_in_raw[i] ~ std_normal();
}// Normal likelihood on analytical effects
```

```
for(i in 1:nobs_in){
y_in[i] ~ normal(G_in[Subject_in[i]] + E_in[Subject_in[i]] ,sigma_e);
}
}
```

As with the pre-study Stan model, while prior distributions are specified for the pre- and in-study σ and ν parameters, log transformations of these parameters are ultimately saved in the R code as described below, posterior samples of the untransformed parameters can always be recovered by exponentiation.

6.3.6 Fitting the SSCP Comparison Stan Model in R

Code snippet D will execute the SSCP Stan model in snippet C and provide a fit to data from both a pre and a respective in-study. The in-study data has no within subject replication so the estimate for analytical variability, σ_e comes from the pre-study data. The justification for this is that the same assay is used in the same laboratory to analyze both studies. The code below assumes that analytical and biological outliers have been identified and removed by the Rosner and INRQP methods, respectively.

```
# D. Fit SSCP Stan model to both pre- and in-study data
# Define data for Stan
dataList = list(
nobs_pre = length(y_pre), # number of pre-study observations
nsubjects_pre = length(unique(Subject_pre)), # number of pre-study subjects
y_pre = y_pre, # vector of Pre-study log(S/N) assay responses
Subject_pre=Subject_pre, # vector of pre-study subject IDs
nobs_in = length(y_in), # number of in-study observations
nsubjects_in = length(unique(Subject_in)), # number of in-study subjects
y_in = y_in, # vector of in-study log(S/N) assay responses
Subject_in=Subject_in, # vector of in-study subject IDs
k=3 # prior discount factor
)
# Define the parameters for Stan
parameters = c("mu_pre","lsigma_pre","lnu_pre","sigma_e","mu_in",
               "lsigma_in","lnu_in" )
# Translate model to C++ and compile to DSO (takes about 1 minute):
StabDSO <- stan_model( 'SSCP model.stan' )
# Generate posterior sample of n.chains*(iter - warmup)/thin MCMC draws
options (mc.cores = n.chains)
stanFit <- sampling( object=StabDSO ,
pars=parameters,
data = dataList ,
chains = 4 ,
iter = 8000 ,
warmup = 4000 ,
thin = 1,verbose=TRUE , control=list(
adapt_delta=0.995, max_treedepth=15))
# Examine the quality of the fit
stan.sum<-summary(stanFit)
stan.sum$summary
```

6.4 Case Study

The ADA screening bioassay considered in this case study was designed to detect antibodies in human serum directed against an experimental humanized monoclonal antibody drug intended to target and block the growth of cancer stem cells. The screening assay was based on Electrochemiluminescence technology. The assay result is a log-transformed ratio of luminescence counts of the sample (S) relative to that from a pooled negative control (N).

Below we illustrate CP estimation for this bioassay from a pre-study (study "I") and SSCP comparisons in 2 corresponding in-studies (studies "I-1" and "I-2") using the Bayesian hierarchical models described above. Because CP estimation is intimately dependent on the methodology used for preliminary outlier identification, we also briefly describe the novel the methods we prefer for identification and removal of analytical and biological outliers prior to CP estimation and SSCP comparisons.

6.4.1 Study Descriptions

Table 6.1 displays study designs and outlier identification for pre-study I and corresponding in-studies I-1 and I-2.

TABLE 6.1
Study characteristics and the number of outliers identified by various procedures.

Study	N	IDs	Reps	n.Grubbs	n.Rosner	n.boxplot	n.INRQP
I	150	50	3	7	0	4	2
I-1	51	51	1	0	0	4	4
I-2	47	47	1	0	0	4	2

In pre-study I, three replicate results (Reps) were obtained from each of 50 normal human sera (IDs) for a total of 150 responses. The 3 replicates were obtained from different runs and plates within a run. Three total runs with 3 plates per run were performed for a total of 9 plates. Drug naive (day zero) clinical phase 1 clinical subjects from in-studies I-1 and I-2 were tested in singlicate in separate runs and plates. The case study data can be downloaded from `https://github.com/BayesCMC/Book`.

6.4.2 Use of Rosner's Test to Identify Analytical Outliers

Analytical outliers are sometimes identified by applying the Grubbs test (Grubbs, 1950) to each pre-study subject replicate set. A two-sided Grubbs test, which presumes normality, can be implemented using the `grubbs.test()` function of the outliers R package as shown in code snippet E below. While not an outlier strategy we would recommend, we compare the Grubbs test to Rosner's test in the assessment of analytical outliers in the case study described below.

```
# E. Grubbs test
require(outliers)
```

```
IDs <- unique(ID) # vector of unique subject IDs
Grubbsout <- rep(FALSE,length(y)) # initialize all
                                  # observations to FALSE
for(i in c(1:length(IDs)){
  n_notNA <- length(which(!is.na(y[ID==IDs[i]])))
  if(n_notNA >= 3){ # at least 3 nonmissing replicates required
    temp <- grubbs.test(y[ID==IDs[i]],two.sided=TRUE)
    if(temp$p.value<0.05){ # alpha = 0.05
    temp2<-round(y[which(ID==IDs[i])],6)==
    round(as.numeric(strsplit(temp$alternative, " ")[[1]][3]),6)
   Grubbsout[ID==IDs[i]] <- temp2
  }
 }
}
```

Code snippit E takes as input y, a numeric vector of nobs pre-study $\log(S/N)$ results, and ID a character vector of nobs respective subject identifiers. It outputs Grubbsout, a logical vector of length nobs giving the Grubbs test outcome (TRUE=outlier). While not an outlier strategy we would recommend, we compare the Grubbs test to Rosner's test (see code snippit I) in the assessment of analytical outliers in the case study described below.

Devanarayan (2017) has emphasized the value of identifying analytical outliers globally as conditional residuals from latent subject means through mixed-effects modeling. Our approach tests ANOVA residuals using Rosner's outlier test to manage the Type I error rate. Rosner's test (Rosner, 1975) can identify multiple outliers (up to a maximum of k), while accounting for multiplicity. Rosner's test is based on a generalized extreme Studentized deviate to detect one or more outliers in a univariate data set that follows an approximately normal distribution. A primary limitation of tests such as the Grubbs test is that the suspected number of outliers must be specified exactly to assure a pre-specified type I error rate. Rosner's test only requires that an upper bound for the number of suspected outliers be specified.

In code snippet F, we pre-specify a Type I error of 0.05 in detecting up to $k = 10$ suspected outliers in pre-study I ANOVA residuals. Rosner's test is implemented using the rosnerTest() function of the EnvStats R package.

```
# F. Identify analytical outliers using Rosner's test
#                                on ANOVA residuals
require(EnvStats)
fit1 <- lm(y ~ as.factor(ID),mydata)
# Up to 10 suspected outliers at alpha = 0.05
ros <- rosnerTest(fit1$residuals,k=10,alpha=0.05)$all.stats
outliers <- ros$Obs.Num[ros$Outlier==TRUE]
mydata$Outlier <- FALSE
mydata$Outlier[outliers] <- TRUE
mydata$residual <- fit1$residuals
```

Initially, the data frame mydata includes y, the vector of $\log(S/N)$ assay results and ID, a vector identifying the pre-study subject for each observation. The above code adds a logical variable Outlier which has the value TRUE for identified outliers. A variable residual is also added which gives the deviation from the subject mean. Rosner's test was applied only once to all pre-study I ANOVA residuals. For comparison, Grubbs test ($\alpha = 0.05$) was separately applied to each subject replicate set.

In Table 6.1, the number of analytical outliers identified by the Grubbs (n.Grubbs) or Rosner's (n.Rosner) tests are indicated for each study. Rosners test, which found no analytical outliers, appears less liberal than the Grubbs test, which identified 7 outliers. Identification of analytical outliers in pre-study I is also illustrated in Figure 6.1. This scatter plot was produced using the `geom_boxplot()` function of the `ggplot2` R package. ANOVA residuals are plotted as gray points. Residuals identified as outliers by Grubbs' test are indicated by black circles. Notice that some outliers identified by the Grubbs test actually have negligible ANOVA residuals.

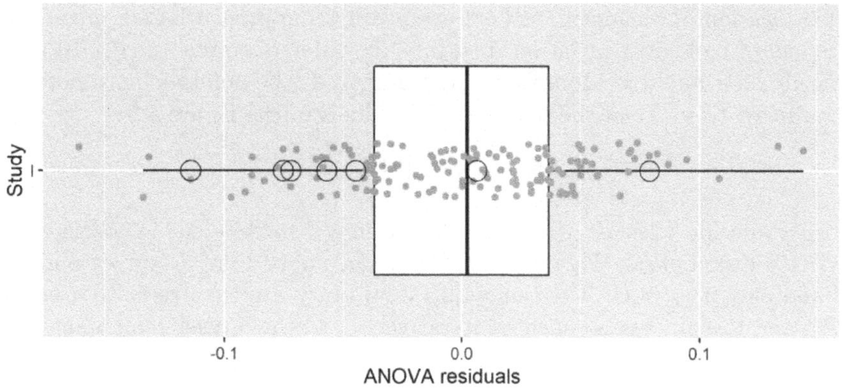

FIGURE 6.1
Identification of analytical outliers in pre-study I. Circles indicate outliers identified by Grubbs test.

No analytical outliers were identified in pre-study I results by Rosner's test. The results from Rosner's test, which adjusts for multiplicity, was considered definitive. Therefore no analytical outliers were removed from pre-study I. Analytical outlier tests could not be performed for in-studies I-1 and I-2 which lack within-subject replicate testing.

6.4.3 Iterated-Normalized-Residual-Quantile-Plot (INRQP) Approach for Identification of Biological Outliers

Code snippit G implements a traditional version of the box plot for detection of biological outliers. Symmetric limits are often taken for outlier identification as a distance of $1.5 \times IQR$ below $Q1$ or above $Q3$, where $IQR = Q3 - Q1$, and $Q1$ and $Q3$ are the 25th and 75th empirical percentiles of the sample. While we do not recommend the use of the box plot procedure for identifying biological outliers, we compare this procedure to one based on a non-normal distribution model in the case study described below.

```
# G. Box plot identification of biological outliers

# conservative factor of 3 used
LL<-quantile(ymean,p=0.25)-3*IQR(boxdat)
```

```
UL<-quantile(ymean,p=0.75)+3*IQR(boxdat)
boxout <-ymean>UL | ymean<LL
```

The input variable ymean is a vector of subject mean $\log(S/N)$ responses. For pre-studies, analytical outliers are assumed previously identified and removed using Rosner's test. For in-studies there is no intra-subject replication so ymean is a vector of individual responses. The code below generates a logical vector boxout whose value is TRUE if the corresponding response is identified as a biological outlier. While we do not recommend the use of the box plot procedure for identifying biological outliers, we compare this procedure to one based on a non-normal distribution model as described below.

For identification of biological outliers, we prefer an approach based on the parametric working model of biological variation. Let $\mathbf{y}$ be an ordered sample of $n > 10$ independent and identically distributed random values. Let $\hat{\mu}$, $\hat{\sigma}$, and $\hat{\nu}$ be point estimates of an exGAUS distribution fitted to $\mathbf{y}$. Then the normalized residuals of the fit are

$$\mathbf{r} = \Phi^{-1}(\text{pexGAUS}(\mathbf{y}|\hat{\mu}, \hat{\sigma}, \hat{\nu})). \tag{6.13}$$

We wish to decide whether the largest value in $\mathbf{y}$, namely y_n, is consistent with the fitted exGAUS distribution. Therefore we define an upper limit U on r_n and remove y_n from $\mathbf{y}$ if and only if $r_n > U$. The remaining values in $\mathbf{y}$ are then re-fit to a new exGAUS distribution and the process is repeated iteratively until the largest remaining value in r is $\leq U$.

At each iteration, with m values remaining in $\mathbf{r}$, we re-establish U as follows: Assuming $\mathbf{y}$ is a sample from an exGAUS distribution, the values in $\mathbf{r}$ should be normally distributed with sample mean $\bar{r}$ and population standard deviation s. With this in mind, we define U as the upper limit of a two-sided 95% confidence band of a normal quantile plot of q_i^{th} sample quantiles r_i vs corresponding expected quantiles $T_{q_i} = \bar{r} + s \times \Phi(q_i)$ where $q_i = (i - 0.5)/m$. The required upper bound is then $U = \hat{r}_m + \Phi^{-1}(0.975) \times SE_m$ where $\hat{r}_m = a + b \times T_{P_m}$, $P_m = (m - 0.5)/m$, $b = (Q_{\mathbf{r},0.8} - Q_{\mathbf{r},0.2})/(T_{0.8} - T_{0.2})$, $a = Q_{r,0.8} - b \times T_{0.8}$, and

$$SE_m = \frac{ab}{\phi(P_m)}\sqrt{\frac{P_m(1 - P_m)}{m}}. \tag{6.14}$$

This iterative process is easily automated in using the qqplotr R package (Almeida et al., 2018) which also provides diagnostic normal quantile plots. The pth sample quantile of the vector $\mathbf{y}$ is based here on the default R quantile function (type 7, Hyndman and Fan (1996)) and is indicated as $Q_{\mathbf{y},p}$.

We refer to this approach as an iterated-normalized-residual-quantile-plot (INRQP) approach.The INRQP procedure thus iteratively identifies and removes the most extreme values that exceed the 95band of a normalized residual quantile plot. As described below, the INRQP procedure takes into account the presumed exponential Gaussian distribution of biological effects and therefore, we consider the INRQP outlier identification definitive.

INRQP can be automated in R using functions gamlssML() of the R package gamlss and the functions stat_qq_band(), stat_qq_line(), and stat_qq_point() of the R package qqplotr. In code snippet H, the data frame meandata variable SB_means is a vector of subject mean $\log(S/N)$ responses and ID is a corresponding subject identifier. For pre-studies, analytical outliers are assumed previously identified and removed using Rosner's test. For in-studies there is no intra-subject replication so SB_means is a vector of individual responses.

The `while{}` statement iterates as long as the variable `outside = TRUE`. With each iteration, the most extreme result is tested. If it is identified as a biological outlier, the data frame `meandata` variable `outside_np` is set to `TRUE`, and is removed from future iterations. Iterations continue until the most extreme normalized residual falls within the exGAUS quantile plot confidence band. The algorithm generates a new variable `outside_np` which has a value of `TRUE` if the subject is identified as a biological outlier.

```
# H. INRQP identification of biological outliers
require(gamlss)
require(ggplot2)
require(qqplotr)
meandata$outside_np <- FALSE # Initialize biological outlier indicator
outside <- TRUE # iterate while TRUE
iteration <- 0 # iteration counter
while(outside){
iteration <- iteration + 1
meandata2 <- meandata[!meandata$outside_np,] # retain only outside_np==FALSE
# Fit an exGAUS distribution
exGAUSfit.pre <- gamlssML(meandata2$SB_means,family=exGAUS)
# match normalized residuals with ID (assume same sort order??)
resids <- tibble(resids=exGAUSfit.pre$residuals,
ID=meandata2$ID)
# need to sort by resids because ggplot::qplotr() sorts data
resids <- arrange(resids,resids)
# Examine normalized residuals via normal quantile plot
gg <- ggplot(data = resids, mapping = aes(sample = resids)) +
stat_qq_band(qprobs=c(0.2,0.8)) +
stat_qq_line(qprobs=c(0.2,0.8)) +
stat_qq_point() +
labs(x = "Theoretical Quantiles", y = "Sample Quantiles")
# extract the xy values for labeling
gg_data <- ggplot_build(gg)
xy <- gg_data$data[[3]][,1:2] # x (theoret) and y (observed) quantiles
ub <- gg_data$data[[1]][,4:5] # upper and lower (CI bounds for the y values)
print(gg + geom_text(aes(x=xy$x,y=xy$y,label=ID),nudge_x=-.1))
# Test if maximum normalized residual is beyond confidence band
nr_max <- xy[nrow(xy),2] # maximum normalized residual
ci_bounds <- ub[nrow(xy),] # CI limits for the maximum normalized residual
outside <- FALSE # re-initialize the while indicator
outside <- !(nr_max >= ci_bounds[2] & nr_max <= ci_bounds[1])
                                            # if TRUE-> outlier
if(outside){ # if an outlier
ID_out <- resids$ID[nrow(xy)] # the ID that is not representative
# add the indicator to meandata and alldata4
meandata$outside_np[meandata$ID==ID_out] <- TRUE
}
} # end of while
```

Figure 6.2 illustrates the INRQP approach to identification of biological outliers in study I. The 50 subject $\log(S/N)$ means were fit to an exponential Gaussian distribution and the residuals of that fit (differences between empirical and theoretical cumulative probabilities) were normalized by a inverse cdf transform. The resulting normalized residuals are displayed on each of the 3 plots along with a 95% confidence band. Because the highest sample quantile (subject 12, upper left plot) is not contained within the confidence band, it was identified as an outlier (not belonging to the negative population) and removed. Upon re-analysis, the result from subject 26 was similarlyidentified as a biological outlier and removed (upper right plot). Upon re-analysis (right graph) the most next highest sample quantile (subject 25, lower plot) is contained within the confidence band so no further iterations were performed.

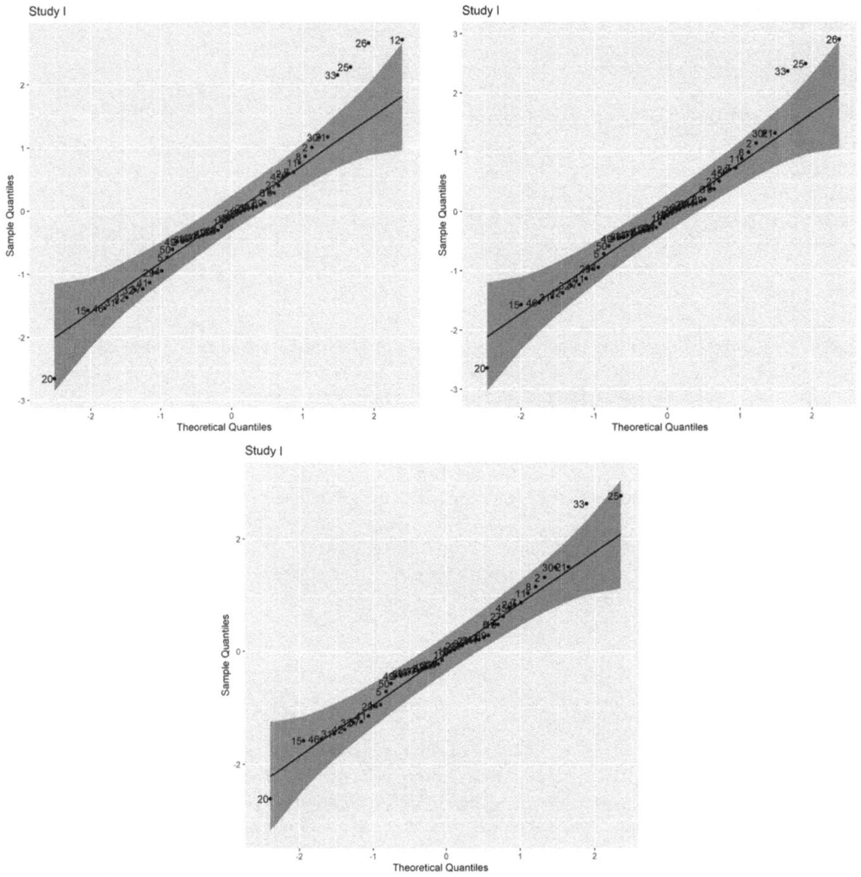

FIGURE 6.2
Illustration of INRQP biological outlier identification for pre-study I.

Biological outliers were similarity assessed by INRQP in studies I-1 and I-2 based on individual $\log(S/N)$ results. For comparison, the boxplot procedure was also employed for all 3 studies. In Table 6.1, the number of biological outliers identified by Tukey's boxplot (n.boxplot) or INRQP (n.INRQP) tests are indicated for each study. The boxplot procedure identified 4 biological outliers in each study. The INRQP procedure was more conservative in identifying only 2 biological outliers for studies I and I-2.

Figure 6.3 illustrates the observations identified as biological outliers by either the boxplot (circles) or INRQP (triangles). In in-study I-1, both procedures identified the same 4 results as biological outliers. In pre-study I and in-study I-2, the INRQP procedure only identified the 2 most extreme boxplot outliers. The boxplot outlier procedure, even using $3.0 \times IQR$, can lead to excessive outlier rejections from real data. Table 6.1 suggests that the INRQP may be less liberal relative to the boxplot procedure.

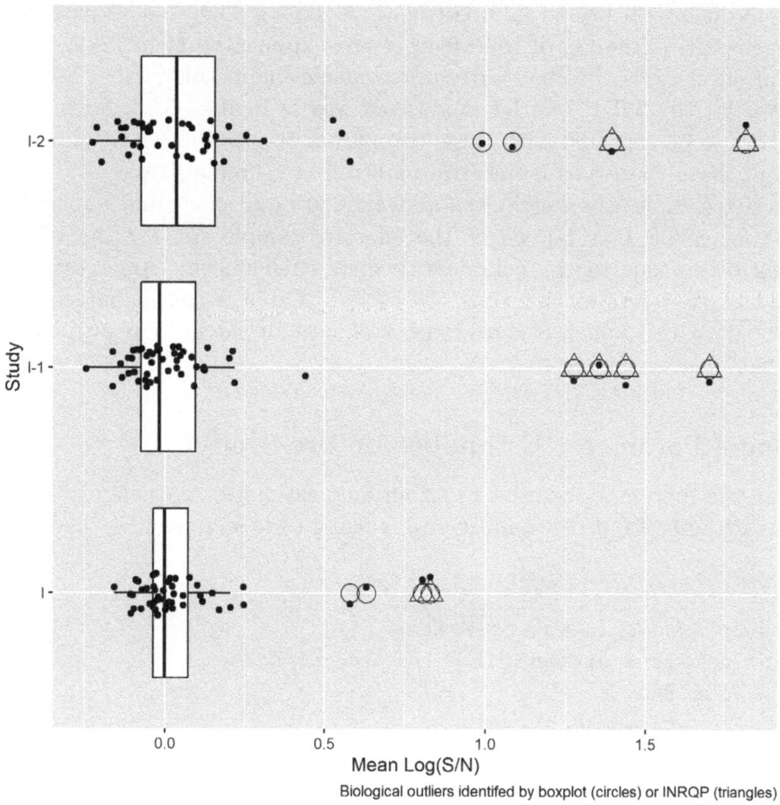

FIGURE 6.3
Identification of biological outliers in 10 pre-studies and 4 in-studies.

6.4.4 Model Parameters Estimation in Stan

Below model parameter posterior estimates are shown for 3 analyses:

1. Pre-study I (CP estimation),
2. SSCP (CP comparison: pre-study I vs in-study I-1), and
3. SSCP (CP comparison: pre-study I vs in-study I-2).

These analyses are performed using Hamiltonian Monte-Carlo by the R package `rstan` and the respective Stan model and R codes described above. For each analysis, 4 independent 4,000 draw chains (after a discarded 4,000 draw warm-up) are generated for a total of 16,000 MCMC draws from the posterior distributions of model parameters. Prior to these analyses, analytical, and then biological, outliers were identified and removed from each study by Rosner's test, followed by the INRQP procedure, respectively.

6.4.5 Convergence Diagnostics

As noted previously, diffuse prior distributions with discount factor $k \geq 3$ were employed and the value of k was found to have no discernible impact on the posterior distributions. Trace plots of the 4 chains revealed excellent mixing. No cases of divergent transitions or exceeding maximum tree depth were reported. The R-hat convergence metric was within 0.002 of 1.0 in all cases. The standard errors of the posterior means of all model parameter estimates were all less than 3% of the standard deviation of their posterior distributions.

Pairs plots did reveal low to mild correlations among some model parameters, particularly between $\log(\nu)$ (the log of the mean of the exponential effect) and μ (the mean of the Gaussian effect). The Pearson correlation coefficient in this latter case was generally ¡0.53, however for the SSCP I vs I-1 analysis it was as high as 0.73. Such levels of multi-colliniearity are to be expected with these two parameters as the relative impact of each on the true result mean ($= \mu + \nu$) is uncertain given finite sample sizes.

The effective sample size metric was above 1,880 in all cases and above 2,400 in most cases except for SSCP I vs I-1 where the effective sample size for the I-1 study $\log(\nu)$ was only 992 (likely due to the colliniearity mentioned above). An effective sample size of 992 would allow determination of a 5% FPR tail area within a percentage margin of $100/\sqrt{992 \times 0.05} = 14\%$ which is considered adequate for the present purposes considering the limited sample sizes involved.

6.4.6 Model Parameter Estimates for Pre-Study

Samples from the marginal posterior distributional estimates of pre-study I model parameters can be extracted from the stanFit object using code snippet I.

```
## I. posterior sample for pre=study I
mcmc <- as.data.frame(stanFit)
mcmc.mu <- mcmc$mu
mcmc.sigma <- exp(mcmc$lsigma)
mcmc.nu <- exp(mcmc$lnu)
mcmc.sigma_e <- mcmc$sigma_e
n.draws<- length(mcmc.mu)
```

Similarly, samples from the marginal posterior distributional estimates of either the I-1 or I-2 SSCP comparison model parameters can be extracted using code snippet J.

```
# J. posterior sample for in-studies I-1 and I-2
mcmc <- as.data.frame(stanFit)
mcmc.mu_pre <- mcmc$mu_pre
mcmc.sigma_pre <- exp(mcmc$lsigma_pre)
mcmc.nu_pre <- exp(mcmc$lnu_pre)
mcmc.mu_in <- mcmc$mu_in
mcmc.sigma_in <- exp(mcmc$lsigma_in)
mcmc.nu_in <- exp(mcmc$lnu_in)
mcmc.sigma_e <- mcmc$sigma_e
n.draws<- length(mcmc.mu)
```

Figures 6.4 to 6.6 illustrates kernel density estimates from the posterior samples of model parameters in the pre-study I, SSCP (I vs I-1), and SSCP (I vs I-2) analyses, respectively.

Figures 6.4 to 6.6 were produced using the function `ggplot()` and default settings of the `geom_density()` function from the R package `ggplot2`. These functions take as input 16,000 draws from the posterior distribution and 1,600,000 random samples from the prior distribution of each model parameter. The solid and dashed lines indicate the kernel density

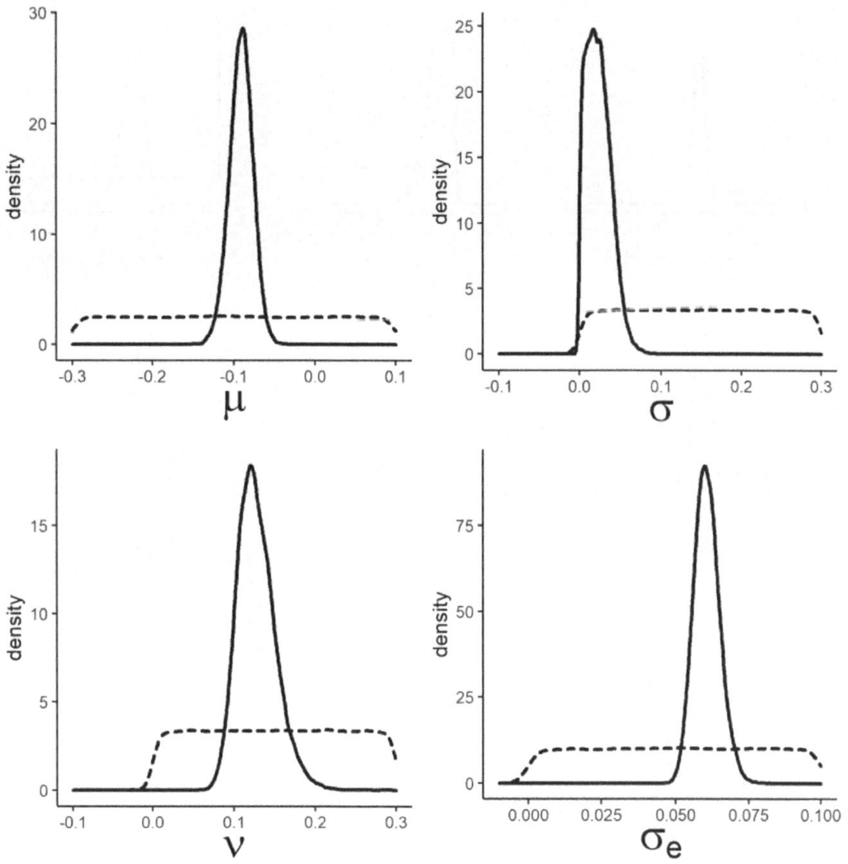

FIGURE 6.4
Kernal density plots of samples from the posterior distributions of model parameters estimated for study I.

estimates of the posterior and prior distributions, respectively. The kernel densities displayed are based on draws/ random samples whose values fall within the plot limits. Consequently the prior kernel densities of the prior appear artificially rounded near truncation points such as the plot extremes and (in the case of σ, ν or σ_e) near zero. In fact the prior densities extend well beyond the plot extremes.

To facilitate comparisons, the horizontal axes in Figures 6.5 and 6.6 are the same for pre-study (top row) and in-study (middle row). The bottom rows in these Figures (σ_e posterior distribution) is essentially identical to the corresponding distribution in Figure 6.4. This is to be expected since the posteriors for σ_e is derived in all 3 analyses solely from the replication present in pre-study I.

The prior densities in Figures 6.4 to 6.6 appear diffuse over the region of the respective posterior mass. This confirms that the prior choices have minimal impact on the posterior estimates. Most of the posterior distributions appear mono-modal, reasonably smooth, and well defined. However, the in-study posterior distributions of σ exhibit shouldering that may indicate that the relative contributions of Gaussian (i.e., σ) and exponential (i.e., ν) sources of variance are not well defined in these smaller data sets. However, the posterior densities of ν are well defined above zero in all cases. This suggests that biological effects in

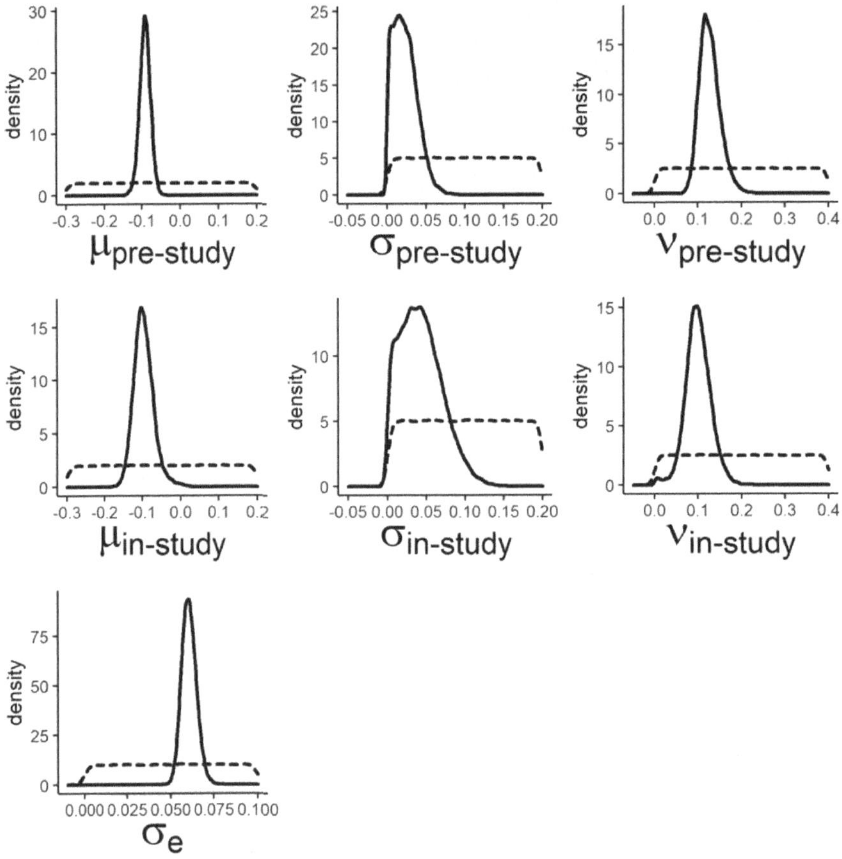

FIGURE 6.5
Kernal density of parameter posterior densities from SSCP analysis I-1 compared with pre-study I.

all 3 studies are not normally distributed and exhibit a positive skewness captured by the parametric exponential Gaussian model.

The ν posterior mode is higher for in-study I-2 than for in-study I-1 and the posterior mode for the I-2 σ is correspondingly lower than for I-1. The posterior distribution of the I-2 ν is clearly higher than that for pre-study I. This suggests that a greater portion of the variance in I-2 reportable results is due to positive skewness than is the case with either pre-study I or in-study I-1.

Figures 6.4 to 6.6 thus provide a visual diagnostic tool that is unavailable with non-Bayesian modeling. The presence of shouldering in posterior distributions can be diagnostic of model uncertainty. In addition, the exponential Gaussian model ν parameter provides a model-based, interpretable metric of positive skewness present in the underlying population, even after log transformation of the reportable response and the removal of suspected unrepresentative analytical and biological outliers. Posterior estimates of ν parameter can be compared across populations as part of the SSCP decision process.

Table 6.2 lists, for each of the 3 studies, posterior sample mean estimates of the four model parameters. Symbolizing these posterior mean estimates as $\hat{\mu}, \hat{\sigma}, \hat{\nu}$, and $\hat{\sigma}_e$ respectively, plug-in estimates of the mean (`mean`), standard deviation (`stddev`), and moment skewness (`skewness`) of the estimated exponential Gaussian distributions are obtained as

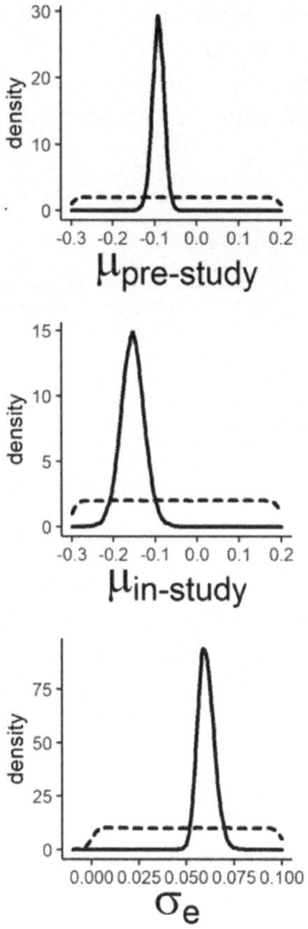

FIGURE 6.6
Kernal density of parameter posterior densities from SSCP analysis I-2 compared with pre-study I.

follows (see also the formulae given in Section 6.2):

$$\text{mean} = \hat{\mu} + \hat{\nu} \tag{6.15}$$

$$\text{stddev} = \hat{\sigma}^2 + \hat{\nu}^2 \tag{6.16}$$

$$\text{skewness} = 2 \times (1 + \hat{\sigma}^2/\hat{\nu}^2)^{-3/2} \tag{6.17}$$

The point estimates of skewness are well above zero in all cases suggesting that the distribution of biological effects is non-normal and right skewed in all 3 studies.

The last column (anal.pct) lists the percentage of overall variance in individual assay $\log(S/N)$ response that is due to analytical variance,

$$\text{anal.pct} = \frac{\hat{\sigma}_e^2}{\hat{\sigma}^2 + \hat{\nu}^2 + \hat{\sigma}_e^2} \times 100. \tag{6.18}$$

It is notable that the analytical variance is a considerable portion of total variance for pre-study I (the estimates of anal.pct for in-studies comes entirely from study I replication since in-study testing includes only a single test for each subject).

While not part of this case study, samples from posterior distributions of these 4 metrics could be easily obtained by applying the above formulae to each posterior draw. Such information could be used to assess the extent of non-normality and better judge the number of replicates needed to adequately power future pre-studies using this screening assay.

TABLE 6.2
Posterior mean parameter estimates and other metrics from 3 studies.

Study	$\hat{\mu}$	$\hat{\sigma}$	$\hat{\nu}$	$\hat{\sigma}_e$	mean	stddev	skewness	anal.pct
I-1	−0.096	0.043	0.100	0.061	0.003	0.109	1.554	23.741
I-2	−0.154	0.042	0.252	0.060	0.098	0.256	1.919	5.280
I	−0.091	0.023	0.128	0.061	0.037	0.130	1.909	17.951

6.4.7 CP Estimate for Pre-Study I

Assuming that analytical and biological outliers have been identified and removed from a $\log(S/N)$ data vector SB, a traditional approach to CP estimation, based on a function kindly provided by Zhang et al. (2013), can be implemented in R simply as in code snippit K.

```
# K. Traditional CP estimation
cutpoint<-function(data,alpha=0.05)
{
SB<-data$SB
Normal <- shapiro.test(SB)$p.value>0.05
if(Normal){cutpoint=exp(mean(SB)+qnorm(1-alpha)*sd(SB))
} else {cutpoint=exp(quantile(SB, p=1-alpha))
}
list(Normal=Normal,CP=cutpoint)
}
```

Here, the decision whether to use a parametric or nonparametric CP is based on a Shapiro-Wilk test of normality conducted at an $\alpha = 0.05$ level. The output includes a logical variable, Normal, which indicates whether normality was accepted as well as a CP estimate, CP, on the original (S/N) scale. The traditional approach to CP determination relies heavily on outlier elimination and either "force fits" a normal distribution model or defaults to a less efficient non-parametric model. Bayesian modeling offers a more principled alternative.

Following tradtion, We define the CP as the 0.95^{th} quantile of the posterior distribution of individual in-study test results. Therefore analytical variability needs to be factored in. This is done by adding in σ_e so that the posterior distribution reflects the quantile of an individual result rather than a subject mean. CP is thus a fixed function of the four parameters μ, σ, ν, and σ_e. A 16,000 draw sample from the posterior distribution of CP is obtained using the R package gamLSS function qexGAUS() as shown in code snippet L.

```
# L. posterior sample of CP for pre-study I
mcmc.CP <- rep(NA,n.draws)
for(i in 1:n.draws){
mcmc.CP[i] <- exp(qexGAUS(0.95,
mu=mcmc.mu[i],
sigma=sqrt(mcmc.sigma[i]^2 + mcmc.sigma_e[i]^2),
nu=mcmc.nu[i]))
}
mean(mcmc.CP)
quantile(mcmc.CP,probs=c(0.1,0.5,0.9))
```

Figure 6.7 illustrates a model based CP estimation for pre-study I that is created by code snippet M (note this code presumes a CP `CPtrad` was obtained using the traditional CP estimation method illustrated in code snippet K previously).

```
# M. Illustrate Bayesian model based CP estimation for pre-study I
# Capture the key posterior estimates in TradCP
mu.post.mean <- mean(mcmc.mu)
mu.post.sd <- sd(mcmc.mu)
sigma.post.mean <- mean(mcmc.sigma)
sigma.post.sd <- sd(mcmc.sigma)
nu.post.mean <- mean(mcmc.nu)
nu.post.sd <- sd(mcmc.nu)
sigma_e.post.mean <- mean(mcmc.sigma_e)
sigma_e.post.sd <- sd(mcmc.sigma_e)
CP.post.q025 <- quantile(mcmc.CP,probs=c(0.025))
CP.post.q50 <- quantile(mcmc.CP,probs=c(0.5))
CP.post.q975 <- quantile(mcmc.CP,probs=c(0.975))
topl <- tibble(log_SN = y) # individual results for histogram
pdf_range <- seq(min(y),max(y),0.001) # range for plot
n_pdf_range <- length(pdf_range)
CPtrad <- log(CPtrad) # traditional CP on the log scale
CPpost <- log(CP.post.q50)# posterior median CP on the log scale
CP_dat <- tibble(CPpost = CPpost,CPtrad = CPtrad)
CP.dens <- density(log(mcmc.CP))
CP.post <- tibble(log_SN = CP.dens$x, density = CP.dens$y)
# lower plot of posterior of individual results
p <- ggplot(topl, aes(x=log_SN)) +
geom_histogram(aes(y=..density..), bins=30,colour = "white",fill="grey75") +
geom_vline(aes(xintercept=CPtrad), CP_dat, col="black") +
geom_vline(aes(xintercept=CPpost), CP_dat, col="red", linetype=2) +
geom_segment(x=log(CP.post.q025), y=0,
xend=log(CP.post.q975), yend=0, size=3,color="red") +
labs(title=paste("Posterior for individual results based on Study",
     studies[i_stud]),
x="log transformed individual signal to noise response") +
theme_classic()
for (i in 1:100){ # add 100 random posterior realizations
p = local({
draw <- sample(1:n.draws, 1, replace=T)
pdf <- dexGAUS(pdf_range,
mu= mcmc.mu[draw],
sigma= sqrt(mcmc.sigma[draw]^2 + mcmc.sigma_e[draw]^2),
nu= mcmc.nu[draw])
```

```
# kernal density of one draw from the posterior of individual results
dens <- tibble(log_SN = pdf_range, density = pdf)
p + geom_line(data=dens, aes(y=density), colour="red", alpha=0.3)
})
}
# Create a visual of the posterior relative to ID means
# topl inlcudes the id means in histogram
topl <- tibble(log_SN = meandata$SB_means[meandata$Study == studies[i_stud] &
!meandata$outside_np])
pdf_range <- seq(min(y),max(y),0.001)
n_pdf_range <- length(pdf_range)
# upper plot of posterior of biological effects (subject means)
p2 <- ggplot(topl, aes(x=log_SN)) +
geom_histogram(aes(y=..density..),bins=30,colour = "white", fill="grey75") +
labs(title=paste("Posterior of mean responses based on Study",
     studies[i_stud]),
x="ID mean of log transformed individual signal to noise response") +
theme_classic()
for (i in 1:100){ # add 100 random posterior realizations
p2 = local({
draw <- sample(1:n.draws, 1, replace=T)
pdf <- dexGAUS(pdf_range,
mu= mcmc.mu[draw],
sigma= mcmc.sigma[draw],
nu= mcmc.nu[draw])
# dens is kernal density of random postetior realizations of ID means
dens <- tibble(log_SN = pdf_range, density = pdf)
p2 + geom_line(data=dens, aes(y=density), colour="red", alpha=0.3)
})
}
grid.arrange(p2, p, nrow = 2) # display figure
```

The upper panel of Figure 6.7 is based on the mean responses of the 48 subjects in pre-study I classified as naive by the INRQP process which are plotted as a histogram. The curves are 100 random samples from the posterior distribution of mean responses. These 100 curves give a visual impression of the uncertainty in estimating the biological effect distribution from only 48 subjects. The strong right skewness of this biological distribution is clearly evident.

The lower panel of Figure 6.7 is based on the 144 individual results remaining after analytical and biological outlier removal which are plotted as a histogram. The curves are 100 random samples from the posterior distribution of expected independent individual values. While some right skewness is still evident, it is tempered by the addition of analytical deviations to the biological effects. The vertical dashed line and wide horizontal bar indicate the posterior median and 95% central credible interval estimates of the CP on the $\log(S/R)$ scale, respectively. For reference, the traditional CP estimate obtained using code snippet K is shown as a vertical black line. The Bayesian CP estimate is slightly higher than that of the traditional.

Table 6.3 provides a comparison of untransformed CP point estimate determined by either a traditional (CPtrad) or posterior median and 95% central credible interval estimates (CP.post.q50, -.q025, and -.q975, respectively) based on posterior estimates of the parameters of the exponential Gaussian model. Using the traditional approach, normality (Normal) was assessed, by a Shapiro-Wilk test with $\alpha = 0.05$, after removal of outliers using the Grubbs and boxplot tests. Notice that normality was rejected (`FALSE`) for all 3 studies even after outlier removal using traditional approaches.

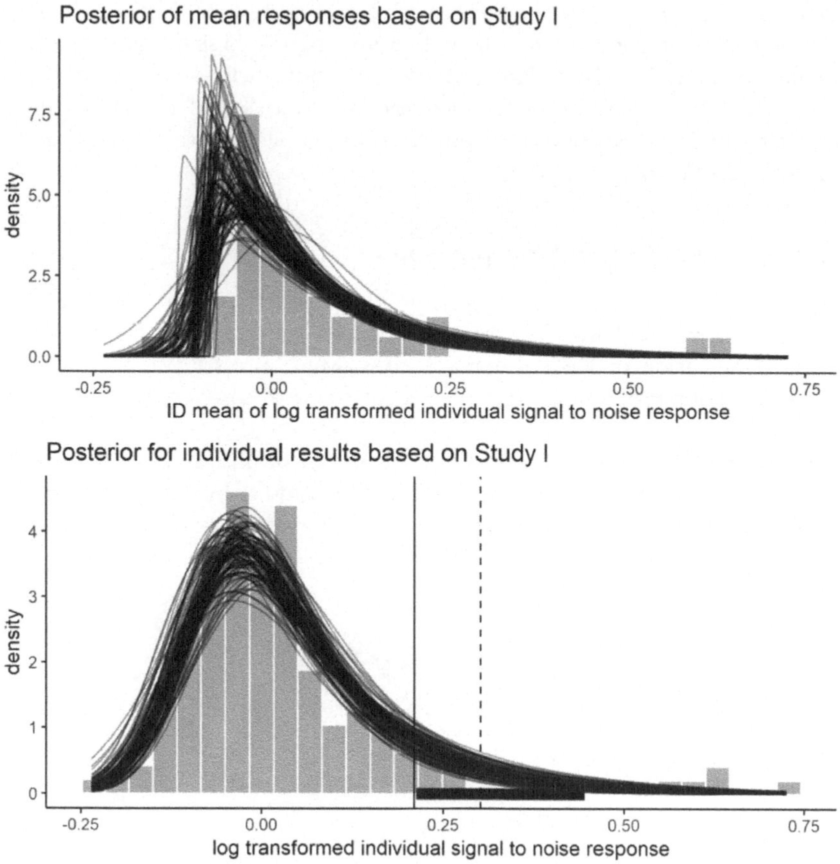

FIGURE 6.7
CP estimation for pre-study I.

TABLE 6.3
CP determination (on the untransformed scale) by both traditional and posterior predictive approaches.

Study	Normal	CPtrad	CP.post.q50	CP.post.q025	CP.post.q975
I-1	FALSE	1.232004	1.258504	1.167962	1.443901
I-2	FALSE	1.657142	1.822992	1.505845	2.466611
I	FALSE	1.233517	1.352324	1.237362	1.562409

Such displays as Figure 6.7 are readily generated and provide useful diagnostics of the agreement between the model and data. The random samples of density curves from the joint posterior gives an intuitive visual feel for estimation uncertainty relative to either the observed subject mean responses (top panel) and individual responses (lower panel). For this case study the agreement appears relatively good. While observed values appear extreme relative to the fitted model, the impact of such extreme values on the estimated CP should be less than with a normal model which cannot accommodate skewness. As Table 6.3 shows, traditional methods default to less sensitive non-parametric CP estimation which cannot provide parametric diagnostics such as Figure 6.7. While in this case study, the CPs estimated using the Bayesian modeling are slightly higher than those determined via traditional methods, the Bayesian estimates are fully justified based on the definition of the CP as the 0.95^{th} quantile of the posterior distribution of individual in-study test results. Further, the Bayesian approach provides a credible interval estimate not available using traditional methods.

6.4.8 Study Specific CP Comparisons

Code snippet N estimates a joint sample from the posterior distribution of CP for both prestudy, `mcmc.CP_pre`, and in-study, `mcmc.CP_in`, on the untransformed scale as well as the posterior distribution of their difference (in-study – pre-study), `mcmc.CP.diff`, and estimates the posterior probability that the CP of the in-study is greater than that of the pre-study.

The CP is defined as the 0.95^{th} quantile of the posterior of individual test result. Therefore analytical variability needs to be factored in. This is done by adding in `sigma_e` so that the posterior distribution reflects the quantile of an individual result rather than a subject mean.

```
# N. posterior sample of CP (untransformed scale)
#     SSCP studies I vs I-1 or I-2
mcmc.CP_pre <- rep(NA,n.draws)
mcmc.CP_in <- rep(NA,n.draws)
for(i in 1:n.draws){
mcmc.CP_pre[i] <- exp(qexGAUS(0.95,
mu=mcmc.mu_pre[i],
sigma=sqrt(mcmc.sigma_pre[i]^2 + mcmc.sigma_e[i]^2),
nu=mcmc.nu_pre[i]))
mcmc.CP_in[i] <- exp(qexGAUS(0.95,
mu=mcmc.mu_in[i],
sigma=sqrt(mcmc.sigma_in[i]^2 + mcmc.sigma_e[i]^2),
nu=mcmc.nu_in[i]))
}
# sample from the posterior of CP difference (In - Pre)
mcmc.CP.diff <- mcmc.CP_in - mcmc.CP_pre
# posterior quantiles of CP difference
CP.diff.q025 <- quantile(mcmc.CP.diff,probs=c(0.025))
CP.diff.q50 <- quantile(mcmc.CP.diff,probs=c(0.5))
CP.diff.q975 <- quantile(mcmc.CP.diff,probs=c(0.975))
# posterior probability that CP difference is > 0
Prob.CP.diff.gt.0 <- mean(mcmc.CP.diff > 0)
```

Figures 6.8 and 6.9 illustrate SSCP analyses in which the CP determined from in-studies I-1 and I-2 (bottom panels), respectively are compared to the CP determined from pre-study I (top panels). These Figures are created by the following R code.

```
# 0. Collect the In-study estimates in the following In-study columns:
mu.post.mean <- mean(mcmc.mu_in)
mu.post.sd <- sd(mcmc.mu_in)
sigma.post.mean <- mean(mcmc.sigma_in)
sigma.post.sd <- sd(mcmc.sigma_in)
nu.post.mean <- mean(mcmc.nu_in)
nu.post.sd <- sd(mcmc.nu_in)
# (note sigma_e derived mainly from pre-study)
sigma_e.post.mean <- mean(mcmc.sigma_e)
sigma_e.post.sd <- sd(mcmc.sigma_e)
CP.post.q025 <- quantile(mcmc.CP_in,probs=c(0.025))
CP.post.q50 <- quantile(mcmc.CP_in,probs=c(0.5))
CP.post.q975 <- quantile(mcmc.CP_in,probs=c(0.975))
# (In-study CP - Pre-study CP derived in SSCP analysis)
CP.diff.q025 <- quantile(mcmc.CP.diff,probs=c(0.025))
CP.diff.q50 <- quantile(mcmc.CP.diff,probs=c(0.5))
CP.diff.q975 <- quantile(mcmc.CP.diff,probs=c(0.975))
Prob.CP.diff.gt.0 <- mean(mcmc.CP.diff > 0)
# Create a Visual graphic for the SSCP comparison
# First the individual measurements
pdata1 <- tibble(y = c(y_pre,y_in),
Study = c( rep("I",length(y_pre)), rep("I-1",length(y_in)) ))
# posterior medians
pdata2 <- tibble(CP.q5 = log(c(quantile(mcmc.CP_pre,probs=c(0.5)),
quantile(mcmc.CP_in,probs=c(0.5)))),
Study = c( "I","I-1") )
# 95% credible intervals
pdata3 <- tibble(CP.q025 = log(c(quantile(mcmc.CP_pre,probs=c(0.025)),
quantile(mcmc.CP_in,probs=c(0.025)))),
Study = c( "I","I-1") )
pdata4 <- tibble(CP.q975 = log(c(quantile(mcmc.CP_pre,probs=c(0.975)),
quantile(mcmc.CP_in,probs=c(0.975)))),
Study = c( "I","I-1") )
# range over which to create the posterior expectations
pdf_range <- seq(min(pdata1$y),max(pdata1$y),0.01)
n_pdf_range <- length(pdf_range)
# generate histograms and intervals
p <- ggplot(pdata1) +
geom_histogram(aes( x=y, y=..density..), bins=30, colour = "white",
fill="grey75") +
geom_vline(aes(xintercept=CP.q5), pdata2 , col="black", linetype=2) +
geom_vline(aes(xintercept=CP.q025), pdata3 , col="black", linetype=2) +
geom_vline(aes(xintercept=CP.q975), pdata4 , col="black", linetype=2) +
facet_wrap(~Study,nrow=2) +
xlab("Individual Signal to Noise results on log scale") +
theme_classic()
# overlay 100 random posterior realizations
for (i in 1:100){
p = local({
draw <- sample(1:n.draws, 1, replace=T)
pdf_pre <- dexGAUS(pdf_range,
mu= mcmc.mu_pre[draw],
sigma= sqrt(mcmc.sigma_pre[draw]^2 + mcmc.sigma_e[draw]^2),
nu= mcmc.nu_pre[draw])
draw <- sample(1:n.draws, 1, replace=T)
pdf_in <- dexGAUS(pdf_range,
mu= mcmc.mu_in[draw],
sigma= sqrt(mcmc.sigma_in[draw]^2 + mcmc.sigma_e[draw]^2),
nu= mcmc.nu_in[draw])
dens <- tibble(log_SN = rep(pdf_range,2),
density = c(pdf_pre,pdf_in),
Study = c( rep("I",n_pdf_range), rep("I-1",n_pdf_range)))
```

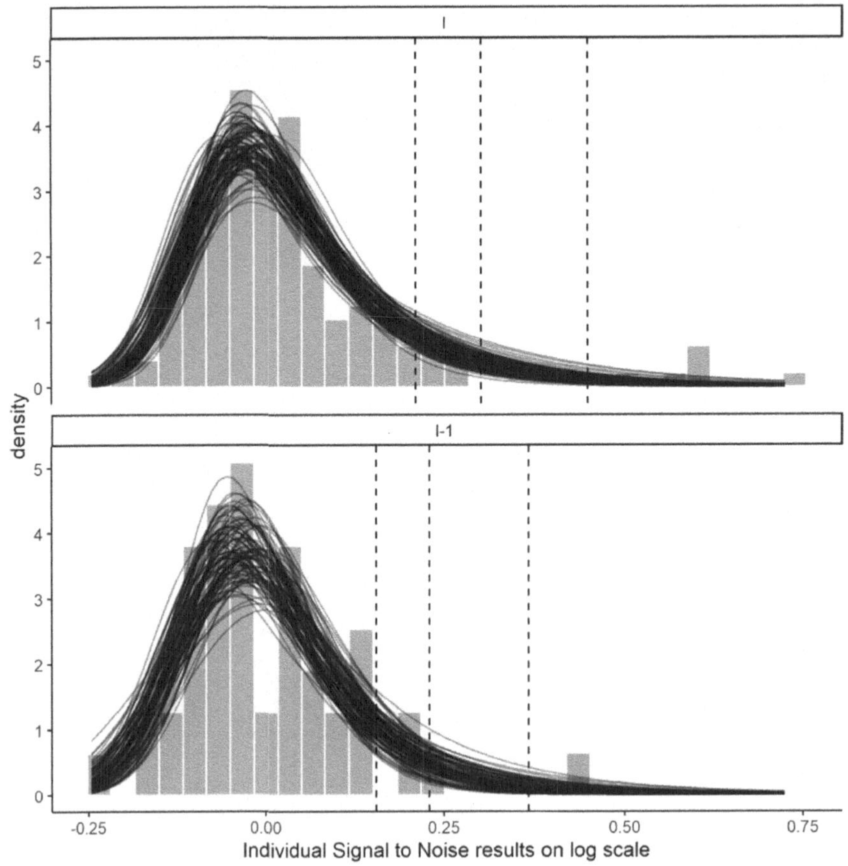

FIGURE 6.8
SSCP comparison for in-study I-1 compared with pre-study I.

```
p + geom_line(data=dens, aes(x=log_SN, y=density), colour="red",alpha=0.3)
})
}
print(p)
```

Each panel in Figures 6.8 and 6.9 includes 3 features:

1. A histogram of individual $\log(S/R)$ values. Note that the pre-study (top panel) individual values are not independent because each ID has 3 replicates. So the histogram is provided here merely for reference.
2. One hundred realizations of the posterior distribution of individual $\log(S/R)$ reportable results. Each realization is generated from a single parameter draw randomly selected from the posterior sample. These provide a visual impression of the uncertainty associated with this posterior distributional estimate.
3. The vertical dashed lines indicate the median and central 95% credible interval of the posterior distribution of the CP determined from each study. A comparison of the location of these lines gives a visual impression of the degree of overlap of

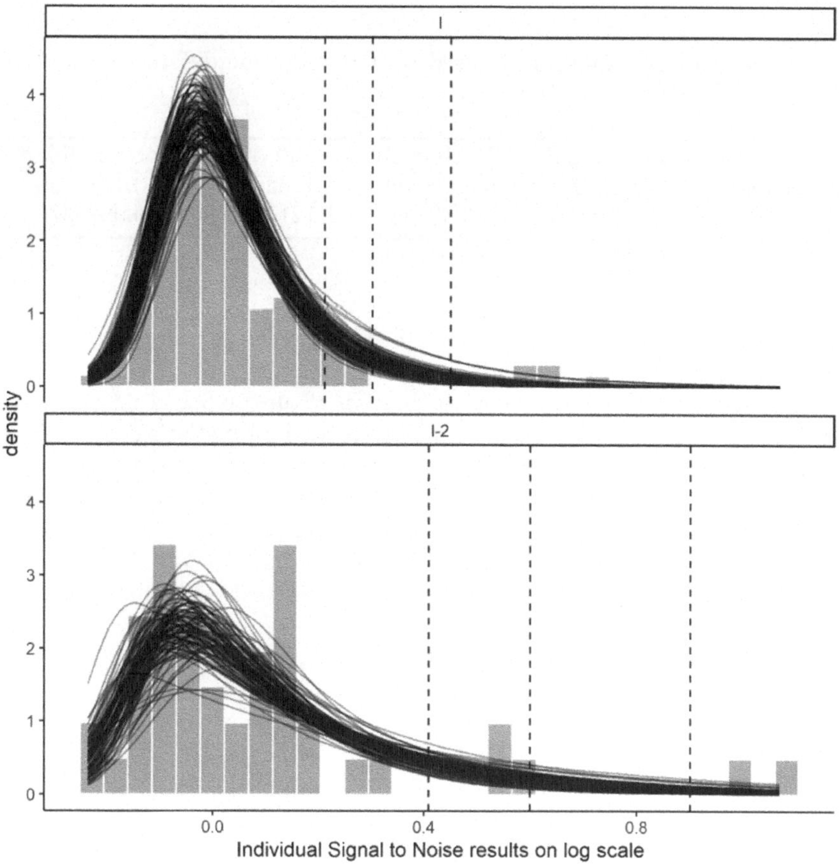

FIGURE 6.9
SSCP comparison for in-study I-2 compared with pre-study I.

the estimates from each study. In particular the median vertical dashed line in each panel serves as a point estimate of the CP for that study (on the log scale), determined to provide an FPR of 5%. The posterior mean CP could also serve as a point estimate, the median allows a risk-based interpretation as the 50th percentile of the posterior distribution.

Figure 6.8 suggests that the I-1 in-study CP may be lower, and Figure 6.9 suggests that the I-2 in-study CP may be greater, than the provisional CP from pre-study I. Table 6.4 presents more quantitative SSCP comparisons based on the estimated posterior difference (in-study minus pre-study) in CP (untransformed scale) for the 4 in-studies relative to their respective pre-studies.

Table 6.4 provides the posterior median (CP.diff.q50) as well as the central 95% credible interval (CP.diff.q0.25, CP.diff.q975) estimates of the CP difference. If the 95% central 95% credible interval excludes zero, there is evidence that the CP determined from the pre-study may not provide the expected FPR of 5% in the in-study. This is the case for in-study I-2, but not for in-study I-1. The last column in Table 6.4 provides the posterior probability that the CP difference is greater than zero (Prob.CP.diff.gt.0). This offers a direct risk-based SSCP decision metric. If Prob.CP.diff.gt.0 deviates importantly from 0.5 (e.g., ≤ 0.05 or

TABLE 6.4
SSCP comparisons for two in-studies based on CP posterior differences (in-study minus pre-study).

Study	CP.diff.q50	CP.diff.q025	CP.diff.q975	Prob.CP.diff.gt.0
I-1	-0.0920719	-0.3208490	0.1262066	0.1811250
I-2	0.4611814	0.0945484	1.1210195	0.9929375

≥ 0.95), a decision to determine an in-study specific CP can be made based on a directly relevant probability metric.

Informative visual comparisons, such as those in Figures 6.8 and 6.9 are not available with traditional CP comparison approaches that depend on statistical hypothesis tests of means and variances. Employing a distributional model that accommodates skewness allows the comparison of model based parameter estimates both visually and quantitatively as in Table 6.3. Further, the Bayesian model provides a sample from the posterior difference of the CPs from two studies as in Table 6.4. This permits an SSCP decision based on posterior probabilities; probabilities for events of interest being a fundamental component of risk-based decision making.

6.5 Discussion

The Bayesian approach to the determination of immunogenicity screening CPs illustrated in this chapter is admittedly more challenging than ad hoc traditional approaches currently advocated in industry and regulatory guidance. Identification of a suitable model for the distribution of biological effects requires a sufficiently large and relevant data set. The algorithms for biological outlier detection and parameter estimation depend on the selected distribution model can be complex and computationally intensive. Bayesian approaches demand the consideration, justification, and expression of prior knowledge about the distributional model parameters. Posterior estimation through MCMC or HMC requires specialized statistical expertise and due diligence. The bioanalytical team tasked with determining immunogenicity screening assay CPs may well ask the question: "Is a Bayesian approach worth the effort?"

We argue for an affirmative answer to that question. The dramatic rise in the number of amazing new biological therapies brings with it an increase risk of serious – even life threatening – side effects from therapies, some of which will inevitably induce ADA in clinical subjects and patients. The predictive value of a result from the screening assay represents the eyes and ears of ADA monitoring. The responsibility to accurately determine the immunogenicity risk of a given therapy, in a given population ultimately falls on the shoulders of the bioanalytical team that determines the pre-study CP and conducts in-study SSCP comparisons. We have found the Bayesian approach to CP estimation and SSCP comparison informative, intuitive, and readily implemented using freely available computing packages.

Attempting to fit a model similar to that described in Sections 6.2 and 6.3 using maximum likelihood, would certainly require arbitrary approximations (e.g., asymptotic normality, linear, plug-ins, degrees of freedom) whose impacts are unknown. In comparison,

Bayesian modeling is intuitive, straightforward, approximation free, and highly informative.

The ADA challenge appears sufficiently impactful to deserve the best statistics has to offer with respect to risk-based decision-making. The underlying immunogenicity mechanisms of biological therapies in different populations can be expected to vary greatly. A one-size-fits-all approach is unlikely to be optimal. A therapy-tailored and fit-for-purpose approach has the potential to offer optimal treatment outcomes. This is the opportunity offered by full probability Bayesian models. Such models properly weight the severity of ADA harm by the posterior probability of occurrence of that harm for a more coherent assessment of risk. In our case study we illustrated the CP posterior median as a point estimate. Depending on the decision risk calculation, a more conservative choice, such as the 5th percentile be taken instead. A proper decision theoretic approach takes into account potential harms of wrong decisions that metrics such as type I error and FPR ignore.

Given limited bioanalytical resources and the need for early SSCP assessments, pre-study and in-study sample sizes used for CP estimation and comparison are generally small. Bayesian models offer the opportunity to leverage relevant and justifiable prior knowledge from pre-clinical or other sources. An example in our case study SSCP comparisons is the assumption of a common analytical standard deviation, σ_e, in both pre- and in-study to incorporated analytical variability into the estimation of the in-study CP. While we used diffuse prior distributions for model parameters, employing justified and relevant informative prior distributions have the potential to increase the power of CP decision making.

The lack of understanding of the causes and mechanisms of ADA development need not prevent us from developing more descriptive and predictive statistical models. Sophisticated tools are available for exploring models less dependent on normality. Our case study illustrates how models, such as the exponential Gaussian, can provide informative descriptive metrics and CP determination that is less dependent on arbitrary outlier rejection, normality, or less powerful nonparametric approaches. Daring to explore beyond familiar simple approaches may be a first step in finding connections between our considerable and growing understanding of the biological components of immunogenicity and our ability to predict its likelihood.

7

Application of Bayesian Hierarchical Models to Experimental Design

Adam P. Rauk and Paul Faya

Eli Lilly and Company

CONTENTS

7.1 Introduction

Experimental design plays an important role in the development of biopharmaceutical molecules. Experimental designs are commonly applied in upstream (e.g., cell culture) and downstream (e.g., purification) manufacturing process characterization and optimization studies as well as formulation development studies (Grangeia et al., 2020). The results of these studies assist with optimizing processes and establishing control strategies that utilize Quality by Design principles, demonstrating enhanced knowledge of product performance. This chapter will cover two applications that typically apply experimental design for biological license application (BLA) supporting work: process parameter classification and formulation attribute robustness.

Multivariate studies serve as key components in defining the control strategy for drug substance unit operations. These statistically designed experiments (DOEs) assess process parameters that may affect product quality and quantify the impact on responses (Amadeo et al., 2014; Yang et al., 2019). Process parameters that affect product quality by a magnitude that exceeds a level of practical importance are classified as critical process parameters that should be monitored and controlled (Finkler and Krummen, 2016). The A-Mab (2009) case study developed by the CMC Biotech Working Group provides several examples of how results from DOEs are used to classify critical process parameters.

For drug product formulation development, the sponsor is expected to identify critical and interacting variables and gain an understanding of how they affect drug product quality (ICH Q8(R2), 2009). The application of experimental design to meet this objective has been widely published. A thorough review of formulation development is provided by Wang and Ohtake (2019). Wurth et al. (2016) and Marjou et al. (2018) provide case studies showing how quality by design principles and the application of experimental design can demonstrate

DOI: 10.1201/9781003255093-7

the robustness of a range of formulation conditions, with a frequentist statistical treatment of the data. Narayanan et al. (2021) uses a Bayesian technique to inform sequential design, using the posterior distribution from earlier experiments as the source of prior belief for future studies.

When several molecules are taken through the development activities described above, the same factors are often assessed repeatedly. This provides an opportunity to distil the cumulative results into platform knowledge that offers an understanding of similarities between molecules. Bayesian hierarchical models are well-suited for quantifying platform knowledge for a few reasons. First, the hierarchical model provides a mechanism to quantify typical performance as well as to assess how much the model parameter effects vary between molecules. Second, the Bayesian framework can directly incorporate prior knowledge and empirical data into a single model. While frequentist approaches can also leverage platform knowledge, they typically rely on an "all-or-nothing" proposition; either enough platform knowledge exists such that a factor is negligible and can be excluded from the design, or the factor receives the same treatment as other factors. That is, either there is enough knowledge to justify full understanding of a given process, or new data are collected. On the other hand, Bayesian analysis offers a mechanism to leverage any amount of prior knowledge – even incomplete knowledge – and supplements such knowledge with information gained from additional data.

The remainder of this chapter is structured as follows. In Section 7.2, we define the single-study statistical model that relates the responses to the factors. Section 7.3 describes how the single-study results can be pooled into a hierarchical model to build platform understanding of factor effects. Two case studies are given in Section 7.3 to demonstrate the design and analysis of the platform modeling methodology. Section 7.4 extends one of the case studies to serve as the basis for informative priors. Some concluding remarks and discussion are given in Section 7.5.

7.2 Single-study Model Definition

Consider the following linear model relating the p effects (terms) to the y_i responses for each of the $i = 1, ..., n$, DOE study runs:

$$y_i = \beta_0 + \beta_1 x_{i1} + ... + \beta_p x_{ip} + \varepsilon_i \tag{7.1}$$

where x_{ij} is the condition (factor) for the ith run of the jth term in the model, $j = 1, ..., p$. The p terms in the model can represent main effects, interactions, or curvature effects derived from the factors in the DOE study, and $\varepsilon_i \sim N(0, \sigma)$ is random error. The parameters $\boldsymbol{\beta} = (\beta_0, ..., \beta_p)$ quantify the effect of the p terms on the response, y_i. For example, y_i may represent the measured host cell protein for a given run in a process development experimental design. An 8-run full factorial experiment may be represented by the example design depicted in Table 7.1. The values in the table are coded variables (Montgomery, 2017, for example), where 1 and -1 denote the high and low settings of the factors, respectively.

For this example, the design in Table 7.1 represents a protein A chromatography experiment that varies column load, bed height, and load flow rate. The design is reflected in columns x_1, x_2, and x_3, respectively, which also correspond to the main effect terms for the three design factors. An interaction term between column load and bed height is included in this example, which is represented by $x_1 x_2 = x_4$. In this example, β_0 measures the baseline level of host cell protein (intercept), β_1 quantifies the main effect term for column load,

TABLE 7.1
3-Factor example.

Factor	Intercept	x_1	x_2	x_3	x_4
Parameter	β_0	β_1	β_2	β_3	β_4
	1	−1	−1	−1	1
	1	1	−1	−1	−1
	1	−1	1	−1	−1
	1	1	1	−1	1
	1	−1	−1	1	1
	1	1	−1	1	−1
	1	−1	1	1	−1
	1	1	1	1	1
	Baseline	Column Load	Bed Height	Flow Rate	Column Load × Bed Height Interaction

β_2 the main effect term for bed height, β_3 the main effect term for flow rate, and β_4 the interaction term between column load and bed height.

After the study is executed, the model in (7.1) can be fit using traditional least-squares estimates for the model parameters. Alternatively, Bayesian methods can be used to obtain posterior distributions for the model parameters. Although analysis of a single DOE study is outside the scope of this chapter, straightforward methods to fit such models using Bayesian methods are available by using free software such as the `brms` (Bayesian regression models using STAN) package Bürkner et al. (2021) in R (R Core Team, 2021).

7.3 Hierarchical Model

A hierarchical (or multilevel) analysis expands the basic model in (7.1) by allowing the parameters, $\boldsymbol{\beta}$, to differ between molecules. That is, each parameter is treated as a random value drawn from a normal distribution with some center and variance. For instance, rather than estimating a single value for β_0, the intercept, all intercepts are modeled as normally distributed with a center at μ_{β_0} and standard deviation at σ_{β_0}. That is, $\beta_{0,k} \sim N(\mu_{\beta_0}, \sigma_{\beta_0})$, where $k = 1, ..., m$ molecules. More generally, the effect of the jth term is normally distributed with a center at μ_{β_j} and variance $\sigma^2_{\beta_j}$:

$$\beta_{j,k} \sim N(\mu_{\beta_j}, \sigma_{\beta_j}) \tag{7.2}$$

for all p terms in the DOE model. For Bayesian inference, prior distributions are required on each of the p set of hyperparameters, $(\mu_{\beta_j}, \sigma_{\beta_j})$, as well as on the residual error term, σ. Let $\boldsymbol{\theta} = (\mu_{\beta_1}, ..., \mu_{\beta_p}, \sigma_{\beta_1}, ..., \sigma_{\beta_p}, \sigma)$ denote the vector of parameters to estimate. Following Bayes' theorem, the joint posterior distribution for $\boldsymbol{\theta}$ is

$$\pi(\boldsymbol{\theta}|\boldsymbol{D}) \propto L(\boldsymbol{D}|\boldsymbol{\theta})\pi(\boldsymbol{\theta}), \tag{7.3}$$

where $\pi(\cdot)$ denotes the prior, $L(\cdot)$ denotes the likelihood function, and $\boldsymbol{D}$ denotes the DOE study results across the molecules. In terms of the choice of prior distributions for $\boldsymbol{\theta}$, we recommend flat, relatively non-informative distributions such that posterior inference is driven by the data. In the `brms` package, prior distributions for the standard deviation terms, σ_{β_k}, are by default selected to be weakly informative, using half Student-t distributions with

3 degrees of freedom and large scale parameters relative to the spread of the data. These prior distributions help to improve sampling and other model properties (e.g., shrinkage) (see Bürkner et al. (2021) for more details). For the center parameters, $\mu_{\beta_0}, \mu_{\beta_1}, ..., \mu_{\beta_p}$, `brms` assigns by default non-informative flat priors, where likelihood for any real number is proportional to 1. We adopt the `brms` default priors for $\boldsymbol{\theta}$ in the two case studies presented in this chapter. Note that the `brms` package also permits the user to specify the prior for each parameter. In Section 7.4, we given an example of specifying informative priors based on posterior distributions obtained from previous studies.

An important assumption for hierarchical models is exchangeability (see Bernardo and Smith (2009)). Similar to the frequentist assumption that observations are independent and identically distributed, the model is based on the notion that the molecule-specific parameters follow a distribution that describes future molecules. The population within the dataset that is used to construct the model must be representative of future molecules for which inference will be applied. Platform knowledge from molecules using one modality cannot simply apply to a new modality. Significant process changes may result in subgroups that should be recognized as a covariate in the model. This does not mean, however, that the model cannot incorporate molecules with some variation. Rather, inference from the hierarchical model must take into consideration the scope represented in the underlying data set. If the data contain very consistent processes and molecule structures, the scope of inference is limited to the same process and similar molecules. If molecules span different processes and more highly varied structures, inference applies more broadly.

7.3.1 Example 1: Protein A Purification

In the first example, the protein A capture step is characterized for ten molecules using statistically designed experiments that evaluate the effect of column load (load), bed height (bh), and flow rate (fr) on residual levels of host cell protein (HCP) transformed to the logarithmic scale. This platform-level characterization is an important input for determining the criticality of a process parameter for future molecules. Indeed, for a new molecule, the purpose of the DOE is to quantify the impact of the factors on levels of host cell protein to determine whether the process is robust within the tested range or if the magnitude of the effect exceeds a level that is practically meaningful (i.e., it is a critical process parameter). For the purpose of this example, the practical threshold will be set at logarithmic difference of 0.3 and all factors are scaled to a range of −1 to 1. Figure 7.1 depicts the predicted HCP levels across 10 different molecules as a function of the three factors studies. These prediction profiles are based on a least-squares fit of the model in (7.1), where the interaction term is between load and bh. The raw data from this example are provided in Table 7.2.

TABLE 7.2
Example 1 data showing log(HCP) for each DOE run for ten molecules.

Run	Load	bh	fr	mab01	mab02	mab03	mab04	mab05	mab06	mab07	mab08	mab09	mab10
1	−1	0	0	2.05	2.08	1.98	1.96	1.82	1.50	2.89	1.74	2.62	2.29
2	−1	−1	−1	2.07	1.80	1.85	1.97	1.81	1.51	2.82	1.58	2.47	2.21
3	1	−1	−1	1.89	1.76	1.75	1.70	1.76	1.42	2.60	1.30	2.80	2.59
4	1	0	0	1.97	1.64	1.87	1.62	1.65	1.63	2.81	1.66	2.62	2.40
5	−1	1	−1	2.00	2.03	1.99	2.09	1.98	1.52	2.93	1.93	2.75	2.57
6	0	−1	0	1.94	1.68	1.79	1.84	1.93	1.44	2.87	1.67	2.64	2.22
7	0	1	0	2.05	1.69	1.87	1.79	1.78	1.43	2.97	1.66	2.86	2.56
8	1	1	−1	2.09	1.62	2.00	1.70	1.60	1.40	2.77	1.76	2.74	2.09
9	−1	−1	1	1.98	1.69	1.70	1.82	1.81	1.39	2.77	1.58	2.63	2.19
10	0	0	−1	2.02	1.79	1.94	1.81	1.88	1.48	2.73	1.75	2.73	2.23
11	0	0	1	1.87	1.74	1.76	1.65	1.64	1.66	3.03	1.72	2.60	2.32
12	1	−1	1	1.91	1.59	2.00	1.92	1.77	1.67	2.85	1.58	2.65	2.48
13	−1	1	1	2.12	1.98	2.05	1.99	1.84	1.57	3.26	1.74	2.58	2.18
14	0	0	0	2.09	1.74	1.86	2.00	1.63	1.31	2.78	1.74	2.73	2.30
15	1	1	1	1.99	1.58	1.67	1.59	1.66	1.50	2.47	1.77	2.79	2.32
16	0	0	0	1.95	1.70	1.85	1.82	1.75	1.49	2.84	1.46	2.71	2.30

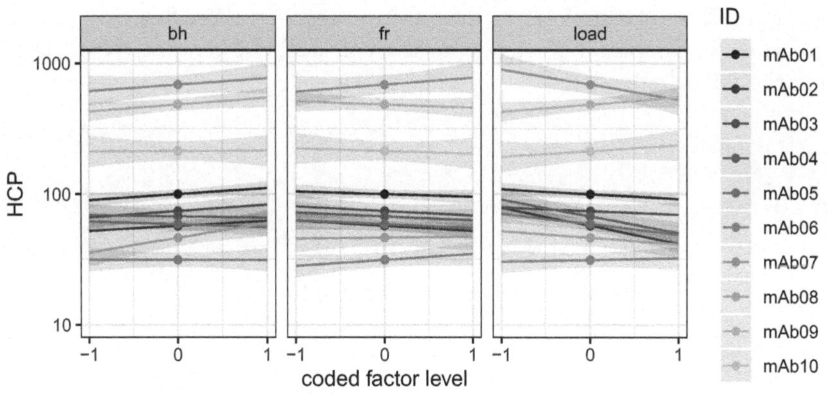

FIGURE 7.1
Univariate relationships between HCP and three unit operation factors (bed height, flow rate, and load) for ten molecules.

For analysis, the data shown in Table 7.2 is represented in the `data.frame` object `sim1`, arranged with a single response column, `y`, and a column that denotes the molecule, `mAb` (see Table 7.3).

TABLE 7.3
Example 1 data in `data.frame` format.

Run	Load	bh	fr	mAb	y
1	−1	0	0	mab01	2.05
2	−1	−1	−1	mab01	2.07
3	1	−1	−1	mab01	1.89
⋮	⋮	⋮	⋮	⋮	⋮

The hierarchical model used to fit the data in Table 7.2 is specified using the `brms` package as follows:

```
data(sim1)
fit_brm1 <- brm(y ~ load + bh + fr + load:bh +
                (1 + load + bh + fr + load:bh||mAb),
                data=sim1)
```

The model `fit_brm1` includes main effect terms for load (`load`), bed height (`bh`), and flow rate (`fr`) as well as an interaction term between load and bed height (`load:bh`). Molecule (`mAb`) is defined as a grouping factor, with group-level effects for all terms in the model, including the intercept (`1`). The syntax `||` excludes correlations between group-level effect from inclusion in the model. For all terms in the model, including the intercept, molecule-specific parameters will be estimated, while at the same time distributions for each term quantifies variation between molecules.

The brms package uses a default of four Markov chains, with a burn-in of 1000 iterations followed by applying 1000 sample iterations. Convergence was verified using the diagnostic methods described in Chapter 3. Such diagnostics can easily be generated from the fit_brm1 object using the following code.

```
summary(fit_brm1)
#>  Family: gaussian
#>   Links: mu = identity; sigma = identity
#> Formula: y ~ load + bh + fr + load:bh + (1 + load + bh + fr + load:bh || mAb)
#>    Data: sim1 (Number of observations: 160)
#> Samples: 4 chains, each with iter = 2000; warmup = 1000; thin = 1;
#>          total post-warmup samples = 4000
#>
#> Group-Level Effects:
#> ~mAb (Number of levels: 10)
#>               Estimate Est.Error l-95% CI u-95% CI Rhat Bulk_ESS Tail_ESS
#> sd(Intercept)     0.52      0.15     0.32     0.89 1.00     1116     1567
#> sd(load)          0.08      0.03     0.04     0.14 1.00     1279     2166
#> sd(bh)            0.03      0.02     0.00     0.07 1.00     1224     1786
#> sd(fr)            0.02      0.02     0.00     0.06 1.00     1383     2125
#> sd(load:bh)       0.04      0.02     0.00     0.09 1.00     1200     1438
#>
#> Population-Level Effects:
#>           Estimate Est.Error l-95% CI u-95% CI Rhat Bulk_ESS Tail_ESS
#> Intercept     2.03      0.17     1.68     2.38 1.01      558      967
#> load         -0.05      0.03    -0.10     0.01 1.00     1784     2220
#> bh            0.03      0.01     0.00     0.06 1.00     2948     2624
#> fr           -0.01      0.01    -0.04     0.02 1.00     3508     2636
#> load:bh      -0.05      0.02    -0.09    -0.02 1.00     2190     2187
#>
#> Family Specific Parameters:
#>       Estimate Est.Error l-95% CI u-95% CI Rhat Bulk_ESS Tail_ESS
#> sigma     0.10      0.01     0.09     0.12 1.00     2718     2691
#>
#> Samples were drawn using sampling(NUTS). For each parameter, Bulk_ESS
#> and Tail_ESS are effective sample size measures, and Rhat is the potential
#> scale reduction factor on split chains (at convergence, Rhat = 1).
```

As the R output shows, convergence is confirmed with Rhat values near 1 for all parameters. Additionally, there is sufficiently low autocorrelation for effective sample sizes that are large enough to draw meaningful conclusions. Plots of the posterior samples show smooth distributions, and trace plots depict adequate mixing (Figure 7.2).

Magnitudes for the group-level variability effects provide estimates for differences between molecules. Aside from baseline magnitude differences between intercepts, the load main effect varies most between studies (sd = 0.07). The population effects have 95% credible intervals that span zero or have small magnitudes compared to the group-level variability. The load effect, for example, is estimated at -0.05, with a 95% credible interval of $(-0.10, 0.01)$.

The posterior distributions for each molecule-specific load effect, for example, can be displayed with the command below, using the tidybayes, dplyr, ggplot2, and ggdist packages. The resulting plots are provided in Figure 7.3.

```
fit_brm1 %>%
  tidybayes::spread_draws(b_load,r_mAb[mAb,parameter]) %>%
  dplyr::filter(parameter=="load") %>%
  dplyr::transmute(load=b_load+r_mAb) %>%
```

```
ggplot2::ggplot(aes(load, mAb))+
theme_bw()+
tidybayes::stat_halfeye()
```

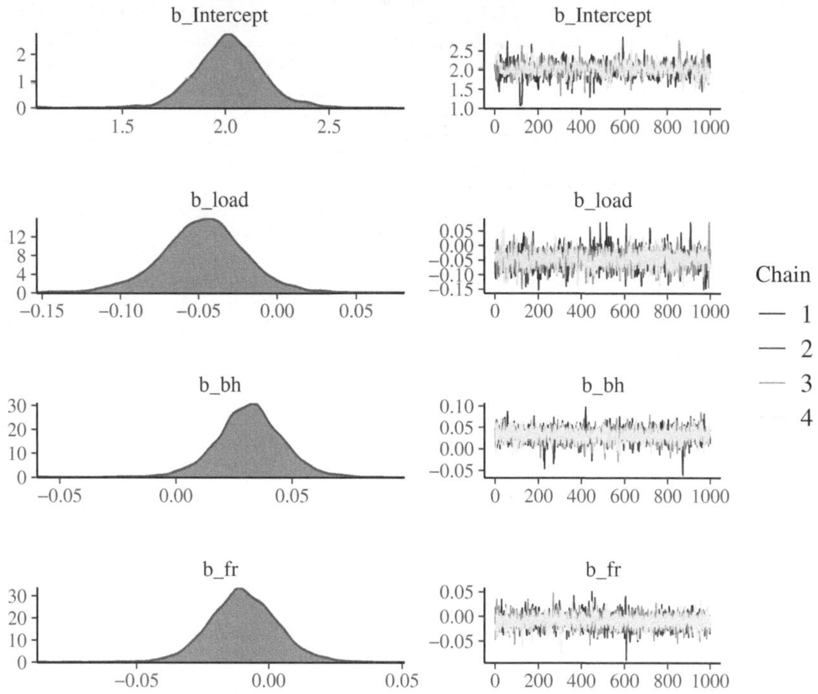

FIGURE 7.2
Posterior distributions for the group-level means of the main effects.

We also provide a more customized depiction of the posterior distributions for the molecule-specific effects in Figure 7.3. The same molecule-specific posterior distributions that are shown in Figure 7.4 are depicted as vertical lines that extend to the 95% credible interval, with dots showing the posterior median. The group level mean posterior distribution is displayed as a gradient for each term (load, bh, fr, and load:bh). We find this visualization useful because it clearly shows the population level effects, group-level variability, and how these parameters were informed by results from ten separate studies. The load effect stands out as showing evidence for the most variation between studies, with slightly greater tendency for a negative relationship. For the interested reader, the code to generate the plot in Figure 7.4 can be found in this book's Github repository.

When setting up a control strategy, this model enables a data-driven assessment of the risk that a process parameter exceeds a magnitude of practical importance. This may supplement the risk assessment that identifies process parameters to take forward to empirical experimentation or serve as a basis for quantified prior knowledge. As this example illustrates, the variation between molecules provides valuable insight to fully characterize the Protein A capture process across the platform. Even though the average of the parameter estimates for load is near zero, there is notable variation between molecules. While there is

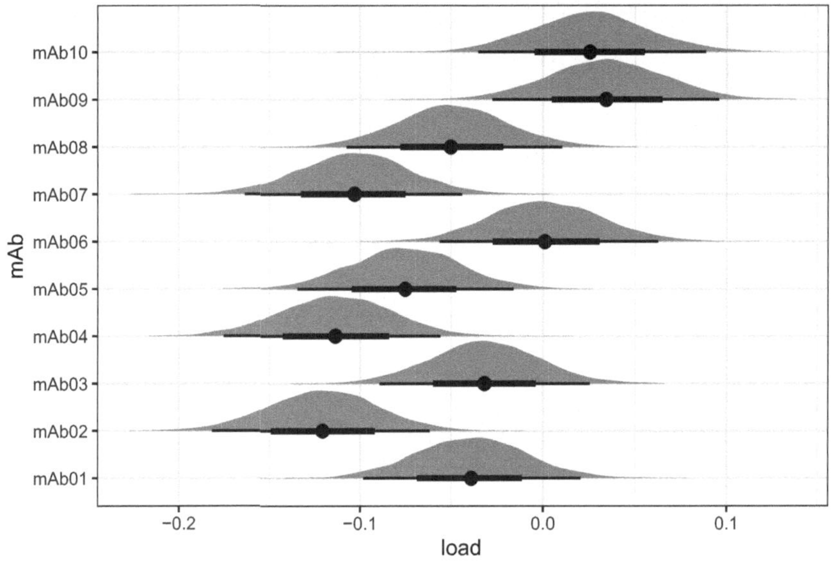

FIGURE 7.3
Posterior distributions for molecule-specific load effect.

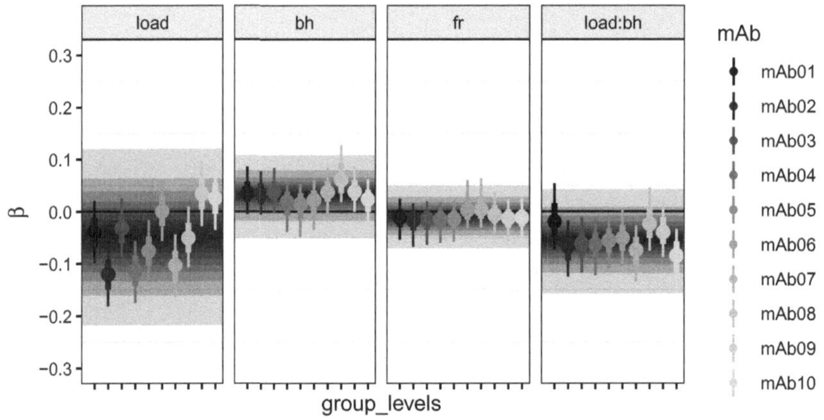

FIGURE 7.4
Circles represent parameter estimates (posterior median) for each molecule and factor, with 95% credible intervals (tails extending from each dot). Group-level mean posterior distribution is displayed in grayscale horizontal regions.

no consistent directional impact on levels of HCP, there are many instances where the effect is convincingly different from zero, as indicated by the credible intervals. Bed height and flow rate show much more consistency between molecules as compared to load. Bed height consistently demonstrates a positive relationship, with taller bed heights corresponding to higher levels of HCP.

Recall that the purpose of the studies is to determine which parameters should be classified as critical. For illustration purposes, this example sets the practical impact magnitude at 0.3 (log scale). Since the group-level mean posterior distribution (gray region) is entirely contained within the limit of practical importance, the analysis shows that there is low probability that future molecules will exceed this level. Not only are the outcomes from all previous studies within 0.3, but the variability between studies is sufficiently low to provide assurance that future experiments will not exceed this level. Such assurance can be used as justification to reduce the size of future DOE studies or eliminate them altogether for molecules that are within the platform. Indeed, the data provide platform-wide evidence that all effects are at low risk of exceeding a magnitude of practical importance.

7.3.2 Example 2: Formulation Robustness

For the second example, we explore an example relevant to determining robustness with respect to formulation attributes. The purpose of the experiment is to demonstrate that the target formulation is robust to potential variation in the factors studied, such as concentration, pH, and NaCl. The response represents the product purity at some relevant time point and temperature (e.g., shelf-life at the long-term storage condition, 1-month at 30°C, etc.). After repeating this experiment for multiple molecules (raw data are provided in Table 7.4), the least-squares fits of model (1) for each molecule are overlaid in Figure 7.5.

TABLE 7.4
Example 2 data showing purity at a given formulation condition for ten molecules.

Run	conc	pH	NaCl	mab01	mab02	mab03	mab04	mab05	mab06	mab07	mab08	mab09	mab10
1	0	1	−1	96.0	95.4	96.0	96.3	95.7	94.5	95.4	94.7	96.3	94.7
2	0	−1	1	94.7	96.3	96.6	97.4	95.9	95.2	96.3	95.9	96.9	95.7
3	−1	0	−1	96.1	98.0	97.1	97.0	97.3	96.6	97.6	97.0	98.4	96.9
4	1	0	1	94.8	95.9	95.4	95.6	95.6	95.3	96.3	94.7	96.4	94.8
5	−1	−1	0	94.7	96.2	96.7	97.5	96.2	96.0	96.5	96.4	96.9	96.2
6	1	1	0	95.0	94.4	94.6	94.9	94.5	93.3	94.3	93.2	94.3	93.2
7	−1	1	1	96.3	95.9	96.2	96.3	96.0	94.1	95.4	94.6	95.8	94.2
8	1	−1	−1	93.6	94.9	95.5	96.5	95.3	94.6	95.1	94.7	95.8	95.1
9	0	0	0	96.7	97.5	96.5	97.1	97.0	96.2	97.3	96.3	97.9	96.4

As with Example 1, the data used for analysis is arranged with a single response column, y, and a column that denotes the molecule, `mAb`. The object `sim2` is a `data.frame` as depicted in Table 7.5.

The hierarchical model is implemented using `brms`, estimating main effect terms for concentration (conc), pH, and sodium chloride (NaCl), and quadratic terms for concentration (`I(conc`^{2}`)`) and pH (`I(pH`^{2}`)`), which were identified by the experimenter as impactful effects that warrant inclusion in the model.

```
data(sim2)
fit_brm2 <- brm(y ~ conc + pH + NaCl +
                  I(conc^2) + I(pH^2) +
                  (conc + pH + NaCl + I(conc^2) + I(pH^2)||mAb),
                  data=sim2)
```

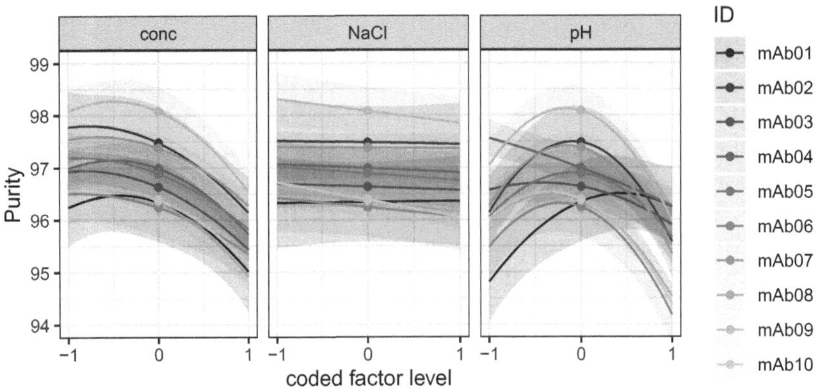

FIGURE 7.5
Relationship between purity and three formulation factors (concentration, sodium chloride, and pH).

TABLE 7.5
Example 2 data in `data.frame` format.

Run	conc	pH	NaCl	mAb	y
1	0	1	−1	mab01	96.0
2	0	−1	1	mab01	94.7
3	1	0	−1	mab01	96.1
⋮	⋮	⋮	⋮	⋮	⋮

Convergence was verified using the diagnostic methods described in Chapter 3 using the `fit_brm2` object. Plots of the posterior samples show smooth distributions, and trace plots depict adequate mixing (Figure 7.6).

```
summary(fit_brm2)
#>  Family: gaussian
#>   Links: mu = identity; sigma = identity
#> Formula: y ~ conc + pH + NaCl + I(conc^2) + I(pH^2) + (conc + pH + NaCl +
#>          I(conc^2) + I(pH^2) || mAb)
#>    Data: sim2 (Number of observations: 90)
#> Samples: 4 chains, each with iter = 2000; warmup = 1000; thin = 1;
#>          total post-warmup samples = 4000
#>
#> Group-Level Effects:
#> ~mAb (Number of levels: 10)
#>               Estimate Est.Error l-95% CI u-95% CI Rhat Bulk_ESS Tail_ESS
#> sd(Intercept)     0.65      0.19     0.39     1.10 1.00     1305     1942
#> sd(conc)          0.07      0.05     0.00     0.18 1.00     1186     1324
#> sd(pH)            0.51      0.15     0.30     0.87 1.00     1317     2356
#> sd(NaCl)          0.08      0.05     0.01     0.19 1.00     1041     1262
#> sd(IconcE2)       0.08      0.06     0.00     0.23 1.00     1907     2157
#> sd(IpHE2)         0.57      0.18     0.33     1.02 1.00     1420     2113
#>
#> Population-Level Effects:
#>           Estimate Est.Error l-95% CI u-95% CI Rhat Bulk_ESS Tail_ESS
#> Intercept    96.88      0.23    96.43    97.34 1.00      837     1441
```

```
#> conc        -0.71      0.04     -0.78     -0.63 1.00     3642     2710
#> pH          -0.41      0.17     -0.75     -0.07 1.00      803     1183
#> NaCl        -0.13      0.04     -0.21     -0.05 1.00     2974     2476
#> IconcE2     -0.53      0.06     -0.64     -0.42 1.00     5070     3211
#> IpHE2       -1.07      0.19     -1.47     -0.69 1.00      992     1773
#>
#> Family Specific Parameters:
#>       Estimate Est.Error l-95% CI u-95% CI Rhat Bulk_ESS Tail_ESS
#> sigma     0.21      0.02     0.16     0.26 1.01     1376     2386
#>
#> Samples were drawn using sampling(NUTS). For each parameter, Bulk_ESS
#> and Tail_ESS are effective sample size measures, and Rhat is the potential
#> scale reduction factor on split chains (at convergence, Rhat = 1).
```

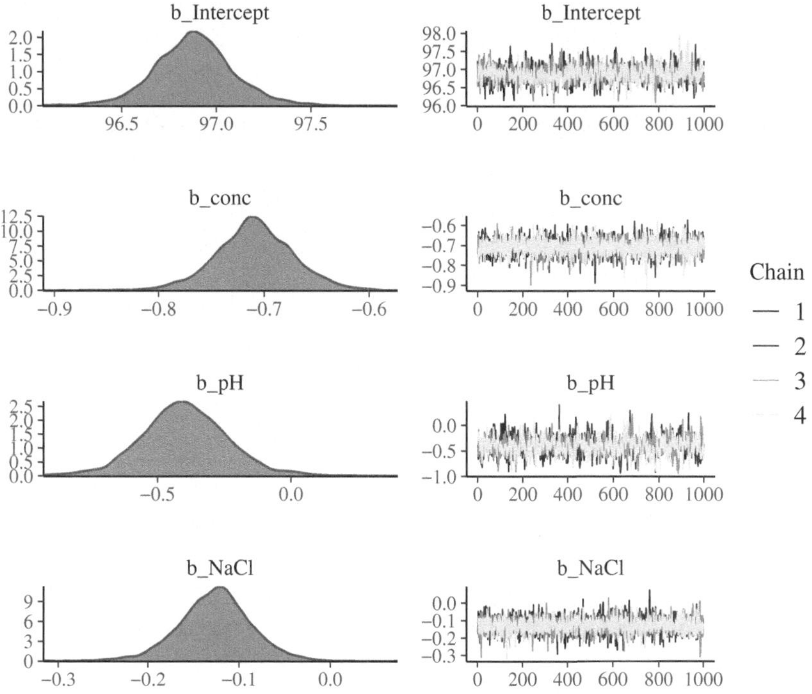

FIGURE 7.6
Posterior distributions and trace plots for the main-effect parameters.

While high level conclusions about typical formulation performance can be drawn by simply fitting the DOE results independently as shown in Figure 7.5, the hierarchical model offers distributions for the hyper-parameters (μ_{β_j}'s and σ_{β_j}'s) that quantify the typical impact on purity as well as variation between molecules. As seen in Figure 7.7, there is a general negative pH relationship with negative curvature. The concentration and NaCl terms show high agreement between studies. The consistency for the concentration and NaCl effects is so great, in fact, that there is little evidence of true molecule differences.

Again, the hierarchical model offers a clear picture of the similarities among molecules. Moreover, the model enables the dissimilarities to be quantified through the group-level effects, which may serve to inform the prior distribution for analyses of future molecules. While there is much more variation in the effect of pH in the current example compared

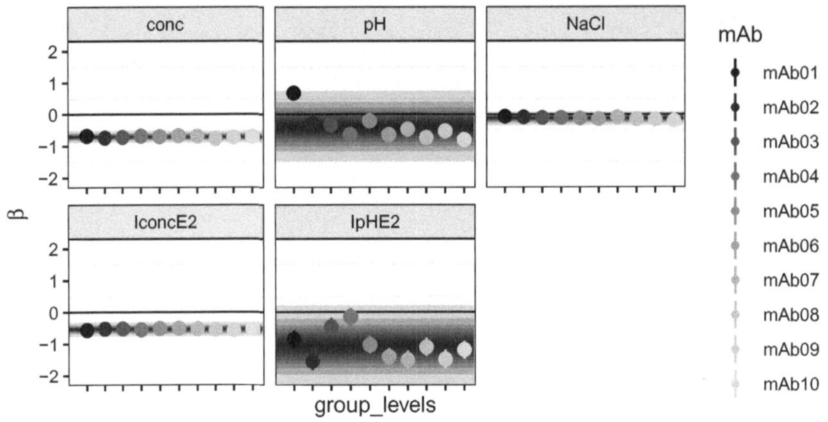

FIGURE 7.7
Parameter estimates (circle) for each molecule and factor, with 95% credible intervals (tails extending from each dot). Group-level mean posterior distribution is displayed in greyscale horizontal regions.

to concentration and NaCl, the experimenter can conclude that there is low probability that the absolute value of the effect magnitude exceeds 2. Because the concentration and NaCl effects are so consistent, accurate predictions are possible from prior knowledge alone. However, the pH relationship must rely more heavily on molecule-specific data.

7.4 Informative Priors

The previous examples show how multiple studies can be analyzed in a hierarchical model to quantify platform knowledge. In this section, we continue with Example 2 to illustrate how platform knowledge gleaned from the hierarchical model can serve as prior distributions for subsequent analyses.

Since no correlation was included for the group effect, `(...||mAb)`, group-level mean posterior distributions can be generated using the following code:

```
brm2_draws <- fit_brm2 %>%
  tidybayes::spread_draws(
              b_conc,sd_mAb__conc,
              b_IconcE2,sd_mAb__IconcE2,
              b_NaCl, sd_mAb__NaCl,
              sigma) %>%
  dplyr::mutate(
    conc=rnorm(nrow(.), mean=b_conc, sd=sd_mAb__conc),
    conc2=rnorm(nrow(.), mean=b_IconcE2, sd=sd_mAb__IconcE2),
    NaCl=rnorm(nrow(.), mean=b_NaCl, sd=sd_mAb__NaCl)
  )
```

The object brm2_draws contains posterior samples for the hyper-parameters (μ_{β_j}'s and σ_{β_j}'s) for concentration, NaCl, and concentration curvature, plus group-level mean posterior samples (conc, conc2, and NaCl). These distributions are summarized by calculating the mean and standard deviation, as shown below.

```
brm2_draws %>%
  summarise(
    conc_mean=mean(conc), conc_sd=sd(conc),
    conc2_mean=mean(conc2), conc2_sd=sd(conc2),
    NaCl_mean=mean(NaCl), NaCl_sd=sd(NaCl)
  )

# A tibble: 1 x 6
   conc_mean conc_sd conc2_mean conc2_sd NaCl_mean NaCl_sd
       <dbl>   <dbl>      <dbl>    <dbl>     <dbl>   <dbl>
      -0.710  0.0897     -0.530    0.114    -0.126   0.103
```

As an illustrative example, consider a new molecule that screens pH at the same levels as above, with observed purities of 97.0, 96.5, and 95.0 for the levels −1, 0, and 1, respectively. Informative prior distributions are constructed from the mean and standard deviation of the group-level mean distributions above. The student-*t* distribution with 3 degrees of freedom is selected to give additional credence to parameter magnitudes that extend toward the tails of the distribution. The prior distribution for sigma is centered at the estimate from the hierarchical model (0.2) but selected to be more diffuse than the prior data suggest (0.1).

```
fit_brm3 <- brm(y~conc+pH+NaCl+I(conc^2)+I(pH^2),
                prior = c(
                  prior("student_t(3, -0.71, 0.09)", class="b", coef="conc"),
                  prior("student_t(3, -0.53, 0.12)", class="b", coef="IconcE2"),
                  prior("student_t(3, -0.13, 0.10)", class="b", coef="NaCl"),
                  prior("normal(0.2, 0.1)", class="sigma")
                  ),
                 data=data.frame(pH=c(-1,0,1),
                                 conc=0,
                                 NaCl=0,
                                 y=c(97,96.5,95)))
```

Note that the model no longer contains a hierarchical component. While the prior distributions were informed from multiple studies, the current analysis applies to data for a single study.

With very little experimental data combined with platform knowledge in the form of informative prior distributions, the model fit_brm3 provides predictions across the full operating space. In the code below, the posterior predictive samples are processed to determine the probability that observed purity is greater than 95 percent, gt95. The resulting probability estimates incorporate uncertainty from variability between molecule concentration and NaCl effects, model uncertainty that stems from limited data, and random analytical variability between individual observations. Figure 7.8 provides a visual depiction of the probability that observed purity is greater than 95% as a function of concentration and pH across the two NaCl levels.

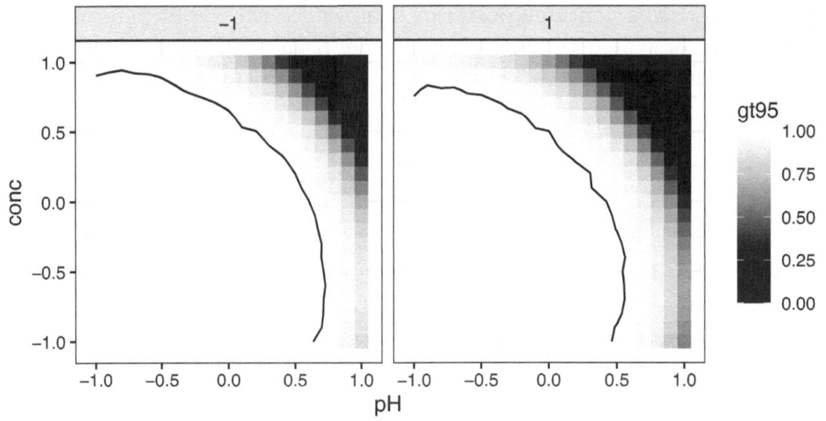

FIGURE 7.8
Probability that observed purity exceeds 95% at a given concentration and pH, shown at low and high NaCl. The black contour line shows the 99% boundary.

```
pred_grid <- expand.grid(
  pH=seq(-1,1,0.1),
  conc=seq(-1,1,0.1),
  NaCl=c(-1,1)
)

pred_vals<-brms::posterior_predict(
      fit_brm3,
      newdata=pred_grid
    )

pred_grid$gt95 <- apply(pred_vals, 2, function(x){mean(x>95)})
```

The summarized posterior results, pred_grid, can be visualized using the ggplot2 package.

```
pred_grid %>%
  ggplot2::ggplot(aes(pH, conc, z=gt95, fill=gt95))+
  geom_tile()+
  geom_contour(breaks=0.99, color="black")+
  scale_fill_gradient(low="black",high="white",limits=c(0,1))+
  facet_grid(.~NaCl)+
  theme_bw()
```

7.5 Discussion

Design differences (factor/effect sparsity)

For simplicity, the examples in this chapter maintain the same experimental designs for multiple molecules. However, over time, it is not uncommon for designs to vary from one molecule to the next. This is particularly prevalent as platform understanding matures and non-impactful factors are dropped from the standard design and are instead kept constant. While this scientific knowledge is incorporated in risk assessments that inform the experimental design, holding non-influential factors constant can produce data sparsity which may be problematic in the hierarchical model when combined with non-informative priors (this can also be problematic for least-squares estimation). As opposed to excluding the factor effect entirely, informative priors may be considered to reflect this scientific knowledge. For example, variability between studies (i.e. σ_{β_j}) for factors that were found to be small and varied infrequently may be defined as a distribution with high density near zero (e.g. half-normal, with high precision) to assume consistency between molecules.

Differences in designs can also result in sparsity for higher order terms. For instance, screening designs efficiently evaluate many effects, but at the cost of resolving some higher order terms, such as interactions and quadratic effects. If combined with response surface designs, variation in the complexity of parameters that can be estimated for a given molecule will arise. While response surface designs can support a large number of interactions and quadratic terms, screening designs may not provide enough data to reliably quantify higher-order terms to support the hierarchical model. As with factor sparsity, this may be an opportunity to consider prior information as an alternative to simply excluding the effect altogether. For example, variability between main effects may offer a reasonable upper bound on differences that are plausible between interaction terms. In Example 1, for instance, the load main effect showed the greatest variation between studies. This variability may provide a useful prior distribution for higher-order effects that would otherwise result in model instability, and such approach is consistent with the hierarchy principle (Montgomery, 2017).

Importance of parameter variability

In Example 2, concentration has the largest effect on the response, but the magnitude is very consistent among the studies. When considering where experimental resources should be placed, intuition leads to greater focus on how molecules respond to pH due to higher variability. This exposes a limitation to strictly data-driven mathematical models. That is, the largest effects may not require the most experimental investment if they are more predictable. This is where the Bayesian hierarchical approach offers tremendous benefit. The scientist need not be limited between two mutually exclusive choices of "platform knowledge" vs "experimental" characterization. Instead, the scientist can adopt a flexible strategy that uses a combination of both prior knowledge and experimental data in a quantitative and probabilistic fashion to form a holistic understanding of the process.

Factor scaling considerations

If the factor ranges are reasonably consistent among the studies included in the hierarchical analysis, then the factor levels may not require any scaling prior to fitting the model. In the event that factor ranges are inconsistent between molecules, differences between the overall quality attribute levels for a given molecule may become colinear with estimates of the factor effect. If the factor ranges do not fundamentally alter the effect on the quality attributes, scaling may be considered. By scaling the factor ranges for a given molecule (i.e. center each range at 0), the model interpretation is changed to reflect plausible effect magnitudes when varying the factor from a given molecule's target. This interpretation may be particularly helpful in cases where the factor effect is typically small and there is interest in estimating plausible upper limits on the magnitude under diverse sets of molecules. Another advantage to this approach is that factors that were not varied experimentally for a given molecule can simply be assigned a value of zero, the target for that study, eliminating the need to retrospectively enter the data for factors that where simply held constant.

8

Bayesian Prediction for Staged Testing Procedures

Katherine E.D. Giacoletti

Merck & Co., Inc.

Tara Scherder

SynoloStats LLC

CONTENTS

8.1 Introduction

Dissolution of a drug (the release of the drug from a dosage form into solution) affects bioavailability and hence therapeutic effectiveness and safety. Consequently, many pharmaceutical dosage forms specify an extent and rate of dissolution in their quality target product profile (QTPP). In-vitro dissolution (drug release) testing is designed to provide an indication of in-vivo dissolution, assure ongoing batch-to-batch consistency, and confirm post-approval activities do not affect product performance.

The acceptance criteria for these analytical tests, whether compendial or product-specific, are often multi-staged with limits for individual dosage units, the average of the batch, and/or the range of dosage units varying by testing stage. Examples include compendial tests applicable to the dissolution of oral solid dosage forms (immediate or modified release), and the in-vitro release of injectable biologics, transdermal and ophthalmic products (USP, General Chapter < 711 >, 2011; USP, General Chapter < 1711 >, 2016; USP, General Chapter < 724 >, 2018). A staged approach is also applied in other common product quality tests including content uniformity of dosages within a batch and the delivered dose uniformity of inhaled products (USP, General Chapter < 905 >, 2014; USP, General Chapter < 724 >, 2018).

In addition to the conditional nature of acceptance at consecutive stages, and possibly consecutive time points for modified release products, modeling is further complicated by application of specific criteria to a combination of dosage unit measurements (e.g., individual, average, and range). These complexities, in addition to multiple variance components, present obvious modeling challenges using typical frequentist methods, potentially resulting in poor estimates of the risk of failure, i.e., process capability. Also, classical methods cannot provide a reasonable metric that succinctly describes the expected product performance derived from this type of multi-staged test. In this chapter, we present

DOI: 10.1201/9781003255093-8

two examples illustrating the use of a Bayesian approach to not only manage the modeling complexities, but also to provide the very useful performance metric of the probability of meeting both individual stage and overall acceptance criteria. These success probabilities also provide insight into the discriminating power of the test to performance changes that could affect bioavailability.

The remainder of the chapter is structured as follows: In Section 8.2, we detail the Bayesian statistical model used, and in Section 8.3 these models are applied in cases studies. The concluding section includes a summary of advantages and challenges of a Bayesian approach for staged testing scenarios, along with a brief discussion of Bayesian solutions to other common manufacturing process performance questions.

8.2 Statistical Model

Oral Solid Dosage (OSD) forms are the most common way to administer drugs and are the focus of the examples in this chapter; however, the statistical model and general approach are readily generalizable to the in-vitro release tests for other dosage forms. Further discussion of a Bayesian approach to model dissolution testing, including dissolution similarity, can be found in Mockus and LeBlond (2020).

Dissolution testing of immediate-release OSD products is performed in 3 stages as described in the following table (Table 8.1) extracted from USP, General Chapter $< 711 >$ (2011).

TABLE 8.1
USP, General Chapter $< 711 >$ (2011) Acceptance Table 1.

Stage	Number Tested	Acceptance Criteria
S_1	6	Each unit is not less than $Q + 5\%$.
S_2	6	Average of 12 units ($S_1 + S_2$) is equal to or greater than Q, and no unit is less than $Q - 15\%$.
S_3	12	Average of 24 units ($S_1+S_2+S_3$) is equal to or greater than Q, not more than 2 units are less than $Q - 15\%$, and no unit is less than $Q - 25\%$.

The quantity Q is the amount of dissolved API specified in the individual product specifications or monograph, expressed as the percentage of labeled content (referred to as "% label claim" or "%LC"). Modified-release products have similar testing procedures with criteria at multiple time points over the intended release period. For simplicity, the focus of this chapter will be on modeling and prediction for immediate-release products, though the same concepts apply to modified-release products (see, for example, Lebrun et al. (2015)).

The specific statistical model depends on the scenario under which the data were generated. For samples taken from multiple representative product batches, with no purposeful variation in process or test method parameters (such that the batches may be considered a random sample of batches from a manufacturing stream), the data can be fit to a hierarchical model such as:

$$y_{ij} \sim N\left(\mu + \lambda_i, \sigma^2_{\varepsilon_{ij}}\right), \tag{8.1}$$

where y_{ij} is the jth tablet measurement from the ith batch, μ is the process mean, $\lambda_i \sim N(0, \sigma^2_{\varepsilon_{ij}})$ are the individual batch-to-batch variations, and $\sigma^2_{\varepsilon_{ij}}$ is the residual tablet variability. This model can be extended to include factors for process or test method parameters affecting the mean, or more or fewer sources of random variation, as appropriate. Such modifications to the basic model will be discussed further in each case study discussed below.

If a non-informative approach is preferred or no prior information is available, a reasonable option is to use "flat" or very weak priors for fixed effects, e.g., $\mu \sim N(0, 10^{10})$, and residual variability $\sigma^2_{\varepsilon_{ij}} \sim$ Inverse-Gamma(0.5, 0.5), but to use a weakly informative prior centered at the frequentist variance component estimate ($\widehat{\text{Var}L}$) for the between-batch variance (or other relevant variance components other than the residual, as discussed for each case study). The latter choice for hierarchical variance components may improve model convergence, while still focusing the model inference on the current data ($\lambda_i \sim$ Inverse-Gamma$(0.5, (\widehat{\text{Var}L})/2)$).

The non-informative approach described above was used in the case studies presented in this chapter (using the `MCMCglmm` package (Hadfield, 2010) in R (R Core Team, 2021)), with the joint posterior distribution of each model comprised of $\geq$ 25,000 draws (after burn-in and thinning). The effective sample size and trace plots were examined to assess model convergence for each case study; for further discussion of best practices for Bayesian model diagnostics, see for example (Seaman Jr. et al., 2020) and Chapter 3 of this book. The predicted probability of meeting the USP $< 711 >$ requirements was estimated as follows, accounting for the staged testing per USP $< 711 >$ and resulting correlation among samples from each stage:

1. For each combination of parameters (mean and variance components) in the joint posterior distribution, sample 24 dosage units.
2. Assess the first 6 dosage units in the sample of 24 against the Stage 1 USP $< 711 >$ dissolution criterion.
3. If the Stage 1 USP $< 711 >$ criterion was not met for a sample, then combine the next 6 dosage units from that sample with the first 6 and assess all 12 dosage units against Stage 2 USP $< 711 >$ criteria.
4. If the Stage 2 USP $< 711 >$ criteria were not met for a sample, then assess the full sample of 24 dosage units against Stage 3 USP $< 711 >$ criteria.

The predicted probability of meeting the requirements of a specific Stage of USP $< 711 >$ testing is estimated as the proportion of simulated samples meeting the criteria out of all simulated samples across the entire joint posterior distribution. The predicted probability of meeting *overall* USP $< 711 >$ requirements is estimated as the proportion of simulated samples which meet the criteria of Stage 1, or of Stage 2 given the simulated sample failed Stage 1, or of Stage 3 given the simulated sample failed Stages 1 and 2.

8.3 Case Studies

The two cases studies are drawn from different stages of the process lifecycle (FDA, 2011) and are briefly described as:

- Stage 1 (Process Design): Estimate the design space (defined below) for the probability of meeting staged OSD dissolution requirements across a range of process parameter combinations

- Stage 2 (Process Performance Qualification (PPQ)): Quantify the predicted probability that the process will meet staged testing requirements for dissolution to make decisions about success of PPQ and the need for continued enhanced sampling in Stage 3: Ongoing Process Verification (OPV)/Continued Process Verification (CPV)

8.3.1 Stage 1: Process Design

To establish an effective control strategy for a pharmaceutical process, designed experiments are often conducted to determine which process parameters (PPs) are critical for controlling the variability of quality attributes (QAs) of the product and setting appropriate operating limits for those PPs to ensure the QAs remain within acceptable ranges. Per ICH Q8(R2) (2009), a design space is defined as the "multidimensional combination of input variables ... that have been demonstrated to provide assurance of quality." The following case study uses simulated data but is representative of a real experiment to establish a design space for a tableting process to minimize the probability of failing the USP $< 711 >$ dissolution testing requirements and maintain the probability of testing beyond Stage 1 to be $\leq 5\%$ to reduce product cost.

The drug product in this case study is an immediate release coated tablet with a dissolution specification of $Q = 80\%$ at 15 minutes. The coating is non-functional, but the amount of coating on the tablet has been found to affect the percentage dissolved by 15 minutes. In addition, tablet thickness is known to affect percentage dissolved. A response surface design was implemented to study these two factors, and two tablets were sampled from each of the beginning, middle, and end of each production run (where a "run" corresponds to a unique combination of tablet thickness and coating level) to obtain the six tablets required for USP $< 711 >$ testing. The results are displayed in Figure 8.1 below, which shows percentage dissolved vs the two PPs displayed in their coded form (i.e., the range studied in the experiment scaled to $[-1, 1]$ and centered at 0).

It is clear from the results that both PPs influence the percentage dissolved, and that one or both will need to be controlled within a tighter range than was studied in the experiment to provide the desired assurance of meeting the dissolution specifications. Frequentist methods are capable of determining PP ranges necessary to control average or individual percentage dissolved above the limit, with a target level of confidence, by estimating confidence or prediction intervals, respectively, for each combination of PPs. However, for dissolution testing, with multiple testing stages with varying requirements for both individual measurements and the average, a Bayesian approach is capable of directly estimating the probability of success, while accounting for statistical uncertainty and the correlations among the samples at each stage.

The model used to estimate a design space for these two PPs for percentage dissolved is a version of the hierarchical model described in the Section 1 with additional terms describing the effects of the PPs on the mean percentage dissolved. The two variance components represent between- and within-location variation within a batch, since in this experiment (and very commonly the case for oral solid dosage manufacturing), stratified sampling was performed in each batch, with a single batch used for each combination of experimental conditions. Thus, the model is:

$$y_{ijkl} \sim N(\mu + \beta_1 X_{1i} + \beta_2 X_{2j} + \beta_3 X_{1i} X_{2j} + \beta_4 X_{1i}^2 + \lambda_i, \sigma^2_{\varepsilon_{ijkl}}), \quad (8.2)$$

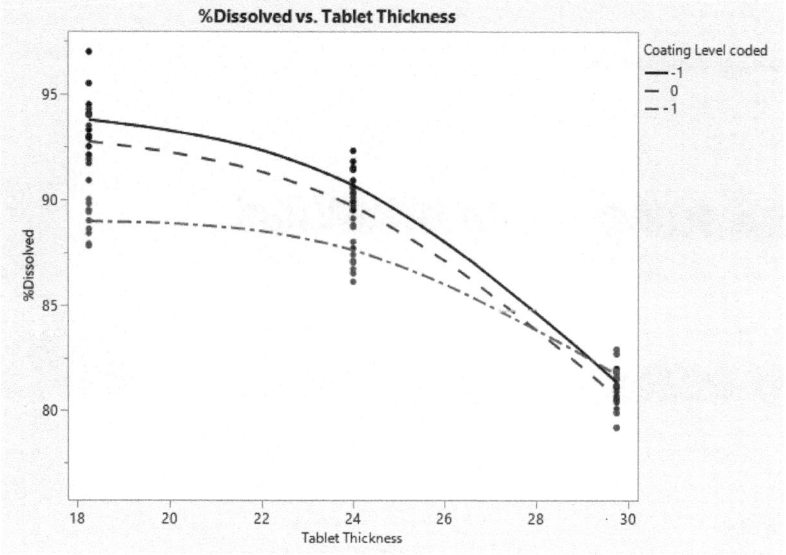

FIGURE 8.1
Percentage dissolved vs tablet thickness by coating level (coded) from process design experiment.

where y_{ijkl} is the kth tablet measurement from the lth sampling location from a batch with the ith (coded) tablet thickness level and j^{th} (coded) tablet coating level, X_{1i} is the ith coded tablet thickness level, X_{2j} is the jth (coded) tablet coating level, μ is the process mean, β_1, β_2, β_3, and β_4 are the coefficients on the tablet thickness main effect, tablet coating main effect, tablet thickness $\times$ tablet coating interaction, and tablet thickness quadratic term effects, respectively, $\lambda_i \sim N(0, \sigma_l^2)$ are the location-to-location variations, and $\sigma^2_{\varepsilon_{ijkl}}$ is the residual tablet variability. The model was fit using the `MCMCglmm` package in R, first fitting a frequentist model to get an estimate of the location-to-location variance for the weakly informative prior for that parameter, as described in Section 8.2:

```
fmod = lmer(y ~ x1 + x2 + I(x1^2) + I(x1*x2) +
            (1|Location), data=d1)
vc=as.data.frame(VarCorr(fmod))

bmod = MCMCglmm(y ~ x1 + x2 + I(x1^2) + I(x1*x2), data = d1,
                random = ~Location,
                nitt = 2503000, burnin = 3000, thin = 100,
prior = list(G = list(G1 = list(V =
                    max(vc$vcov[1],0.000001), nu = 1))))
```

The model summary and trace plots are displayed in Figure 8.2:

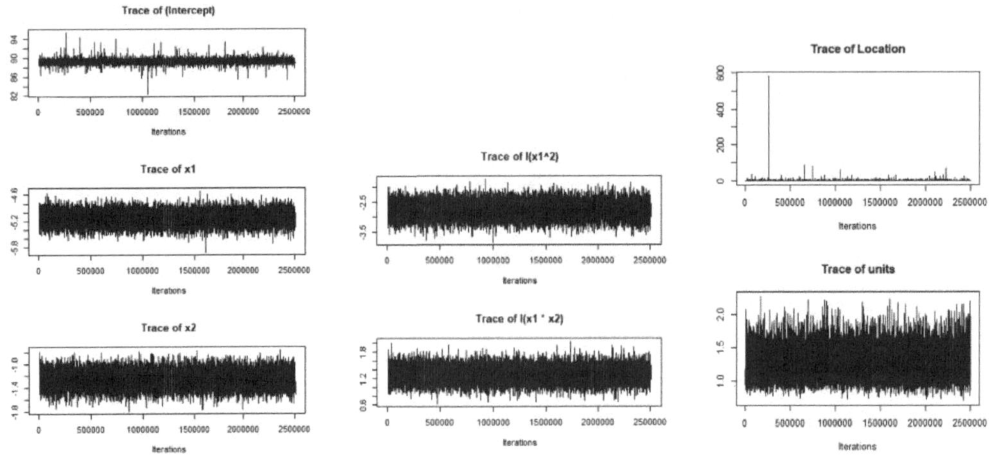

FIGURE 8.2
Trace plots of Markov chains for dissolution DOE model.

```
> summary(bmod)

 Iterations = 3001:2502901
 Thinning interval  = 100
 Sample size  = 25000

 DIC: 282.02

 G-structure:  ~Location

         post.mean l-95% CI u-95% CI eff.samp
Location    0.3209 0.007255   0.8841    25000

 R-structure:  ~units

      post.mean l-95% CI u-95% CI eff.samp
units     1.253   0.8868    1.646    25000

 Location effects: y ~ x1 + x2 + I(x1^2) + I(x1 * x2)

            post.mean l-95% CI u-95% CI eff.samp  pMCMC
(Intercept)    89.277   88.619   89.966    26053 <4e-05 ***
x1             -5.136   -5.410   -4.845    25529 <4e-05 ***
x2             -1.254   -1.517   -1.002    25000 <4e-05 ***
I(x1^2)        -2.779   -3.288   -2.315    25548 <4e-05 ***
I(x1 * x2)      1.294    0.981    1.609    25754 <4e-05 ***
---
Signif. codes:  0 '***' 0.001 '**' 0.01 '*' 0.05 '.' 0.1 ' ' 1
```

```
> par(mfrow = c(3,2))
> traceplot(bmod$Sol[,1:5)
> par(mfrow=c(2,1))
> traceplot(bmod$VCV[,1:2])
```

A key advantage of Bayesian modeling for staged testing is the ability to predict the probability of success at each stage, conditional on results of the previous stage(s), by simulating the sampling procedure and applying any number of acceptance criteria. In this way, correlations among samples across test stages within a batch are inherently incorporated into the predictions, and as with any Bayesian estimation and prediction, uncertainty of the model parameters is also accounted for. In the case of a design space problem, the simulations are performed over a fine grid of combinations of the PP settings and the probability of success is estimated at each point in the grid by fitting the model in (8.2).

Specifically, in this case study, to determine the predicted probability of meeting USP $< 711 >$ staged testing requirements for all combinations of tablet thickness and tablet coating in the experimental ranges tested, the simulation steps described in Section 8.2 were performed for each combination over a fine grid of values: tablet thickness by coating level, using the model of the effects of tablet thickness and coating level on mean percentage dissolved and accounting for variability among locations within a batch and replicates within a location.

```
new.x1 = seq(-1,1,by=0.1)
new.x2 = seq(-1,1,by=0.1)
stage = seq(1,3)

Risk1 = matrix(nrow = length(new.x1), ncol = length(new.x2))
Risk2 = matrix(nrow = length(new.x1), ncol = length(new.x2))
Risk3 = matrix(nrow = length(new.x1), ncol = length(new.x2))
for (i in 1:length(new.x1)){
  for(j in 1:length(new.x2)){
    Nsim=length(bmod$Sol[,1])
    s1samp<-list()
    s2samp<-list()
    s3samp<-list()
    fs1<-logical(length=Nsim) #T/F fail S1
    fs2<-logical(length=Nsim) #T/F fail S2
    fs3<-logical(length=Nsim) #T/F fail S3
    pfail.s1=0 # prob fail stage 1
    pfail.s2=0 # prob fail stage 2
    pfail.s3=0 # prob fail stage 3
    for (m in 1:length(Nsim)){
      s3samp[[m]]=rnorm(24,bmod$Sol[m,1]+
                          bmod$Sol[m,2]*new.x1[i]+
                          bmod$Sol[m,3]*new.x2[j]+
                          bmod$Sol[m,4]*new.x1[j]^2+
                          bmod$Sol[m,5]*new.x1[j]*new.x2[j],
                          sqrt(sum(bmod$VCV[m,])))
```

```
        s2samp[[m]]=s3samp[[m]][1:12]
        s1samp[[m]]=s3samp[[m]][1:6]

        fs1[m]=isTRUE(min(s1samp[[m]])<84.5)

        fs2[m]=isTRUE((fs1[m]=="TRUE") &
                      ((min(s2samp[[m]])<64.5)|
                      (mean(s2samp[[m]])<79.5)))

        fs3[m]=isTRUE((fs2[m]=="TRUE")& (
                     (min(s3samp[[m]])<54.5)|
                     (mean(s3samp[[m]])<79.5)|
                     (s3samp[[m]][[2]]<64.5) ))

      }

      nfs1=length(fs1[fs1==TRUE]) # number failing Stage 1
      nfs2=length(fs2[fs2==TRUE]) # number failing Stage 2
      nfs3=length(fs3[fs3==TRUE]) # number failing Stage 3
      pfail.s1=nfs1/Nsim
      pfail.s2=ifelse(nfs1==0,NA,nfs2/nfs1)
      pfail.s3=ifelse((nfs2==0),NA,nfs3/nfs2)
      pfail.USP711=nfs3/Nsim

      Risk1[i,j] = pfail.s1
      Risk2[i,j] = pfail.s2
      Risk3[i,j] = pfail.s3
    }
  }
```

The predicted probabilities of failing Stage 1 USP $< 711 >$ for all combinations of tablet thickness and coating level are summarized graphically in Figure 8.3, which displays the two PPs using their coded values from low (−1.0) to high (1.0).
A heat map showing the predicted probabilities of failing all 3 stages of USP $< 711 >$, for any combination of the two process parameters studied is displayed in Figure 8.4.

These results together provide specific estimates of patient risk by establishing operating ranges for these two process parameters to provide assurance of meeting dissolution requirements, while minimizing costs by controlling the need for testing beyond Stage 1 of USP $< 711 >$. While frequentist methods could be used to determine operating ranges by comparing a high confidence prediction or tolerance interval to the Stage 1 criterion for 6 individual dosage units, this could result in narrower, unnecessarily conservative operating ranges, because the focus is entirely on the Stage 1 criterion since that is the most feasible approach using frequentist methods (discussed further in the next example). In contrast, a Bayesian approach enables prediction of failure of all stages *while* accounting for statistical uncertainty, thereby protecting patients, while avoiding unnecessarily narrow operating ranges.

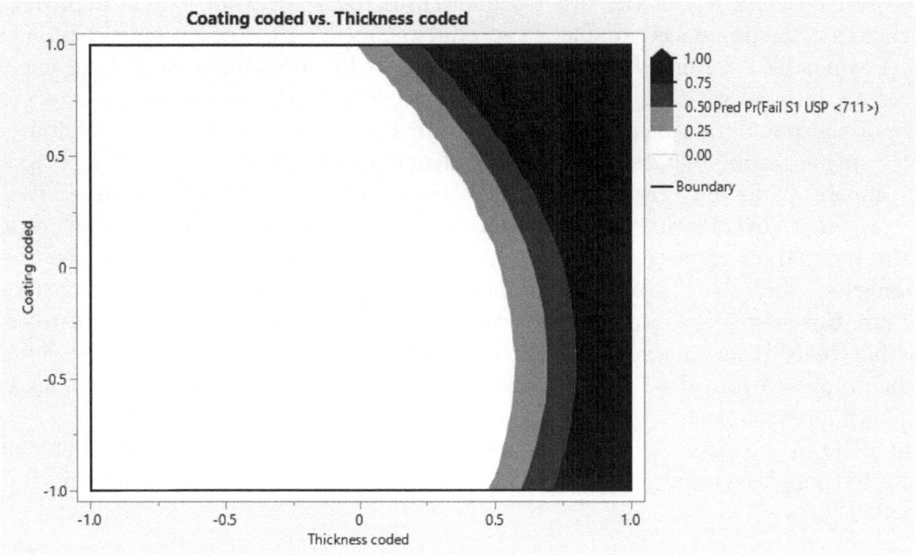

FIGURE 8.3
Heat map of predicted probability of failing stage 1 USP < 711 > criterion by coating level and tablet thickness.

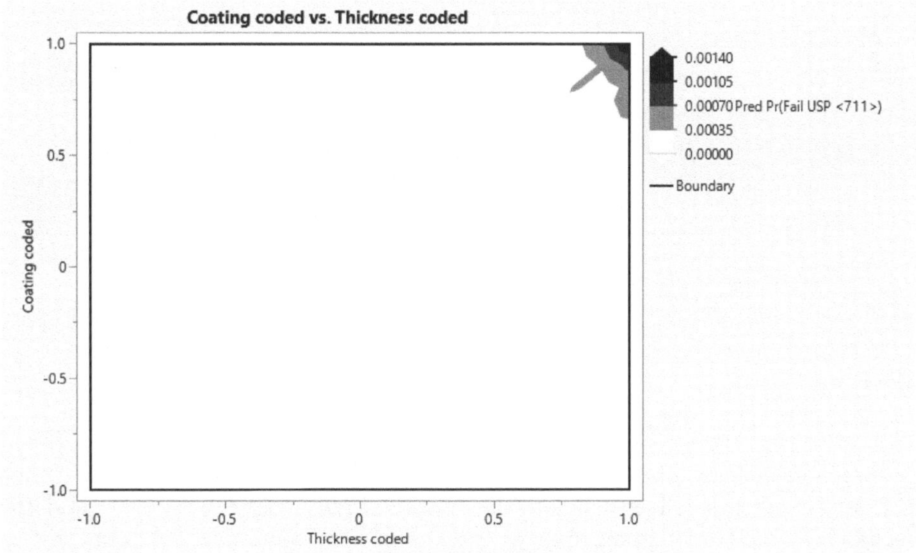

FIGURE 8.4
Heat map of predicted probability of failing all 3 stages of USP <711> criterion by coating level ad tablet thickness.

8.3.2 Stage 2: Process Performance Qualification

The objective of Stage 2 of the process lifecycle is demonstration with a high degree of assurance that the process is capable of reproducibly meeting the acceptance criteria (FDA, 2011). Frequentist tolerance intervals are often used for intra-batch statistical capability analyses; an interval within specification limits provides a high degree of assurance of the quality of the population of dosage units within the batch. For a quality attribute with complex staged testing requirements for the mean and individuals, a conservative approach is to compare a tolerance interval to the Stage 1 requirements for individuals. If a high confidence/high coverage interval is within the Stage 1 limits, there is strong evidence that the population of dosage units within the batch will meet the overall compendial requirements, since the Stage 1 requirement is the most stringent of the staged testing procedure. However, if the interval is not within the Stage 1 limits, this does not necessarily mean that there is an unacceptably high risk of failing the staged testing procedure. A Bayesian approach provides an elegant way to estimate the risk more precisely, as will be shown with an example.

The PPQ in this case study consisted of four batches, with a sample of twelve dosage units tested for dissolution per USP $< 711 >$ in each batch. The data are displayed in Figure 8.5.

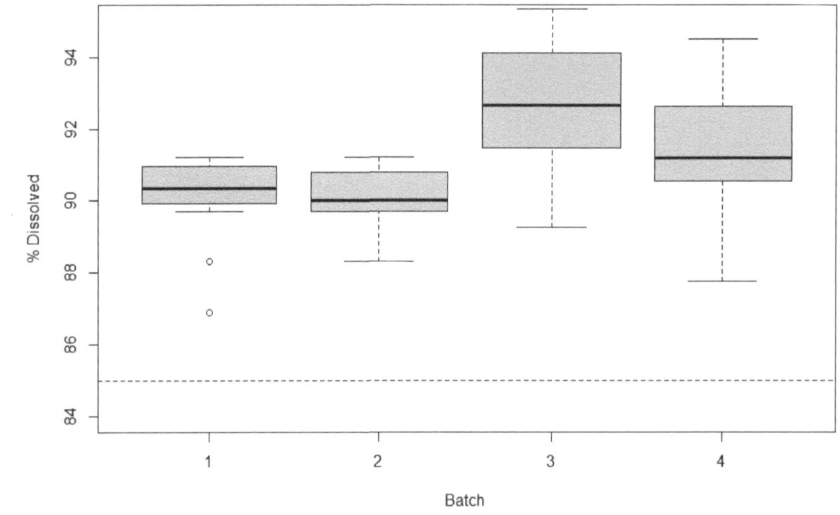

FIGURE 8.5
PPQ dissolution (%) results from 4 batches, $Q = 85\%$ indicated by reference line.

The batch means are all at or above the target of $Q = 85\%$, but clearly the individual values from all batches fall well below the Stage 1 limit of $Q + 5 = 90\%$, and there is non-negligible batch-to-batch variability. Thus, while any statistical intervals will clearly also extend beyond the Stage 1 limits, it is not clear how much risk this translates to with respect to the overall staged testing procedure, and an understanding of the overall process risk requires accounting for both within- and between-batch variability. A Bayesian model provides a straightforward way to address the question: a model can be fit to the data from each batch separately or a process model can be fit to the four batches together, accounting for the variability within and between batches. The latter approach will be described here.

Model 8.1 was fit to the PPQ batch data, using the MCMCglmm package in R, first fitting a frequentist model to get an estimate of the location-to-location variance for the weakly informative prior for that parameter, as described in Section 8.2. The following code fits model 8.1:

```
fmPPQ = lmer( Diss ~ 1 + ( 1 | Batch), data = d)
vcPPQ=as.data.frame(VarCorr(fmPPQ))

bmodPPQ = MCMCglmm( Diss ~ 1, random = ~ Batch, data=d,
                    nitt = 2505000, burnin = 5000,
                    thin = 100,
                    prior = list(G = list(G1 =
                    list(V = max(vcPPQ$vcov[1],1e-10),
                    nu = 1))))
```

The posterior distributions of the model parameters are summarized in Table 8.2.

TABLE 8.2
Posterior parameter estimates (and 95% Credible Intervals) from the Bayesian hierarchical model.

Model Parameter	Median Estimate	95% Credible Interval
Overall Mean	91.0	(89.4, 92.7)
Between Batch SD Mean	1.25	(0.47, 2.82)
Within Batch SD	1.52	(1.24, 1.89)

The model summary and trace plots are displayed in Figure 8.6:

```
> summary(bmodPPQ)

Iterations = 3001:2502901
 Thinning interval  = 100
 Sample size  = 25000

 DIC: 181.6359

 G-structure:  ~Batch

      post.mean l-95% CI u-95% CI eff.samp
Batch     2.746   0.1597    7.761    25000

 R-structure:  ~units

      post.mean l-95% CI u-95% CI eff.samp
units       2.4    1.449    3.478    22733
```

```
 Location effects: Diss ~ 1

            post.mean l-95% CI u-95% CI eff.samp  pMCMC
(Intercept)     91.01    89.35    92.73    24193 <4e-05 ***
---
Signif. codes:  0 '***' 0.001 '**' 0.01 '*' 0.05 '.' 0.1 ' ' 1

> traceplot(bmodPPQ$Sol[,1])
> par(mfrow = c(2,1))
> traceplot(bmodPPQ$VCV[,1:2])
```

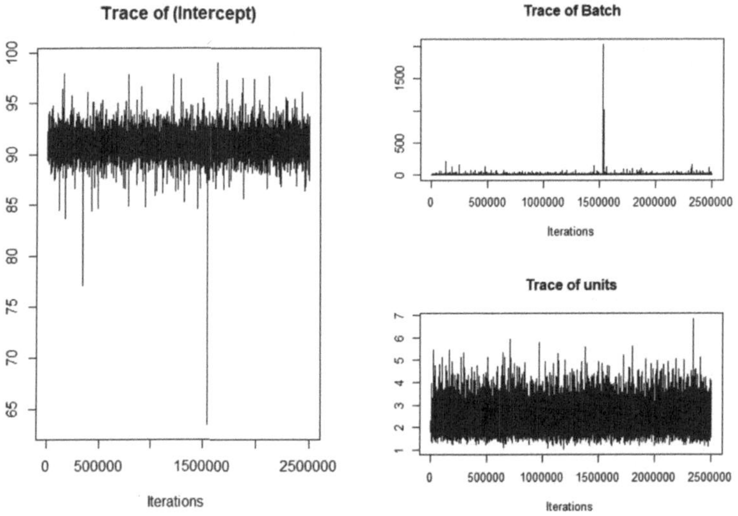

FIGURE 8.6
Trace plots of Markov chains for dissolution PPQ model.

The model provides statistical assurance that the overall process mean will be above the Q value of 85%, since the lower bound of the 95% credible interval for the process mean is 89.4%. Again, an important feature of Bayesian inference is that we are not limited, though, to assessing risk by comparing statistical intervals to limits of interest. Rather, we can directly estimate the probability of meeting requirements. In other words, the results in Table 8.2 are valuable for process understanding and as a summary of the model to validate its fit. However, to understand risk, we can make a simpler and more direct statement. Specifically, in this case, we can use the posterior distribution of the process mean from the model to say that the probability of the mean being less than $Q = 85\%$ is 0.02%. This is a simple reminder of an important motivation for using Bayesian inference: the ability to make direct probability statements regarding patient or process risk.

As emphasized throughout this chapter, evaluating risk for a staged testing procedure is more complex than estimating a probability for a single parameter. As described above in Section 8.2, samples were simulated from a random batch from this process and the predicted probabilities of failing Stage 1 and of failing USP $< 711 >$ overall were estimated to be 76% and 0.02%, respectively:

```
Nsim=length(bmodPPQ$Sol[,1])
s1samp<-list()
s2samp<-list()
s3samp<-list()
fs1<-logical(length=Nsim) #T/F fail S1
fs2<-logical(length=Nsim) #T/F fail S2
fs3<-logical(length=Nsim) #T/F fail S3
pfail.s1=0 # prob fail stage 1
pfail.s2=0 # prob fail stage 2
pfail.s3=0 # prob fail stage 3
for (m in 1:Nsim){
      s3samp[[m]]=rnorm(24,bmodPPQ$Sol[m,1],
                          sqrt(sum(bmodPPQ$VCV[m,1:2])))
      s2samp[[m]]=s3samp[[m]][1:12]
      s1samp[[m]]=s3samp[[m]][1:6]

      fs1[m]=isTRUE(min(s1samp[[m]])<89.5) # Q =  85, Q+5=90

      fs2[m]=isTRUE((fs1[m]=="TRUE")&((min(s2samp[[m]])<69.5)|
                     (mean(s2samp[[m]])<84.5)))

      fs3[m]=isTRUE((fs2[m]=="TRUE")&( (min(s3samp[[m]])<59.5)|
                      (mean(s3samp[[m]])<84.5)|
                      (s3samp[[m]][[2]]<69.5) ))
}

nfs1=length(fs1[fs1==TRUE]) # number failing Stage 1
nfs2=length(fs2[fs2==TRUE]) # number failing Stage 2
nfs3=length(fs3[fs3==TRUE]) # number failing Stage 3
pfail.s1=nfs1/Nsim
pfail.s2=ifelse(nfs1==0,NA,nfs2/nfs1)
pfail.s3=ifelse((nfs2==0),NA,nfs3/nfs2)
pfail.USP711 = nfs3/Nsim
```

In other words, this process will likely require testing beyond Stage 1 but has a negligible chance of failing the full staged testing procedure. A more detailed inspection of the simulations reveals that indeed only 0.07% of simulated samples fail the Stage 2 requirements, so testing is rarely expected to proceed beyond Stage 2. This outcome is substantial evidence of acceptable product quality. Commercial manufacture can proceed with the understanding of the cost implications of the within-batch variability causing the high rate of Stage 1 USP $<$ 711 $>$ failures. This information could also provide the justification to reduce PPQ enhanced sampling to the routine dissolution testing level immediately after PPQ, with plans to address within-batch variability through improvements to the test method, for example. This detailed risk assessment through Bayesian modeling and simulation allows patient-focused and cost-effective decision making.

8.4 Summary and Discussion

There are no known frequentist solutions to the assessment of risk (in terms of process capability) that account for the conditional/correlated structures of the multi-stage testing schemes commonly required to assess product quality. Consequently, typical process capability assessments of these staged tests can be highly erroneous and do not provide an intuitive metric reflecting the risk of failure. This chapter presented two examples of the use of Bayesian methods to enable patient-focused, direct, probabilistic, risk-assessments for these complex, yet common, testing schemes. The second case study also showed how additional variance components (within and between batch variability) can be easily incorporated. And although not illustrated in this chapter's case studies, the use of prior information in the Bayesian model could provide the additional benefit apparent from case studies elsewhere in this book and other literature.

The largest impediment to application of Bayesian methods is the required expertise and skills to model and code the structure. However, an accurate assessment of the risk to fail each testing stage is not the only benefit of investment, potentially avoiding wasteful sampling, testing or controls. An accurate estimate of the probability to pass each stage is also critical to demonstrate whether the test is discriminating, i.e., will identify a change in process performance that could affect bioavailability.

The two case studies reflected situations in the early stages of the process life cycle. The two advantages of the Bayesian approach in these case studies, namely:

1. flexibility to model complex data structures
2. a direct assessment/metric of process performance and hence patient risk, e.g., the likelihood than an individual dosage from future batches will meet acceptance criteria

can be applied to typical problems during Stage 3 of the process life cycle (ongoing commercial manufacture) including, for example:

- Assessment of process capability during the baseline performance stage to determine if enhanced sampling following PPQ can be discontinued.
- Assessment of process capability after a post approval changes to demonstrate acceptable risk to product quality.
- Optimization of processes and analytical methods.
- Establishment of process control limits using both within and between batch components, particularly in early commercial manufacture when the commercial batch data is limited.
- Comparability (of sites/methods/processes) with the possibility to compute the probability of an individual measurement falling outside a distribution of equivalence, instead of equivalence restricted to only means.
- Stability modeling (see Chapter 12).

9

A Bayesian Approach to Multivariate Conditional Regression Surrogate Modeling with Application to Real Time Release Testing

Stan Altan

Janssen Pharmaceutical R&D, LLC. Raritan, NJ

Dwaine Banton

Labcorp Clinical Development, Solna, Sweden

Hans Coppenolle

Janssen Pharmaceutical R&D, LLC. Beerse, Belgium

Martin Kovarik and Martin Otava

Janssen-Cilag s.r.o., Pharmaceutical Companies of Johnson & Johnson, Prague, Czechia

Christian Schmid

Pennsylvania State University, University Park, PA

CONTENTS

DOI: 10.1201/9781003255093-9

9.1 Introduction

The pharmaceutical industry is at the cusp of a revolution in pharmaceutical manufacturing as companies transition from batch processing to continuous manufacturing (CM) processes. The advantages include higher quality, less environmental impact, flexibility in meeting market demand and faster release of drug product to market through a real time release testing (RTRT) strategy. To meet the promise of faster product release to the market, near infrared (NIR) analytical technology has been used for the measurement of critical quality attributes (CQA) such as content and dose uniformity. In this chapter, we propose a statistical approach to provide a surrogate model for dissolution performance or in vitro release (we will use the terms "dissolution" and "in vitro release" interchangeably). The surrogate prediction relies on a NIR measurement at the tablet level, as well as knowledge of the critical process conditions under which the tablets were manufactured. This is an important goal since the laboratory-based analytical method for measuring dissolution performance is time consuming and expensive. There is ample incentive to develop a surrogate measurement method as part of a comprehensive real time release (RTR) strategy. This chapter outlines the essential steps in moving from a comprehensive DoE to a multivariate hierarchical model, where the multivariate response is either: 1) the percentage of dissolution measured at a given time point Q (e.g., $Q30$ denoting 30 minutes specification time point) and the content-by-NIR, or 2) a vector of dissolution measurements at different time points and the content-by-NIR. The response is modeled in relation to critical process factors. The statistical approach leads to a linear estimator relating mean content-by-NIR and manufacturing process effects to a mean dissolution response, for example, dissolution at 30 minutes ($Q30$). We point out the need for a separate validation design as a final confirmation of the accuracy and precision of the predictive surrogate model. In addition, we recommend a Bayesian posterior predictive approach to characterize the surrogate method's analytical performance as part of a qualification exercise in preparation for independent validation. The Bayesian approach provides a flexible way to also update the model during subsequent model maintenance incorporating development phase information with additional commercial production experience. The need to characterize the analytical method performance and ability to incorporate a natural updating of the model with additional information makes the Bayesian approach the preferred way to pursue surrogate model development.

9.2 Statistical Methodology

The essential approach we follow underlying the proposed surrogate model relies on the joint normal distribution of a hard-to-measure variable Y_1 and an easy-to-measure variable Y_2. The assumption can be concisely represented as:

$$Y = \begin{bmatrix} Y_1 \\ Y_2 \end{bmatrix} \sim N\left(\mu = \begin{bmatrix} \mu_1 = X\beta_1 \\ \mu_2 = X\beta_2 \end{bmatrix}, \Sigma = \begin{bmatrix} \Sigma_{11} & \Sigma_{12} \\ \Sigma_{21} & \Sigma_{22} \end{bmatrix}\right) \tag{9.1}$$

where X represents a desired linear combination of important effects, β_1 and β_2. Then, the conditional distribution of the hard-to-measure variable on the observed easy-to-measure variable is the following normal distribution:

$$Y_1^* \equiv (Y_1 | Y_2 = y_2) \sim N\left(\mu_1 + \Sigma_{12}\Sigma_{22}^{-1}(y_2 - \mu_2), \Sigma_{11} - \Sigma_{12}\Sigma_{22}^{-1}\sigma_{21}\right) \tag{9.2}$$

Graybill (1976). We will approach the conditional regression calculation given in (9.2) from a Bayesian perspective. The expected value of the conditional distribution of the hard-to-measure variable, $\mathbb{E}\left[Y_1^*|X, \text{data}\right]$ is estimated from the posterior predictive distribution. This provides a statistical mechanism to establish a surrogate model for a hard-to-measure variable given another easy-to-measure variable.

We introduce the posterior predictive distribution concept in relation to Bayes' rule (Gelman et al., 2013). Let $\pi(\theta)$ represent the probability distribution of the parameters of the model before any experimental information is incorporated, i.e., the prior distribution of the parameters. Let x_n be the length n vector of experimentally observed measurements and let $f(x_n|\theta)$ be the assumed distribution of the experimental data, which provides a basis for deriving the likelihood. We can define the posterior distribution of the parameters and derive the posterior predictive distribution of a new observation as follows:

$$\pi(\theta|x_n) \propto \pi(\theta) f(x_n|\theta) \tag{9.3}$$

and

$$\pi(x|x_n) = \int f(x|\theta)\pi(\theta|x_n)d\theta. \tag{9.4}$$

Smith and Gelfand (1992) showed how the posterior distribution and posterior predictive distributions can be obtained for inferential purposes via simulation. We will follow this approach in this paper. Specifically, using the `rstan` (Stan Development Team, 2021a) package in R (R Core Team, 2021). We will use the STAN software to obtain Hamiltonian Monte Carlo (Stan Development Team, 2021b, see Section 15.1) samples from both the posterior parameter and the posterior predictive distributions. We also note that Y_1 and Y_2 in (9.1) and (9.2) are multivariate vector quantities limited in size only by the design of the experiment.

In summary, the two critical pieces of the statistical methodology used in the surrogate model approach for dissolution are the conditional normal distribution, and the posterior predictive distribution. We will apply this methodology in the context of RTRT, where we wish to predict measurements from a labor-intensive analytical method (i.e., Y_1, the "hard-to-measure" variable), dissolution performance of a solid dosage form at one or more given time points, with an "easy-to-measure" method. One requirement is that the methodology must include knowledge of the experimental conditions of the manufacturing process. The surrogate predictions will rely on the expected value of the conditional posterior predictive distribution, given values of the easy-to-measure variable. In this case, the easy-to-measure variable is the active pharmaceutical ingredient (API) Content-by-NIR, combined with known levels of the fixed process parameters. It is important to note that Content-by-NIR cannot be considered a covariate on the right side of the model equation (9.2), since it is subject to substantial measurement variability. For that reason, the conditional regression approach we discuss in Section 9.3 is preferred.

9.3 Surrogate Modeling for Real Time Release Testing of Dissolution

Conditional regression modeling as an approach to surrogate modeling in the context of RTRT relies heavily on the execution of a properly designed experiment. An experimental design studying the effects of important process parameters, i.e., the critical process parameters (CPPs) and critical materials affecting dissolution, must first be carried out to relate the in vitro dissolution release profile to the CPPs. An important requirement is that tablets manufactured at the various factor combinations of the experiment be measured by NIR spectral analysis, and then followed by either a partial or full in vitro release profile study of each tablet. The choice of a partial or full profile measurement of each tablet will depend on whether the objective is to predict a single in vitro release time point value, or the entire dissolution profile. The latter requires a parametric model relating dissolution to time. If no dissolution-time model is assumed, then a single essential dissolution value will be used (e.g., $Q30$). We will cover the former in the first case study and the latter in the second case study. In the first case study, a partial dissolution profile including say 2 time points could be modeled with a straightforward extension of the method given.

The in vitro release studies should also be carried out according to a design which minimizes the confounding of dissolution run effects (including both the apparatus-dissolution run as well as any associated chemical analytical run effects) and the treatment (combinations of the factors under study, i.e., the CPPs) effects using appropriate blocking and randomization. An example of such a design is a partially or fully balanced Latin square allocation to orthogonalize these confounding factors.

In the case studies discussed in Section 9.4, API Content-by-NIR and percent dissolution data are collected from a 34-run factorial designed experiment. Based on either the individual tablet or the averaged observed percent dissolution at each of 7 timepoints – 5, 10, 15, 20, 30, 45, and 60 minutes – for each run from the experiment, a predictive model for dissolution is derived. In the first case study, we fit a bivariate normal model, predicting in vitro release specifically at a single time point, 30 minutes, denoted as $Q30$. Because only a single time point is predicted, the approach does not require any additional assumptions about the functional relationship between in vitro release and time. In the second case study, the model predicts percent dissolution at any chosen time point, given the values of the process parameters and the averaged value of observed Content-by-NIR from a set of tablets. We recommend the use of an underlying non-linear 3-parameter Weibull model as a descriptor for the true in vitro release profile. We emphasize that this is not based on mechanistic considerations, but rather as an empirical descriptive model, which in our experience works reasonably well in practice. The Weibull model has a long history of application in dissolution studies (Costa and Sousa Lobo, 2001; Dokoumetzidis et al., 2006).

The predictive surrogate model is built in 3 steps:

1. Data preparation step discussed in greater detail in the next section 9.4.

2. The samples drawn from the posterior distribution of the model parameters in Step 1 for Case Study 2 are modeled as a multivariate normal vector, with a linear mean function that depends on the process parameters from the 34-run designed experiment. This 2 or 4-dimensional multivariate normal vector – single time point and measured API Content-by-NIR in the first case study, or three Weibull parameters and averaged Content-by-NIR for the second case study – is the input for the third step.

3. A 1 or 3-dimensional normal random variable is derived, conditional on a given value of average Content-by-NIR and process parameter settings following (9.2). In the first case study, this reduces to a simple linear relationship in a single dimension. In the second case study, the resulting conditional vector of Weibull parameters is used to predict percent dissolution for any given time, based only on the API Content-by-NIR measurement along with process parameter levels. In both cases, a surrogate model for dissolution is derived.

9.4 Case Studies

9.4.1 Data Description

We consider a process characterization study of five process factors (parameters or explanatory variables), following a factorial design plus two center points in 34 runs. We will refer to the factors as Factor 1, Factor 2,..., Factor 5. The data was simulated based on fixed and random effect estimates from a real experiment of a similar design. The simulated data will be used for both case studies. We emphasize that the in vitro release measurements (dissolution percent at the given time point) are the hard-to-measure response variable and the API Content-by-NIR is the easy-to-measure response variable. For each of the 34 runs, these responses are measured from 6 tablets, where the number of tablets from each run is chosen based on experimental requirements and practical considerations.

- Case Study 1: Each tablet's in vitro release is measured at a single time point of interest and augmented with the API Content-by-NIR measurement for that tablet. These data are assumed to have a known independent and identical normal distribution structure with a predefined mean function. The two elements of the response vector are percent dissolution at 30 minutes (Y_1) and API Content-by-NIR (Y_2). These response vectors are directly a part of Step 2 as discussed in Section 9.3 and modeled directly against the process parameters to estimate the process model. Each tablet contributes a response vector in Step 2.
- Case Study 2: The mean function is defined through the 3-parameter Weibull function estimated from the dissolution profile measured at 7 time points (5, 10, 15, 20, 30, 45, 60 min.). The Weibull model fit constitutes the essential piece of Step 1. The response vector being fed into Step 2 are the three Weibull parameter estimates from each individual tablet, augmented with the corresponding individual tablet API Content-by-NIR value.

Preliminary data exploration found only two factors critical to in vitro release, for convenience designated as Factor 1 and Factor 2. This leads to 2^2 combinations plus center point which need to be accounted for in the surrogate model, yielding 5 combinations indexed by k in the data which is available at `https://github.com/BayesCMC/Book`. In practice, many factors and interactions may be found important to include in the process model, but the same general approach would apply regardless of number of terms.

The following R packages are necessary for the analyses that follow:

```
library(tidyverse)
library(readxl)
library(brms)
library(shinystan)
library(rstan)
library(tidybayes)
library(mvtnorm)

# dataCS Read in data
```

9.4.2 Case Study 1

Steps 1, 2

Based on the understanding of the critical process parameters identified at the data exploration phase, the data are modeled as follows:

$$\mathbf{y}_{j(ik)} = \boldsymbol{\mu}_k + \boldsymbol{\lambda}_{i(k)} + \boldsymbol{\varepsilon}_{j(ik)} \tag{9.5}$$

where

- $\mathbf{y}_{j(ik)}$ is a 2-dimensional vector representing $Q30$ and API Content-by-NIR of the jth tablet of the ith run of the kth Factor 1 – Factor 2 combination,
- $\boldsymbol{\mu}_k$ is a 2-dimensional vector representing the mean $Q30$ and API Content-by-NIR at k^{th} Factor 1 – Factor 2 combination, and $\boldsymbol{\mu}_k^t = \mathbf{x}_k^t B$, where $\mathbf{x}_k^t$ is a 1×3 vector of factor levels corresponding to the kth combination: $k = 1 \Rightarrow (1, -1, -1)$, $k = 2 \Rightarrow (1, -1, 1)$, $k = 3 \Rightarrow (1, 0, 0)$, $k = 4 \Rightarrow (1, 1, -1)$, and $k = 5 \Rightarrow (1, 1, 1)$. B is the bivariate coefficient matrix of factor effects:

$$B = \begin{bmatrix} \mu_{Q30} & \mu_{NIR} \\ b_{1,Q30} & b_{1,NIR} \\ b_{2,Q30} & b_{2,NIR} \end{bmatrix}$$

  where, for example, μ_{Q30} represents the process mean $Q30$, $b_{1,Q30}$ and $b_{2,Q30}$ represent the linear effects of factors 1 and 2 on $Q30$, respectively. A similar interpretation applies to the NIR column.

- $\boldsymbol{\lambda}_{i(k)}$ is a 2-dimensional vector representing the random effect of the ith run (batch) nested within the kth Factor 1 – Factor 2 combination, and $\boldsymbol{\lambda}_{i(k)} \sim N(0, \Sigma_\lambda)$,
- $\boldsymbol{\varepsilon}_{j(ik)}$ is a 2-dimensional vector representing the random residual effect (tablet + measurement error) of the $j(ik)^{th}$ sampling unit (tablet), and $\boldsymbol{\varepsilon}_{j(ik)} \sim N(0, \Sigma_\varepsilon)$,
- Σ_λ is a covariance matrix representing random run (manufacturing) effect,

$$\Sigma_\lambda = \begin{pmatrix} \sigma^2_{\lambda,Q30} & \sigma_{\lambda,Q30,NIR} \\ \sigma_{\lambda,Q30,NIR} & \sigma^2_{\lambda,NIR} \end{pmatrix} \tag{9.6}$$

  where the entries in the matrix Σ_λ are defined as follows:

  - $\sigma^2_{\lambda,Q30}, \sigma^2_{\lambda,NIR}$ are the variances of run effect for $Q30$ and NIR, respectively,
  - $\sigma_{\lambda,Q30,NIR}$ is the covariance at run level for $Q30$ and NIR..

- Σ_ε is a covariance matrix representing random dosage unit and analytical measurement uncertainty,

$$\Sigma_\varepsilon = \begin{pmatrix} \sigma^2_{\varepsilon,Q30} & \sigma_{\varepsilon,Q30,NIR} \\ \sigma_{\varepsilon,Q30,NIR} & \sigma^2_{\varepsilon,NIR} \end{pmatrix} \tag{9.7}$$

  where the entries in the matrix Σ_ε are similarly defined as previously given for Σ_λ but applied to the residual error covariance matrix.

In the later development of the conditional regression model, we have several choices for the covariance matrix following (9.1) and (9.2). In the original expressions, only a single covariance matrix is considered, but in actual practice, we have a hierarchical model involving both the batch manufacturing level and the tablet manufacturing level. So conceivably, one could consider:

1. $\Sigma = \Sigma_\lambda$
2. $\Sigma = \Sigma_\varepsilon$
3. $\Sigma = \Sigma_\lambda + \Sigma_\varepsilon$.

We recommend that the first choice be used in practice for the development of the conditional regression model. The reason for this is that choice 2, the covariance matrix at the tablet level is contaminated with uncontrolled sources related to measurement and manufacturing error. The relative contribution of true tablet variance component is generally not measurable at the tablet level. It is likely that the measurement uncertainty is the bulk of the variability at the tablet level, and for that reason, the true correlations would be severely underestimated. On the other hand, the correlation structure at the batch manufacturing level has generally a small component of measurement error and can be understood as the covariances due primarily to the true relationships. In addition, choice 1 can be understood as representing the correlations at a population average level after the joint impact of the DoE factors has been accounted for. Choice 3 is also ruled out for the same reason that the sum of the covariances would be contaminated with an unknown quantity of measurement and uncontrolled error sources. We note that there may be cases where choices 2 or 3 may be sensible, when the measurement error and process controls permit a covariance interpretation mainly attributable to process or manufacturing effects.

We use `brm()`, a function to fit Bayesian generalized linear and nonlinear multivariate models through Stan Development Team (2021b). The formula is denoted in a similar fashion to how model equations are traditionally written in R. The left-hand side represents the response variable(s), in Case Study 1, the 2-dimensional response vector consisting of $Q30$ and the API content, measured by NIR. On the right-hand side of the formula, we have the model's fixed effects (`factor1*factor2`) as well as a random effect (`1|q|runK`). By indicating a 2-dimensional response vector, the function automatically estimates a 2 by 2 covariance matrix. Note that the `brm` function defining the random component for `runK` requires specification of a symbol between the `1` and the `runK` call, which for convenience we have chosen `q`. The reason to include this is to induce correlated random effects.

We use three independent Markov chains (`chains=3`), each running on a separate processing unit (`cores=3`). Each chain consists of a total of 16000 iterations where only every 5th iteration is kept (`thin=5`) after the first 1000 iterations were discarded as burn-in (`warmup = 1000`).

For this model fit we rely on the default priors of the `brm()` function, which means that we assume non-informative priors for the fixed effects ($\mu_k \propto 1$). To understand the priors of the covariance matrix Σ, recall that any covariance matrix can be decomposed as

$$\Sigma = V^{1/2} \Omega V^{1/2} \tag{9.8}$$

where Ω is a correlation matrix and $V^{1/2}$ is a diagonal matrix of standard deviations. We assume each standard deviation to follow a half-t distribution with 3 degrees of freedom, a vaguely informative prior that usually leads to better convergence of the models than most other priors. The correlation matrix Ω is assumed to follow a lkj-distribution (Lewandowski et al., 2009)

$$\text{lkj}(\Omega|\eta) \propto \det(\Omega)^{\eta-1}. \tag{9.9}$$

If $\eta = 1$, all correlation matrices are equally likely a priori. If $\eta > 1$, then extreme correlation matrices become less likely, whereas if $0 < \eta < 1$, extreme correlation matrices become more likely. For the simulation study $\eta = 1$ was chosen, which indicates an uninformative prior distribution. The results and corresponding output from the code below are provided and discussed in the Section 9.5.

```
fitCS1 <- brm(mvbind(md30, NIRc) ~ factor1*factor2 +
           (1|q|runK), data = dataCS,
           iter = 15000, warmup = 1000, chains = 3, thin = 5,
           seed = 1234, cores = 3,
           control = list(adapt_delta = 0.95,
           max_treedepth = 10))

launch_shinystan(fitCS1)
```

Step 3

Step 3 begins with the application of (9.1) to (9.5),

$$y_{ijk} \sim N(\mu_k, (\Sigma \equiv \Sigma_\lambda + \Sigma_\varepsilon)), \text{where } y = \begin{pmatrix} y_{Q30} \\ y_{NIR} \end{pmatrix} \tag{9.10}$$

and the conditional distribution formula (9.2), giving the conditional expectation of the hard-to-measure variable:

$$\mathbb{E}[Y_{Q30}|Y_{NIR} = nir] = \mu_{Q30} + \Sigma_{\lambda,12}\Sigma_{\lambda,22}^{-1}(nir - \mu_{NIR}). \tag{9.11}$$

For the purposes of understanding the surrogate predictive model better, we focus on prediction at the batch/run level:

$$\mathbb{E}[Y_{Q30}|Y_{NIR} = nir, \lambda_{ik}^* = a_i] = (\mu_{Q30} + a_{i,Q30}) + \Sigma_{\lambda,12}\Sigma_{\lambda,22}^{-1}(nir - (\mu_{NIR} + a_{i,NIR})) \tag{9.12}$$

$$= (x_c \times B[,1] + a_{i,Q30}) + \Sigma_{\lambda,12}\Sigma_{\lambda,22}^{-1}(nir - (x_c \times B[,2] + a_{i,NIR})) \tag{9.13}$$

where $\mathbf{x}_c \times B$ represents the appropriate linear combination of process parameters for which a surrogate prediction is desired, and *nir* represents an average API content-by-NIR measurement. The estimator can be written as:

$$\hat{\mathbb{E}}[Y_{Q30}|Y_{NIR} = nir, \lambda_{ik}^* = a_i] = (\hat{\mu}_{Q30} + a_{i,Q30}) + \frac{\hat{\sigma}_{\lambda,Q30,NIR}}{\hat{\sigma}_{\lambda,NIR}^2}(nir - (\hat{\mu}_{NIR} + a_{i,NIR})) \tag{9.14}$$

As an alternative to the usual ratio of covariances, the DoE bivariate regression estimates can be substituted for the usual estimator of the slope in the previous equation, when only 1 process factor is in the predictive model, giving an alternative conditional regression model at the center point as:

$$\hat{\mathbb{E}}[Y_{Q30}|Y_{NIR} = nir, \lambda_{ik}^* = a_i] = (\hat{\mu}_{Q30} + a_{i,Q30}) + \frac{\hat{\beta}_{Q30}}{\hat{\beta}_{NIR}}(nir - (\hat{\mu}_{NIR} + a_{i,NIR})) \tag{9.15}$$

The expectation is with respect to a mean prediction, hence the random batch component does not disappear completely, represented by a_i, an unknown bias common to all individual tablet predictions for a given batch. It can be understood as the unattenuated part of the random batch component unaccounted for by the conditional regression relationship. The intention is to institute sufficiently tight manufacturing controls to minimize this component as well, with the understanding that it may have some small non-zero value. For this reason, it is critical to obtain a design which provides a reasonably precise estimate of Σ_λ. It is essential to apply a Bayesian approach to assess the potential impact of this bias represented by the vector quantity a_i in (9.13) to study the properties of the surrogate estimator.

The above model is a development applicable to a prediction at the run mean level. We mentioned that the batch random component contributes an unexplained bias in the estimate for any given randomly chosen batch. In practice, we can also apply this model to individual tablets. In this case, the unknown tablet random component is also present in (9.15) but given the large number of tablets that is likely to be chosen for sampling, we expect that the random components would sum close to zero so the prediction would be very similar to the prediction from (9.15).

In the code below the `posterior_samples()` command, the posterior samples of the `brm`-object `fitCS1` are extracted. The following lines of code return the mean of the posterior samples of the 2-dimensional response vector μ as well as the diagonal entries of $V^{1/2}$ and the off-diagonal entries of Ω which are needed to obtain the predictive equation in (9.15). Equation (9.16) is the "working" surrogate model as we will use for predictions:

$$\hat{\mathbb{E}}[Y_{Q30}|Y_{NIR} = nir] = \hat{\mu}_{Q30} + \frac{\hat{\beta}_{Q30}}{\hat{\beta}_{NIR}}(nir - \hat{\mu}_{NIR}) \tag{9.16}$$

```
chainsCS1 <- posterior_samples(fitCS1)[,1:14]

## Conditional model at batch level
# mu_Q30
round(mean(chainsCS1[,"b_md30_Intercept"]), 2)

# Sigma
round(mean(chainsCS1[,
      "cor_runK__md30_Intercept__NIRc_Intercept"]*
chainsCS1[,"sd_runK__md30_Intercept"]/
chainsCS1[,"sd_runK__NIRc_Intercept"]), 2)

#mu_NIR
round(mean(chainsCS1[,"b_NIRc_Intercept"]), 2)
```

Its properties were studied through Bayesian simulation, providing estimates of precision for future samples of tablets. Details of the model estimates are given in the Results section. Note the following equation (and respectively for ε): $\rho_{\lambda,Q30,NIR} = \sigma_{\lambda,Q30,NIR}/(|\sigma_{\lambda,Q30}||\sigma_{\lambda,NIR}|)$, where $\rho_{\lambda,Q30,NIR}$ is the true correlation coefficient between the $Q30$ measurement and the corresponding API content by NIR at the run level. This is expressed in this way since the prior distributions are made on the correlations as shown in (9.8).

9.4.3 Case Study 2

Using the same experiment as described in the first case study, the same process parameters given in the first case study determined as critical are used for the modeling in Case Study

2. Case Study 2 provides an approach to estimating the entire in vitro release profile, thus enabling any time point prediction on the profile. Like Case Study 1, the data consists of 34 runs $\times$ 6 tablets/run = 204 rows corresponding to the tablets, and the columns are 1 column for API Content-by-NIR, and 7 columns of %-dissolution corresponding to the 7 time points of the dissolution profile. The 3-step process for deriving the surrogate model are applied as follows:

Step 1

The mean function relating dissolution percent to time is defined in relation to the 3-parameter Weibull. Let $\lambda = \ln(1/(1-\gamma))$, $0 < \gamma < 1$, and

$$\mathbb{E}[Y|t, \theta_1, \theta_2, \theta_3, \lambda] = \theta_1 \left[1 - \exp\left\{-\lambda \left(\frac{t}{\theta_2}\right)^{\theta_3}\right\}\right]. \tag{9.17}$$

The parameter θ_1 can be thought of as a dissolution extent parameter, θ_2 is the time to achieve $\gamma\theta_1\%$ dissolution for given γ, and θ_3 is a shape parameter, which provides sufficient flexibility to provide an empirical description of the observed dissolution profiles. In practice, a form assuming $\lambda = 1$ is used, in which case, θ_2 corresponds to the time when $\gamma = 62.5\%$ of θ_1 is achieved.

The likelihood for the first step of the modeling is:

$$y_{ij}|t_j, \boldsymbol{\theta_i} \sim N\left(\theta_1 \left[1 - \exp\left\{-\lambda \left(\frac{t}{\theta_2}\right)^{\theta_3}\right\}\right], \sigma_d\right), \ \sigma_d > 0. \tag{9.18}$$

Here, $i = 1, ..., 34$ represents each experimental run; $j = 1, ..., 7$ represents each time point for a given run; y_{ij} are the averaged percent dissolution values at each time point for each run; $\boldsymbol{\theta}_i$ is a 3-dimensional vector consisting of the Weibull parameters; and σ_d represents random unexplained variation comprised of uncontrolled manufacturing variability and analytical uncertainty.

Prior to using `brm()` for Case Study 2, we need to obtain the responses: the parameters of Weibull model. Hence, we transform the data into long format and utilize `nls()` function to obtain the fits via frequentist modeling. Note that we must determine starting values for the `nls()`. This can be achieved via a trial-and-error approach, previous experience or running over a grid of suitable values. The aim is to obtain a set of values that lead to good convergence. We fit a Weibull curve for each tablet separately, retaining resulting parameters as responses for further modeling.

```
numTablets <- nrow(dataCS)

# Transpose to long format and convert data types
dataCSLong <- gather(data = dataCS,
                     DissoTime, Value, md05:md60)
dataCSLong$DissoTime <- as.numeric(unlist(str_extract_all(
dataCSLong$DissoTime,"\\(?[0-9,.]+\\)?")))
dataCSLong$Value <- as.numeric(as.character(dataCSLong$Value))

# set seed and starting value
set.seed(1234)
startingValue <- list(theta1 = 100, theta2 = 7, theta3 = 0.8)
```

```
# Estimate Weibull per tablet
res <- pred <- dat <- coefsNew <- NULL

for(i in 1: nrow(dataCS)){
  tablet_i <- dataCSLong[which(dataCSLong$tabx == i),]
  fixedWeibullTablet_i <- nls(Value ~ theta1*(1 -
                              exp(-exp(theta3 *
                                  (log(DissoTime) -
                                  log(theta2))))),
                             data = tablet_i,
                             start = startingValue)
  coefsNew <- rbind(coefsNew, coef(fixedWeibullTablet_i))
}
coefsNew <- as.data.frame(coefsNew)

# save the model estimates in the data frame
dataCS$WUB <- coefsNew$theta1
dataCS$Wlambda <- coefsNew$theta2
dataCS$Wk <- coefsNew$theta3
```

Step 2
Based on results of the first step, and API Content-by-NIR values, the second step is to estimate the parameters of the multivariate process model:

$$\left(\hat{\boldsymbol{\theta}}, NIR\right)_{j(ik)} |X, B \sim \mathrm{MVN}_4(\mathbf{x}^t_{i(jk)}B, \Sigma). \tag{9.19}$$

The corresponding prior distributions are:

$$\begin{aligned} p(B) &\propto 1 \\ L &\sim \mathrm{ljk}(1) \\ \tau &\sim \mathrm{Uniform}(0, \infty). \end{aligned}$$

Here, as in Case Study 1, $k = 1, ..., 5$ represents the combinations of the two process factors, i is the run within that combination and j is the tablet nested within the $i(k)^{th}$ experimental run. "NIR" represents the Content-by-NIR measurement for that given tablet; X is a 204 x 3 model design matrix, a main effects design only: intercept, Factor 1, and Factor 2; $\mathbf{x}_{j(ik)}$ is the row vector from the model matrix corresponding to the jth tablet from run $i(k)$; B is a 3 by 4 effects matrix, where each column represents a "parameter" – $\theta_1, \theta_2, \theta_3$, and Content-by-NIR – and each row represents the effect of the process parameters – intercept (mean value at target), slope of Factor 1, and slope of Factor 2; and Σ_λ and Σ_ε are 4 by 4 variance-covariance matrices at the experimental run and tablets levels for the 4 elements of the response vector. As seen in Case Study 1, we use the fact that $\Sigma = V^{1/2}\Omega V^{1/2} = V^{1/2}LL^TV^{1/2}$, where V represents a diagonal matrix of variances, τ; Ω is a correlation matrix, and L is the corresponding Cholesky factorization of Ω; and ljk represents a distribution function for correlation matrices (Lewandowski et al., 2009). Just as for the first case study, all priors are set as the default priors in `brms`, chosen to be as "non-informative" as possible. These could be updated with more informative priors as additional data are collected in the model maintenance phase.

We again use the brm() function for the Bayesian estimation. The sole difference is that the function requires the specification of a 4-dimensional response vector in comparison to the 2-dimensional response vector of Case Study 1.

```
fitCS2 <- brm(mvbind(WUB, Wlambda, Wk, NIRc)~factor1*factor2 +
                (1|q|runK), data = dataCS,
                iter= 30000, warmup = 10000, chains = 3,
                thin = 5, seed = 1234, cores = 3,
                control = list(adapt_delta = 0.95,
                max_treedepth = 10))

launch_shinystan(fitCS2)
```

The output of the above brm invocation will be given in Section 9.5 with associated interpretation.

Step 3

The distribution of the mean of the conditional distribution of the 3 Weibull parameters, given an average Content-by-NIR measurement and process factor settings, is:

$$\begin{aligned}\mathbb{E}[\boldsymbol{\theta}|NIR = nir, \mathbf{x}_{\text{pred}}, B, \Sigma_\lambda] &= \\ (\mathbf{x}_{\text{pred}} \times B[,1:3])^t + \Sigma_\lambda[1:3,4] \times \Sigma_\lambda^{-1}[4,4] &\times (nir - \mathbf{x}_{\text{pred}} \times B[,4]) = \boldsymbol{\theta}^*\end{aligned} \tag{9.20}$$

where $\mathbf{x}_{\text{pred}}$ is a 1×3 row vector of intercept and process factor conditions at which prediction is to be made (not necessarily one of the conditions of the DoE), and "NIR" is a given average Content-by-NIR value for which a predicted dissolution value is needed. A point estimate of $\boldsymbol{\theta}^*$ can be obtained by using either the means or medians of the posterior distributions of the parameters in the above expectation. Finally, the estimated $\boldsymbol{\theta}^*$ can be plugged back into the expectation of the dissolution model as defined in (9.18) to obtain a point estimate of the mean dissolution at any given time point.

If a credible interval for the point estimate of the mean dissolution at a given point is needed, the entire posterior distribution of $\boldsymbol{\theta}^*$ can be used:

$$y_{\text{pred}}|t, \mathbf{x}_{\text{pred}}, NIR \sim N\left(\theta_1^*\left[1 - \exp\left\{-\lambda\left(\frac{t}{\theta_2^*}\right)^{\theta_3^*}\right\}\right], \sigma_d\right). \tag{9.21}$$

Expression (9.21), the posterior predictive distribution, can be used to obtain predicted values for dissolution at any given time point. One can get a point estimate for the predicted value by using the median values from the posterior distributions of $\boldsymbol{\theta}^*$ and σ_d. If a credible interval of the predicted value is needed then the entire posterior distributions for all parameters in the expression can be used. Using the methods of Smith and Gelfand (1992), one can obtain posterior samples via an appropriate MCMC method, and then plug those samples into the likelihood, and sample from the likelihood to obtain a median, which can be used as a point estimate for percent dissolution. A $(1-\alpha)100\%$ credible interval can be calculated for any chosen α by this procedure. Note that by using samples from the posterior distributions of all unknown parameters, the uncertainty in y_{pred}, represented by its distribution, consists of all the accumulated uncertainty of the parameters used, and unexplained variation in the experiment.

Analogously to Case Study 1, the code below extracts the mean estimates and variance-covariance matrix components that are needed to obtain the predictive equation as in (9.20).

```
chainsCS2 <- posterior_samples(fitCS2)[,1:36]

## Conditional model at batch level
# mu_Q30
round(mean(chainsCS2[,"b_WUB_Intercept"]), 2)
round(mean(chainsCS2[,"b_Wlambda_Intercept"]), 2)
round(mean(chainsCS2[,"b_Wk_Intercept"]), 2)

# theta
round(mean(chainsCS2[,"cor_runK__WUB_Intercept__NIRc_Intercept"]*
chainsCS2[,"sd_runK__WUB_Intercept"]/
chainsCS2[,"sd_runK__NIRc_Intercept"]), 2)
round(mean(chainsCS2[,"cor_runK__Wlambda_Intercept__NIRc_Intercept"]*
chainsCS2[,"sd_runK__Wlambda_Intercept"]/
chainsCS2[,"sd_runK__NIRc_Intercept"]), 2)
round(mean(chainsCS2[,"cor_runK__Wk_Intercept__NIRc_Intercept"]*
chainsCS2[,"sd_runK__Wk_Intercept"]/
chainsCS2[,"sd_runK__NIRc_Intercept"]), 2)

# mu_NIR
round(mean(chainsCS2[,"b_NIRc_Intercept"]), 2)
```

9.5 Results

9.5.1 Case Study 1

9.5.1.1 Model Diagnostics

One way to assess the model's performance is by evaluating the trace plots of each main effect as well as the resulting main effect's posterior distribution. Figure 9.1 visualizes these plots for model (9.5). Trace plots and posterior distributions for model (9.19) look like those of model (9.5) and are therefore omitted from the discussion in Section 9.5.2. In Figure 9.1, we can see that each effect's trace plot has stabilized resulting in an approximately bell-shaped distribution plot, suggesting good convergence to the posterior distributions.

Table 9.1 displays the bulk and tail effective sample sizes of each main effect in model (9.5). The bulk-ESS is a rank-based measure to estimate the efficiency in the bulk of the distribution and relates to the efficiency of mean estimates, while the tail-ESS estimates the efficiency in the tail of the distribution and relates to the efficiency of variance estimates. As a rule of thumb, we propose that if the ESS is 1000 or higher, that is sufficient to characterize the posterior distribution along with reasonably symmetric and smooth trace plots under the assumptions of normality.

The `brm()`-function returns by default the Gelman-Rubin convergence diagnostic (Gelman and Rubin, 1992), also known as the potential scale reduction statistic $\hat{R}$, a criterion which evaluates the between and the within chain variation. As a rule of thumb $\hat{R} < 1.1$

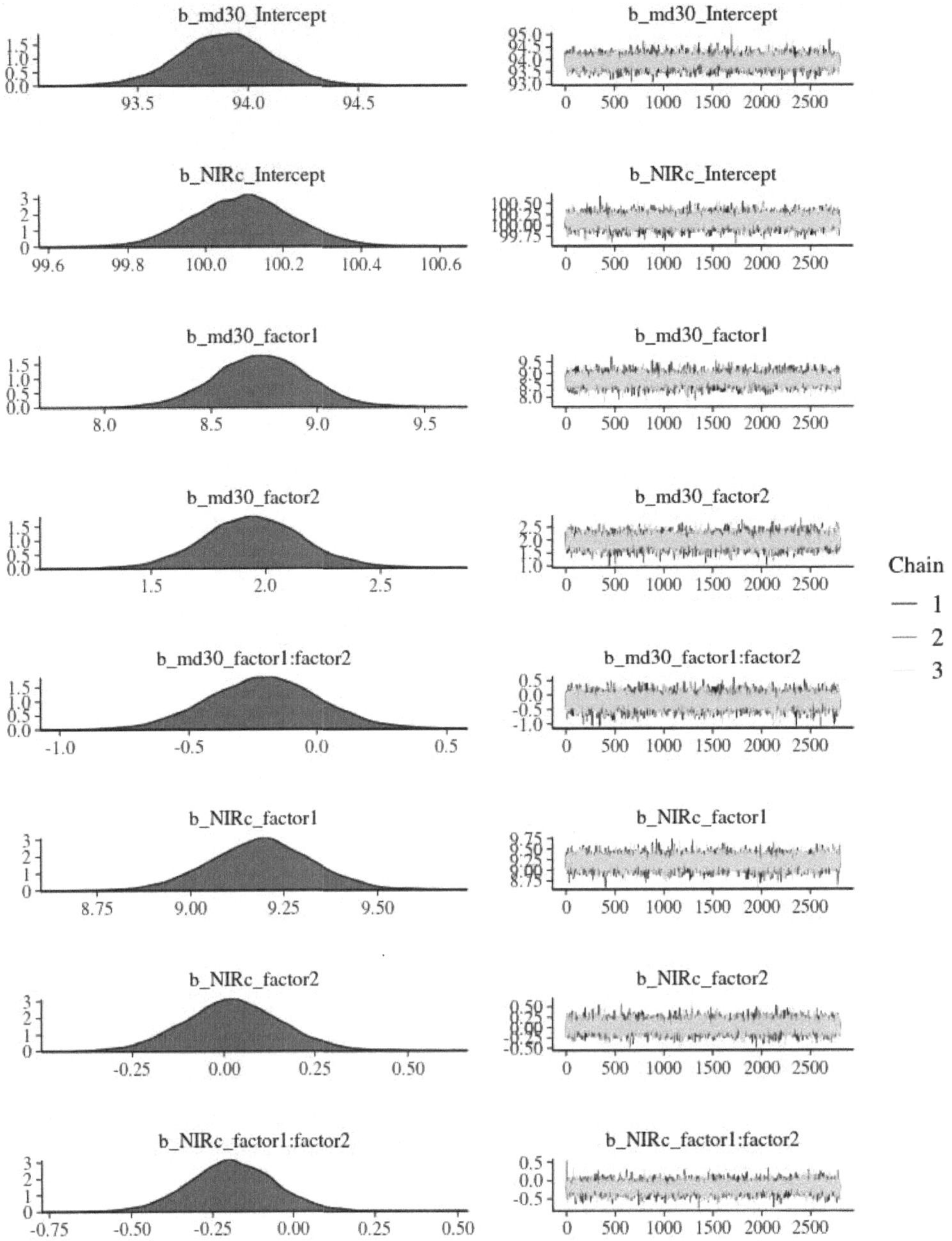

FIGURE 9.1
Posterior distribution and trace plots for the main effects of model (9.5).

is usually used as the threshold, indicating that a chain converged to a stationary target distribution and therefore has passed the Gelman-Rubin criteria. All chains in this model have a potential scale reduction statistic $\hat{R} < 1.1$.

9.5.1.2 Modeling Results

The modeling results of step 1 are shown in Table 9.2.

TABLE 9.1
Bulk estimated sample size and tail estimated sample size for the main parameters of model (9.5).

Model	Parameter	Bulk ESS	Tail ESS
$Q30$ Model	Intercept	7446	7823
	Factor 1	7413	7926
	Factor 2	7536	7505
	Factor 1×Factor 2	7205	7817
NIR Model	Intercept	6803	7216
	Factor 1	7127	7513
	Factor 2	6613	7332
	Factor 1×Factor 2	6976	7787

TABLE 9.2
Results of the Bayesian model.

Parameter Group	Parameter	Posterior Mean	SE	95% Credible Limits
Mean structure: Q30 model	Intercept	93.9	0.2	(93.5, 94.3)
	Factor 1 (F1)	8.7	0.2	(8.3, 9.2)
	Factor 2 (F2)	2.0	0.2	(1.5, 2.4)
	Interaction F1×F2	−0.2	0.2	(−0.7, 0.2)
Mean structure: NIR model	Intercept	100.1	0.1	(99.8, 100.4)
	Factor 1 (F1)	9.2	0.1	(8.9, 9.5)
	Factor 2 (F2)	0.02	0.1	(−0.3, 0.3)
	Interaction F1×F2	−0.2	0.1	(−0.5, 0.1)
Variance components: Σ_λ	$\lvert\sigma_{\lambda,Q30}\rvert$	1.1	0.2	(0.8, 1.6)
	$\lvert\sigma_{\lambda,NIR}\rvert$	0.7	0.1	(0.5, 1.0)
	$\rho_{\lambda,Q30,NIR}$	0.2	0.2	(−0.2, 0.6)
Variance components: Σ_ε	$\lvert\sigma_{\varepsilon,Q30}\rvert$	0.9	0.1	(0.7, 1.0)
	$\lvert\sigma_{\varepsilon,NIR}\rvert$	0.4	0.03	(0.3, 0.4)
	$\rho_{\varepsilon,Q30,NIR}$	0.3	0.1	(0.1, 0.5)

9.5.1.3 Calculation of Surrogate Model Parameters

Based on the data from the 34-run experiment, the following predictive model is derived at target setpoint of factor 1 and factor 2 for a future $Q30^*$, given an observed API Content-by-NIR mean, $\bar{x}_{\text{NIR}}$:

$$Q30^* = 93.9 + 0.4(\bar{x}_{NIR} - 100.1) \tag{9.22}$$

The predictive model cannot account for the random batch effect on $Q30$. It is essentially independent of the random batch effect on API Content as can be seen from the covariance patterns in Table 9.2. Consequently, the uncertainty in the prediction will come from two independent sources: 1) the random $Q30$ batch effect, which cannot be observed in this setup for any given future batch, and 2) the uncertainty in the parameter estimates in the predictive model. The standard errors of the parameter estimates from the experiment are given in Table 9.2. These give a sense of how much model uncertainty contributes to the prediction error. However, since the experiment has provided a reasonable estimate of the magnitude of the $Q30$ random component at the batch level, it should be possible to estimate uncertainty limits on the predicted $Q30^*$.

Assessing Overall Uncertainty in Predictions

We continue a Bayesian approach to estimate the overall total uncertainty limits on surrogate predictions based on the posterior predictive distribution of the given conditional expression model (9.22) as presented above. The following quantities were generated for each post-warmup iteration to characterize the posterior predictive distribution of $Q30$, thus assessing the uncertainty associated with the conditional predictive model:

- A random run component,
- A posterior predictive mean value for that run,
- 30 random tablet errors for the given run.

The above quantities are generated from a bivariate normal model, considering correlations between API Content-by-NIR and $Q30$. The procedure results in the 30 random tablet API Content-by-NIR and $Q30$ measurements for a given run.

The mean API Content-by-NIR value for the 30 tablets is calculated; this is then used, along with the posterior estimates of the relevant parameters, to generate a value for the expectation of the conditional $Q30$ for a given mean API Content-by-NIR value given by the previously derived expression (9.22): $Q30^* = 93.9 + 0.4(\bar{x}_{NIR} - 100.1)$. Hence, we have one posterior conditional expected value for $Q30$ given mean API Content-by-NIR value for each sampling iteration. We can compare this directly with the posterior batch mean generated at each iteration of the Hamiltonian sampling. Combined across all iterations, this allows us to account for all sources of uncertainty in the estimates of interest, and thus allowing the statement of probability intervals.

The resulting density plots and quantiles comparing the predicted value with the expected value (Figure 9.2) and the difference between the two (Figure 9.3) are given below. These results show that, on average, the difference between the surrogate model and the in vitro release method for Q30 is approximately zero and that both methods are generally within the prespecified acceptable limits of each other when uncertainty is taken into account. The question of a prespecified criterion for acceptability will depend on various factors related to the product and the method. Additionally, the choice of a criterion can be connected to the total variability of the measurement system of the gold standard method, and requirements laid out in the product's analytical target profile.

TABLE 9.3
Posterior distribution summaries.

	Batch Mean	Predicted Dissolution
Median	93.9	93.9
95% credible interval	(91.6, 96.3)	(93.4, 94.5)
99% credible interval	(90.8, 97.0)	(93.2, 94.7)

The code below is utilized to obtain the results presented in figures and tables above. First, we define the predictive equation as given in (9.2) in function predictCS1target which returns expected dissolution at 30 minutes when both factors are set to target and conditionally on measured NIR value. The simulation starts with simulating the batch level means and then 30 individual tablets, using as an input for the parameters of multivariate normal distribution the results of the Bayesian model. Finally, the predicted dissolution is obtained via conditional model (9.2) which can then be visualized and compared with simulated "true" dissolution (the code for the figures and tables are shown in chapter's Appendix). Table 9.3 provides a summary of the posterior predictive distributions of the

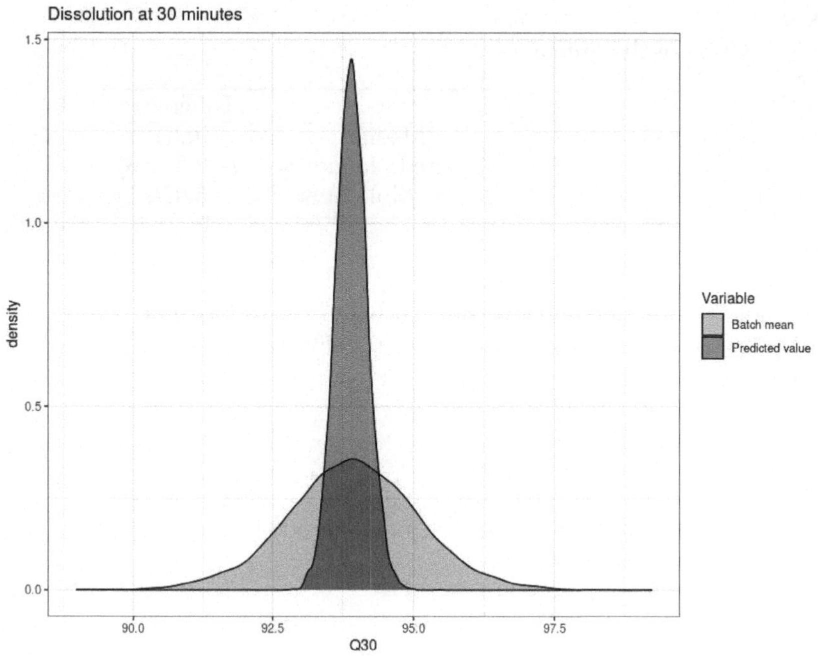

FIGURE 9.2
Comparison of posterior distribution of batch mean for $Q30$ and predicted mean based on 30 randomly sampled tablets.

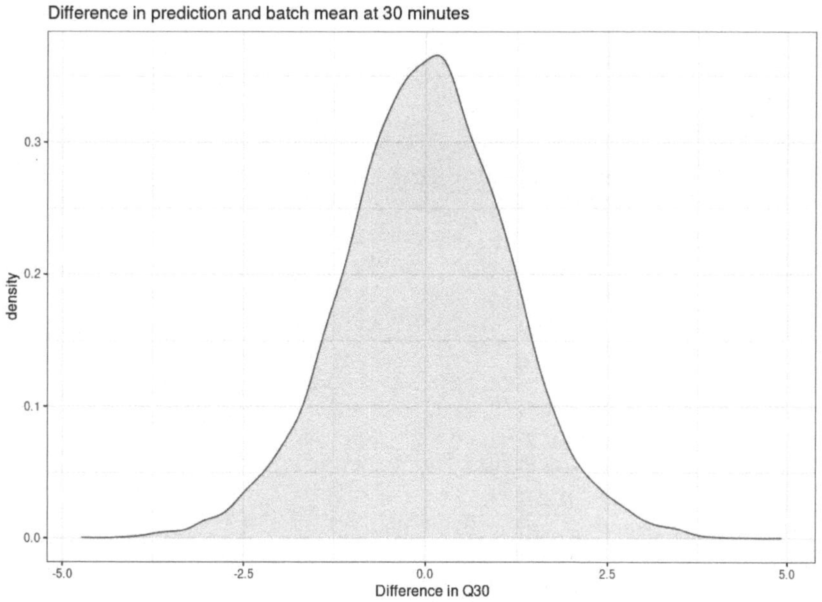

FIGURE 9.3
Posterior distribution of difference between batch mean for $Q30$ and predicted mean based on 30 randomly sampled tablets.

TABLE 9.4
Posterior distribution of the difference.

	Difference
Median	0.02
95% credible interval	(−2.3, 2.3)
99% credible interval	(−3.0, 3.1)

batch means and the surrogate model predicted batch means based on 30 tablets. Table 9.4 provides the 95% and 99% credible intervals for the difference between the batch mean and its surrogate model prediction.

```
predictCS1target <- function(NIRvalue){
round(mean(chainsCS1[,"b_md30_Intercept"]), 2)  +
round(mean(chainsCS1[,"cor_runK__md30_Intercept__NIRc_Intercept"]*
chainsCS1[, "sd_runK__md30_Intercept"]/
chainsCS1[,"sd_runK__NIRc_Intercept"]), 2)*
(NIRvalue - round(mean(chainsCS1[,"b_NIRc_Intercept"]), 2))
}

resultsMean <- matrix(numeric(nrow(chainsCS1)*2), ncol = 2)
colnames(resultsMean) <- c("BatchTrueQ30", "MeanPredQ30mean")

set.seed(12345)
for (i in 1:nrow(chainsCS1)){
sampleBatch <- matrix(rep(
    rmvnorm(1,
    mean = unlist(chainsCS1[i, c("b_md30_Intercept",
                                 "b_NIRc_Intercept")]),
    sigma = matrix( c(
  chainsCS1[i, "sd_runK__md30_Intercept"]^2,
  rep(chainsCS1[i, "sd_runK__md30_Intercept"]*
chainsCS1[i, "sd_runK__NIRc_Intercept"]*
      chainsCS1[i, "cor_runK__md30_Intercept__NIRc_Intercept"], 2),
  chainsCS1[i, "sd_runK__NIRc_Intercept"]^2),
byrow = TRUE, nrow=2)), 30),
byrow = TRUE, nrow = 30)
sampleError <- rmvnorm(30,
mean = c(0,0),
sigma = matrix( c(
   chainsCS1[i, "sigma_md30"]^2,
   rep(chainsCS1[i, "sigma_md30"]*
       chainsCS1[i, "sigma_NIRc"]*
       chainsCS1[i, "rescor__md30__NIRc"], 2),
   chainsCS1[i, "sigma_NIRc"]^2), byrow = TRUE, nrow=2))
sample <- sampleBatch + sampleError
meanDissoPred <- predictCS1target(mean(sample[,2]))
resultsMean[i,] <- c(colMeans(sampleBatch)[1], meanDissoPred)
}
resultsMean <- as.data.frame(resultsMean)
```

9.5.2 Case Study 2

Just as for the first case study we evaluate and verify the model's performance by considering the Gelman-Rubin criteria, main effects' trace plots as well as effective samples sizes. The modeling results of step 1 are shown in Table 9.5.

TABLE 9.5
Results of the Bayesian model.

Parameter Group	Parameter	Posterior Mean	SE	95% Credible Limits
Mean structure: θ_1 model	Intercept	98.8	0.2	(98.5, 99.1)
	Factor 1	9.9	0.2	(9.6, 10.2)
	Factor 2	2.5	0.2	(2.2, 2.8)
	Interaction F1×F2	0.1	0.2	(−0.2, 0.4)
Mean structure: θ_2 model	Intercept	7.8	0.1	(7.7, 7.9)
	Factor 1	0.4	0.1	(0.3, 0.5)
	Factor 2	0.4	0.1	(0.1, 0.3)
	Interaction F1×F2	0.03	0.1	(−0.1, 0.1)
Mean structure: θ_3 model	Intercept	0.8	0.0	(0.8, 0.8)
	Factor 1	0.0	0.0	(0.0, 0.0)
	Factor 2	0.0	0.0	(0.0, 0.0)
	Interaction F1×F2	0.0	0.0	(0.0, 0.0)
Mean structure: NIR model	Intercept	100.1	0.1	(99.8, 100.4)
	Factor 1	9.2	0.1	(8.9, 9.5)
	Factor 2	0.0	0.1	(−0.2, 0.3)
	Interaction F1*F2	−0.2	0.1	(−0.5, 0.1)
Variance components: Σ_λ	$\lvert\sigma_{\lambda,\theta_1}\rvert$	0.6	0.2	(0.2, 1.0)
	$\lvert\sigma_{\lambda,\theta_2}\rvert$	0.3	0.1	(0.2, 0.4)
	$\lvert\sigma_{\lambda,\theta_3}\rvert$	0.0	0.0	(0.0, 0.0)
	$\lvert\sigma_{\lambda,NIR}\rvert$	0.7	0.1	(0.6, 0.1)
	$\rho_{\lambda,\theta_1,NIR}$	0.0	0.3	(−0.5, 0.5)
	$\rho_{\lambda,\theta_2,NIR}$	−0.3	0.2	(−0.6, 0.1)
	$\rho_{\lambda,\theta_3,NIR}$	0.5	0.2	(0.1, 0.7)
Variance components: Σ_ε	$\lvert\sigma_{\varepsilon,\theta_1}\rvert$	1.0	0.1	(0.9, 1.2)
	$\lvert\sigma_{\varepsilon,\theta_2}\rvert$	0.2	0.0	(0.2, 0.3)
	$\lvert\varepsilon, \sigma_{\theta_3}\rvert$	0.0	0.0	(0.0, 0.0)
	$\lvert\sigma_{\varepsilon,NIR}\rvert$	0.4	0.0	(0.3, 0.4)
	$\rho_{\varepsilon,\theta_1,NIR}$	0.3	0.1	(0.0, 0.5)
	$\rho_{\varepsilon,\theta_2,NIR}$	−0.1	0.1	(−0.3, 0.2)
	$\rho_{\varepsilon,\theta_3,NIR}$	0.0	0.1	(−0.2, 0.3)

9.5.2.1 Calculation of Surrogate Model Parameters

Based on the data from the 34-run experiment, the following predictive model is derived at target setpoint of factor 1 and factor 2 for future Weibull parameters, given an observed API Content mean, $\bar{x}_{NIR}$:

$$\begin{aligned}\theta_1^* &= 98.8 - 0.01(\bar{x}_{NIR} - 100.1)\\ \theta_2^* &= 7.8 - 0.01(\bar{x}_{NIR} - 100.1)\\ \theta_3^* &= 0.8 + 0.02(\bar{x}_{NIR} - 100.1)\end{aligned} \tag{9.23}$$

Analogously to Case Study 1, we only work at the level of run (batch) mean when conducting the prediction via a conditional model. First, the Weibull parameters are predicted and then those predicted parameters substituted into the Weibull model are used to obtain specific dissolution time point predictions.

9.5.2.2 Assessing Overall Uncertainty in Predictions

To assess the prediction, we proceed analogously to Case Study 1. We have available full profile predictions, but for comparison purposes, we evaluate the prediction at 30 minutes. We start with a multivariate model for API Content-by-NIR and three Weibull parameters, obtain the batch specific Weibull parameters and obtain dissolution at 30 minutes specific to that batch. We compare this batch specific dissolution with dissolution based on predicted Weibull parameters obtained as prediction for the average API Content-by-NIR of 30 tablets.

The resulting density plots and quantiles comparing the predicted value with the expected value (Figure 9.4) and the difference between the two (Figure 9.5) are given below. These results show that, on average, the difference between the surrogate model and the in vitro release method for $Q30$ is approximately zero and that both methods are within acceptable limits of each other at the batch run level when uncertainty is taken into account. The acceptance criterion must be prespecified at the time of experimental planning or possibly rely on requirements in the original analytical target profile driving a fit for purpose consideration. it is important to keep in mind that the hard to measure method is subject to both sampling variation and analytical method uncertainty that will, in general, be quite different than the surrogate estimator.

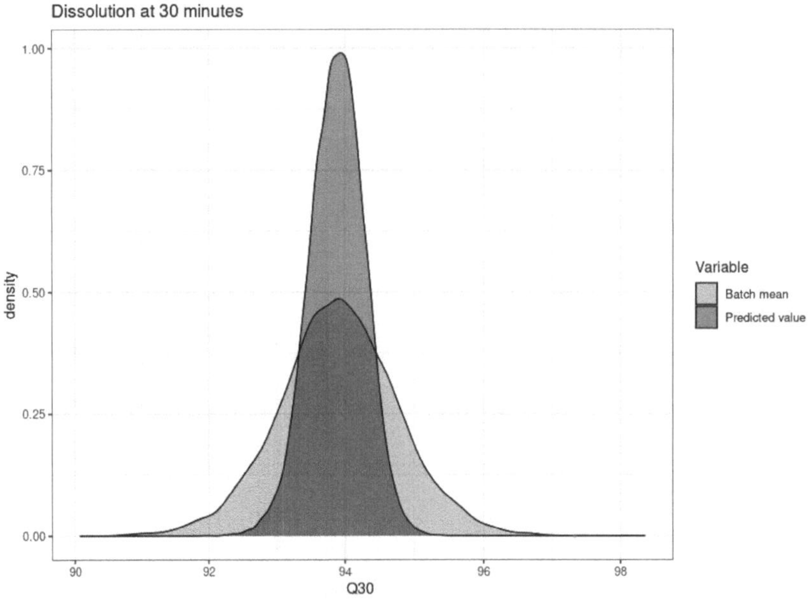

FIGURE 9.4
Comparison of posterior distribution of batch mean for $Q30$ and predicted mean based on 30 randomly sampled tablets based on full profile modeling.

As in Case Study 1, we show the code to obtain the results for visualization above. Firstly, Weibull function is defined to obtain the dissolution at 30 minutes from the set of predicted Weibull parameters. Then, the `predictCS2target` function is constructed to predict dissolution based on model (9.23) for given NIR value and for factors set to target.

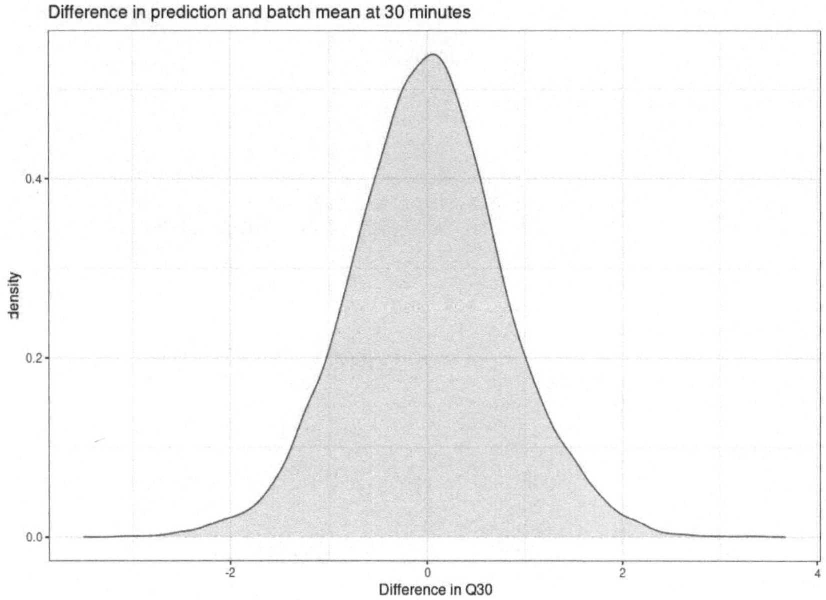

FIGURE 9.5
Posterior distribution of difference between batch mean for $Q30$ and predicted mean based on 30 randomly sampled tablets based on full profile modeling.

Then, the batch means, and 30 individual tablets are simulated, and dissolution is predicted for each of them. Table 9.6 provides the mean and 95% and 99% credible intervals for the batch means and surrogate model predicted means based on 30 tablets. Table 9.7 provides the 95% and 99% credible intervals for the difference between the batch mean and its surrogate model prediction. Finally, the predicted dissolution can be compared with the simulated "true" dissolution at the batch level. Codes for tables and figures are shown in the chapter's appendix.

TABLE 9.6
Posterior distribution of $Q30$ based on full profile modeling.

	Batch Mean	Predicted Dissolution
Median	93.9	93.9
95% credible interval	(92.1, 95.6)	(93.1, 94.6)
99% credible interval	(91.5, 96.2)	(92.8, 94.9)

TABLE 9.7
Posterior distribution of the difference based on full profile modeling.

	Difference
Median	0.01
95% credible interval	(−1.5, 1.6)
99% credible interval	(−2.2, 2.1)

```
weibullF <- function(wub, wl, wk, t){
wub*(1-exp(-exp( wk*(log(t)-log(wl)))))
}

predictCS2target <- function(NIRvalue){
  wub = round(mean(chainsCS2[,"b_WUB_Intercept"]), 2) +
    round(mean(chainsCS2[,"cor_runK__WUB_Intercept__NIRc_Intercept"]*
    chainsCS2[,"sd_runK__WUB_Intercept"]/
    chainsCS2[,"sd_runK__NIRc_Intercept"]), 2)*
    (NIRvalue - round(mean(chainsCS2[,"b_NIRc_Intercept"]), 2))
  wl = round(mean(chainsCS2[,"b_Wlambda_Intercept"]), 2) +
    round(mean(chainsCS2[,"cor_runK__Wlambda_Intercept__NIRc_Intercept"]*
    chainsCS2[,"sd_runK__Wlambda_Intercept"]/
    chainsCS2[,"sd_runK__NIRc_Intercept"]), 2)*
    (NIRvalue - round(mean(chainsCS2[,"b_NIRc_Intercept"]), 2))
  wk = round(mean(chainsCS2[,"b_Wk_Intercept"]), 2) +
    round(mean(chainsCS2[,"cor_runK__Wk_Intercept__NIRc_Intercept"]*
    chainsCS2[,"sd_runK__Wk_Intercept"]/
    chainsCS2[,"sd_runK__NIRc_Intercept"]), 2)*
    (NIRvalue - round(mean(chainsCS2[,"b_NIRc_Intercept"]), 2))
t30pred <- weibullF(wub, wl, wk, t = 30)
return(t30pred)
}

resultsMean <- matrix(numeric(nrow(chainsCS2)*2), ncol = 2)
colnames(resultsMean) <- c("BatchTrueQ30", "MeanPredQ30ind")
set.seed(12345)

for (i in 1:nrow(chainsCS2)){
  sampleBatch <- matrix(rep(rmvnorm(1,
         mean = unlist(chainsCS2[i, c("b_WUB_Intercept",
                                      "b_Wlambda_Intercept",
                                      "b_Wk_Intercept",
                                      "b_NIRc_Intercept")]),
         sigma = matrix( c(
           chainsCS2[i, "sd_runK__WUB_Intercept"]^2,
           chainsCS2[i, "sd_runK__WUB_Intercept"]*
             chainsCS2[i, "sd_runK__Wlambda_Intercept"]*
             chainsCS2[i, "cor_runK__WUB_Intercept__Wlambda_Intercept"],
           chainsCS2[i, "sd_runK__WUB_Intercept"]*
             chainsCS2[i, "sd_runK__Wk_Intercept"]*
             chainsCS2[i, "cor_runK__WUB_Intercept__Wk_Intercept"],
           chainsCS2[i, "sd_runK__WUB_Intercept"]*
             chainsCS2[i, "sd_runK__NIRc_Intercept"]*
             chainsCS2[i, "cor_runK__WUB_Intercept__NIRc_Intercept"],
           chainsCS2[i, "sd_runK__WUB_Intercept"]*
             chainsCS2[i, "sd_runK__Wlambda_Intercept"]*
             chainsCS2[i, "cor_runK__WUB_Intercept__Wlambda_Intercept"],
           chainsCS2[i, "sd_runK__Wlambda_Intercept"]^2,
           chainsCS2[i, "sd_runK__Wlambda_Intercept"]*
             chainsCS2[i, "sd_runK__Wk_Intercept"]*
             chainsCS2[i, "cor_runK__Wlambda_Intercept__Wk_Intercept"],
           chainsCS2[i, "sd_runK__Wlambda_Intercept"]*
             chainsCS2[i, "sd_runK__NIRc_Intercept"]*
             chainsCS2[i, "cor_runK__Wlambda_Intercept__NIRc_Intercept"],
           chainsCS2[i, "sd_runK__WUB_Intercept"]*
             chainsCS2[i, "sd_runK__Wk_Intercept"]*
             chainsCS2[i, "cor_runK__WUB_Intercept__Wk_Intercept"],
           chainsCS2[i, "sd_runK__Wlambda_Intercept"]*
             chainsCS2[i, "sd_runK__Wk_Intercept"]*
             chainsCS2[i, "cor_runK__Wlambda_Intercept__Wk_Intercept"],
```

```
          chainsCS2[i, "sd_runK__Wk_Intercept"]^2,
          chainsCS2[i, "sd_runK__Wk_Intercept"]*
            chainsCS2[i, "sd_runK__NIRc_Intercept"]*
            chainsCS2[i, "cor_runK__Wk_Intercept__NIRc_Intercept"],
          chainsCS2[i, "sd_runK__WUB_Intercept"]*
            chainsCS2[i, "sd_runK__NIRc_Intercept"]*
            chainsCS2[i, "cor_runK__WUB_Intercept__NIRc_Intercept"],
          chainsCS2[i, "sd_runK__Wlambda_Intercept"]*
            chainsCS2[i, "sd_runK__NIRc_Intercept"]*
            chainsCS2[i, "cor_runK__Wlambda_Intercept__NIRc_Intercept"],
          chainsCS2[i, "sd_runK__Wk_Intercept"]*
            chainsCS2[i, "sd_runK__NIRc_Intercept"]*
            chainsCS2[i, "cor_runK__Wk_Intercept__NIRc_Intercept"],
          chainsCS2[i, "sd_runK__NIRc_Intercept"]^2
        ), byrow = TRUE, nrow=4)), 30), byrow = TRUE, nrow = 30)

sampleError <- rmvnorm(30, mean = c(0,0,0,0),
        sigma = matrix( c(
          chainsCS2[i, "sigma_WUB"]^2,
          chainsCS2[i, "sigma_WUB"]*
            chainsCS2[i, "sigma_Wlambda"]*
            chainsCS2[i, "rescor__WUB__Wlambda"],
          chainsCS2[i, "sigma_WUB"]*
            chainsCS2[i, "sigma_Wk"]*
            chainsCS2[i, "rescor__WUB__Wk"],
          chainsCS2[i, "sigma_WUB"]*
            chainsCS2[i, "sigma_NIRc"]*
            chainsCS2[i, "rescor__WUB__NIRc"],
          chainsCS2[i, "sigma_WUB"]*
            chainsCS2[i, "sigma_Wlambda"]*
            chainsCS2[i, "rescor__WUB__Wlambda"],
          chainsCS2[i, "sigma_Wlambda"]^2,
          chainsCS2[i, "sigma_Wlambda"]*
            chainsCS2[i, "sigma_Wk"]*
            chainsCS2[i, "rescor__Wlambda__Wk"],
          chainsCS2[i, "sigma_Wlambda"]*
            chainsCS2[i, "sigma_NIRc"]*
            chainsCS2[i, "rescor__Wlambda__NIRc"],
          chainsCS2[i, "sigma_WUB"]*
            chainsCS2[i, "sigma_Wk"]*
            chainsCS2[i, "rescor__WUB__Wk"],
          chainsCS2[i, "sigma_Wlambda"]*
            chainsCS2[i, "sigma_Wk"]*
            chainsCS2[i, "rescor__Wlambda__Wk"],
          chainsCS2[i, "sigma_Wk"]^2,
          chainsCS2[i, "sigma_Wk"]*
            chainsCS2[i, "sigma_NIRc"]*
            chainsCS2[i, "rescor__Wk__NIRc"],
          chainsCS2[i, "sigma_WUB"]*
            chainsCS2[i, "sigma_NIRc"]*
            chainsCS2[i, "rescor__WUB__NIRc"],
          chainsCS2[i, "sigma_Wlambda"]*
            chainsCS2[i, "sigma_NIRc"]*
            chainsCS2[i, "rescor__Wlambda__NIRc"],
          chainsCS2[i, "sigma_Wk"]*
            chainsCS2[i, "sigma_NIRc"]*
            chainsCS2[i, "rescor__Wk__NIRc"],
          chainsCS2[i, "sigma_NIRc"]^2
        ), byrow = TRUE, nrow=4))
  sample <- sampleBatch + sampleError
  dissoPred <- predictCS2target(sample[,4])
  resultsMeanCS2[i,] <- c(weibullF(sampleBatch[1,1],sampleBatch[1,2],
```

```
                              sampleBatch[1,3], 30),
                        mean(dissoPred)) #
}
resultsMean <- as.data.frame(resultsMean)
```

9.6 Summary

A method for surrogate modeling in the context of real time release testing based on near infrared spectral method technology was presented. The method essentially relates an easy-to-measure Content-by-NIR measurement, combined with important information about the manufacturing conditions, to the hard-to-measure, in vitro release value. The linear relationship between the easy-to-measure and the hard-to-measure variables are established through a multivariate conditional regression approach. The conditional regression leads to a straightforward relationship that can be used to characterize the entire dissolution profile, or selected points. Model performance was assessed statistically through a Bayesian simulation of the surrogate predictions compared to the simulated empirical results and shown to fall within acceptable bounds.

Empirical model validation is an important requirement as well, and it is recommended that the surrogate predictions also be validated with independently manufactured batches to confirm their performance, in addition to examining posterior predictive distributions. The Bayesian approach at all stages of the multivariate conditional regression approach discussed in this chapter provides a general framework for efficient estimation, adjusting for both parameter and data uncertainty, as well as providing comprehensive tools for assessing the model performance in a meaningful way.

9.7 Appendix

9.7.1 R Code Case Study 1

Table 2

```
table1 <- matrix(c(round(colMeans(chainsCS1),
                    2)[c(1,3,4,5,2,6:14)],
round(apply(chainsCS1, 2, sd),2)[c(1,3,4,5,2,6:14)],
apply(chainsCS1, 2, function(x) paste0("(",
   paste0(round(quantile(x, c(0.025, 0.975)), 2),
collapse = ", "), ")"))[c(1,3,4,5,2,6:14)]),
ncol = 3, byrow = FALSE)
```

Figure 2

```
resultsMean %>%
  select(BatchTrueQ30, MeanPredQ30ind) %>%
  pivot_longer(cols = BatchTrueQ30:MeanPredQ30ind,
names_to = "Variable", values_to = "Q30" ) %>%
  ggplot(aes(x = Q30, fill = Variable)) +
  geom_density(alpha = 0.4) +
  scale_fill_manual(labels=c("Batch mean","Predicted value"),
values = c("dodgerblue", "midnightblue")) +
  labs(x = "Q30",
  title = "Dissolution at 30 minutes") +
  theme_bw()
```

Table 3

```
round(apply(resultsMean, 2, median) , 2)
apply(resultsMean, 2, function(x)
  paste0("(", paste0(round(quantile(x, c(0.025, 0.975)),2),
collapse = ", "), ")"))
apply(resultsMean, 2, function(x)
  paste0("(", paste0(round(quantile(x, c(0.005, 0.995)),2),
collapse = ", "), ")"))
```

Figure 3

```
resultsMeanDiff <- resultsMean %>%
  mutate(Difference = BatchTrueQ30 - MeanPredQ30ind)
resultsMeanDiff %>%
  ggplot(aes(x = Difference)) +
  geom_density(alpha = 0.4, fill="lightskyblue",
               col = "royalblue") +
  labs(x = "Difference in Q30",
       title = "Difference in prediction and batch mean at
                30 minutes") + theme_bw()
```

Table 4

```
round(median(resultsMeanDiff$Difference),2)
paste0("(", paste0(round(quantile(resultsMeanDiff$Difference,
c(0.025, 0.975)),2), collapse = ", "), ")")
paste0("(", paste0(round(quantile(resultsMeanDiff$Difference,
c(0.005, 0.995)),2), collapse = ", "), ")")
```

9.7.2 R Code Case Study 2

Table 5

```
table4 <- matrix(c(round(colMeans(chainsCS2),2)[
c(1,5,6,7,2,8,9,10,3,11,12,13,4,14,15,16,17:20,24:30,34:36)],
round(apply(chainsCS2, 2,sd),2)[
c(1,5,6,7,2,8,9,10,3,11,12,13,4,14,15,16,17:20,24:30,34:36)],
apply(chainsCS2, 2, function(x) paste0("(",
paste0(round(quantile(x, c(0.025, 0.975)), 2),
collapse = ", "),")"))[
c(1,5,6,7,2,8,9,10,3,11,12,13,4,14,15,16,17:20,24:30,34:36)]),
ncol = 3, byrow = FALSE)
```

Figure 4

```
resultsMeanCS2 %>%
  select(BatchTrueQ30, MeanPredQ30ind) %>%
  pivot_longer(cols = BatchTrueQ30:MeanPredQ30ind,
names_to = "Variable", values_to = "Q30" ) %>%
  ggplot(aes(x = Q30, fill = Variable)) +
  geom_density(alpha = 0.4) +
  scale_fill_manual(labels=c("Batch mean","Predicted value"),
values = c("dodgerblue", "midnightblue")) +
  labs(x = "Q30",
  title = "Dissolution at 30 minutes") +
  theme_bw()
```

Table 6

```
round(apply(resultsMeanCS2, 2, median) , 2)
apply(resultsMeanCS2, 2, function(x) paste0("(",
paste0(round(quantile(x, c(0.025, 0.975)),2),
        collapse = ", "), ")"))
apply(resultsMeanCS2, 2, function(x) paste0("(",
paste0(round(quantile(x, c(0.005, 0.995)),2),
        collapse = ", "), ")"))
```

Figure 5

```
resultsMeanCS2Diff <- resultsMeanCS2 %>%
  mutate(Difference = BatchTrueQ30 - MeanPredQ30ind)
resultsMeanCS2Diff %>%
  ggplot(aes(x = Difference)) +
  geom_density(alpha = 0.4, fill="lightskyblue",
               col = "royalblue") +
  labs(x = "Difference in Q30",
       title = "Difference in prediction and batch mean at
                30 minutes") + theme_bw()
```

Table 7

```
round(median(resultsMeanCS2Diff$Difference),2)
paste0("(",paste0(round(quantile(resultsMeanCS2Diff$Difference,
c(0.025, 0.975)),2), collapse = ", "), ")")
paste0("(",paste0(round(quantile(resultsMeanCS2Diff$Difference,
c(0.005, 0.995)),2), collapse = ", "), ")")
```

10

Bayesian Approach for Demonstrating Analytical Similarity

Harry Yang

Fate Therapeutics

Steven Novick

AstraZeneca

CONTENTS

10.1 Introduction

Biotechnology-derived drug products hold great promise for treating various diseases such as cancer and inflammatory diseases. Examples of these products include monoclonal antibodies, proteins, and peptides. In recent years, the expiry of patent protection of many biopharmaceuticals has spawned the development of alternative versions of the products known as biosimilars. With a significant number of best-selling biopharmaceuticals coming off patent soon, biosimilar development has become a fast-growing sector of the industry. The advance in regulatory guidance on biosimilars has further fueled the enthusiasm in biosimilar development. In 2010, the passage of the Biologics Price Competition and Innovation Act of 2009, as part of the Affordable Care Act, provided an abbreviated licensure pathway for biological products demonstrated to be biosimilar to or interchangeable with a reference product (RP). Per U.S. Food and Drug Administration (FDA) guidance, biosimilarity means that the biological product is highly similar to the RP notwithstanding minor differences in clinically inactive components and that there are no clinically meaningful differences between the biological product and RP in terms of safety, purity, and potency of the product (FDA, 2015e). Demonstration of biosimilarity has brought about a host of scientific and regulatory challenges (Chow, 2015).

DOI: 10.1201/9781003255093-10

To assist sponsors in biosimilar development and licensure applications, a series of guidelines have been published by the FDA. Among them are (i) the guidance "Scientific Considerations in Demonstrating Biosimilarity to a Reference Product" (FDA, 2015e); (ii) "Quality Considerations in Demonstrating Biosimilarity to a Reference Protein" (FDA, 2015d); and (iii) "Biosimilars: Questions and Answers Regarding Implementation of the Biologics Price Competition and Innovation Act of 2009" (FDA, 2015c). This last guidance describes the FDA's current thinking on demonstration of biosimilarity and related scientific considerations. Of particular note is the introduction of a stepwise approach to data generation and the evaluation of residual uncertainty FDA (2015e). As depicted in Figure 10.1, the approach begins with assessment of analytical similarity, which includes comparisons of structural and functional attributes between the biosimilar and RP. Animal studies are conducted to address any remaining uncertainties concerning the proposed biosimilar product before clinical testing of the product in human subjects is initiated. The stepwise approach continues with clinical studies including assessment of immunogenicity and pharmacokinetics or pharmacodynamics to establish safety and efficacy equivalency. The extent to which the clinical studies are carried out needs to be scientifically justified.

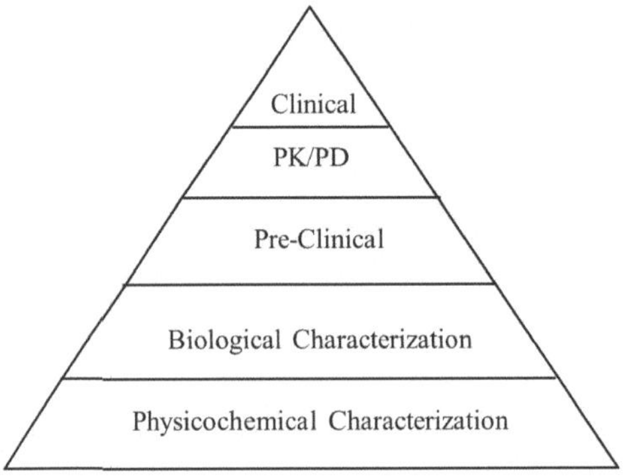

FIGURE 10.1
FDA's stepwise approach to demonstrate biosimilarity.

The FDA guidance clearly states that approval of biosimilar applications is based on the totality of the data and information submitted in the application. In its review, the FDA will use a risk-based approach to evaluating all available data and information submitted (FDA 2015a). The remainder of this chapter is as follows. Section 10.2 provides an outline of the tiered testing approaches. In Section 10.3, various statistical approaches are evaluated for Tier 1 testing. In Section 10.4, based on the work of Yang et al. (2016), we introduce a Bayesian method for demonstrating analytical similarity. The method takes into account the potential correlation among drug product lots as well as critical quality attributes. In Section 10.5, a Bayesian solution is presented for Tier 2 testing. Finally, a concluding discussion is provided in Section 10.6.

10.2 Analytical Similarity Assessment

10.2.1 A Tiered Approach

Demonstration of analytical similarity is the key step in the overall biosimilar development. Although there are many quality attributes (QAs) that can be used to characterize a biological product, their impact on the product safety, efficacy, and quality varies, making it difficult to generalize the testing of QAs for biosimilar equivalence. In addition, due to limited availability of both the proposed test product (TP) and RP lots, it is impractical to ensure sufficient power for testing a large number of QAs. Therefore, consistent with the risk-based product/process development principles in ICH Q9 (2005), ICH Q10 (2009), ICH Q8(R2) (2009), and ICH Q11 (2012), the FDA recommends that an analytical similarity assessment be carried out using a tiered system in which approaches of varying statistical rigor are used. The system begins with a risk assessment of all QAs with regard to their potential impact on activity, pharmacokinetics/pharmacodynamics, safety, and immunogenicity with quality. Considerations are given to both severity and probability of occurrence. Figure 10.2 illustrates a scoring system for determining criticality of QAs. In this particular method, the total risk score is defined as the product of severity and occurrence Yang et al. (2016). The highest risk, middle risk, and lowest risk corresponds to risk scores ≥ 10, $4 \leq$ scores ≤ 9, and scores ≤ 3, respectively.

Severity	5	5	10	15	20	25
	4	4	8	12	16	20
	3	3	6	9	12	15
	2	2	4	6	8	10
	1	1	2	3	4	5
	0	1	2	3	4	5
		Ocurrence				

FIGURE 10.2
Risk ranking based on severity and occurrence (adapted from Yang et al. (2018)).

There are other risk-based assessment tools, such as failure effect mode analysis (FEMA), that can also be used to determine the criticality of QAs (FDA, 2016). Risk ranking is performed in order to justify the relative importance of individual QAs. After a score is assigned to each QA commensurate with its risk, the QA is classified into either Tier 1, 2, or 3, corresponding to the highest risk, middle risk, and lowest risk, respectively.

For particular regulatory applications, the FDA has provided advice on statistical approaches for demonstration of analytical similarity (Chow, 2014; FDA, 2015d). A statistical test of equivalence of means is recommended for Tier 1 QAs. For Tier 2 QAs, a large proportion of individual values of the biosimilar product must fall inside a quality range based on data collected from the RP. For Tier 3 QAs, examination of the data using graphical comparisons is considered appropriate. We now consider statistical issues with the recommended Tier 1 and Tier 2 approaches.

10.2.2 Equivalence Test for Tier 1 QAs

For testing analytical similarity of Tier 1 QAs, the following hypotheses are tested for each QA:

$$H_0 : \mu_R - \mu_T \leq -\delta \text{ or } \mu_R - \mu_T \geq \delta \qquad (10.1)$$
$$H_A : \delta < \mu_R - \mu_T < \delta$$

where μ_R and μ_T denote the means of reference and test (proposed biosimilar) products and δ is the equivalence margin. Similarity of this QA is established if the null hypothesis is rejected.

Under these conditions, the hypotheses in eq. (10.1) may be tested via two one-sided tests (TOST) (Schuirmann, 1987). Let X_{Ri} ($i = 1, ..., N_R$) and X_{Ti} ($i = 1, ..., N_T$) be the test results of reference and test products, respectively. It is assumed that X_{Ri} are independently and identically distributed (i.i.d.) normal random variables with mean μ_R and variance σ_R^2, and X_{Ti} are i.i.d. normal random variables with mean μ_T and variance σ_T^2. A TOST can be used to test eq. (10.1) with test statistics

$$T_L = \frac{\bar{X}_R - \bar{X}_T + \delta}{\mathrm{SE}(\bar{X}_R - \bar{X}_T)} \quad \text{and} \quad T_U = \frac{\bar{X}_R - \bar{X}_T - \delta}{\mathrm{SE}(\bar{X}_R - \bar{X}_T)} \tag{10.2}$$

where $\bar{X}_R$ and $\bar{X}_T$ denote the sample means of the reference and test products, respectively, and $\mathrm{SE}(\bar{X}_R - \bar{X}_T)$ is the estimated standard error of the difference of sample means.

If $\sigma_T \neq \sigma_R$, then $\mathrm{SE}(\bar{X}_R - \bar{X}_T) = \sqrt{S_R^2/N_R + S_T^2/N_T}$ where S_R^2 and S_T^2 denote the sample variances of reference and test product data. The degrees of freedom associated with T_L and T_U are often approximated by the Sattherthwaite method (Satterthwaite, 1946). If $\sigma_T = \sigma_R$, then $\mathrm{SE}(\bar{X}_R - \bar{X}_T) = S_{\text{Pooled}}\sqrt{1/N_R + 1/N_T}$ where $S_{\text{Pooled}} = \sqrt{((N_R - 1)S_R^2 + (N_T - 1)S_T^2)/(N_R + N_T - 2)}$ and the degrees of freedom associated with T_L and T_U are $N_R + N_T - 2$. Operationally, the TOST is equivalent to a confidence interval approach that rejects the null hypothesis in eq. (10.1) with a significance level of 5% when the 90% two-sided confidence interval on $\mu_R - \mu_T$ is entirely contained within $(-\delta, \delta)$ (Chow and Liu, 2008). The two tests mentioned in this section are hereafter referred to as TOST1 ($\sigma_T \neq \sigma_R$) and TOST2 ($\sigma_T = \sigma_R$).

As noted by Yang et al. (2016), the equivalence acceptance criterion (EAC) is a value δ that is practically meaningful within the scientific context of the investigation. Unfortunately, establishment of a scientifically based EAC across all QAs has been elusive. As noted by Shen et al. (2015), there is no clinically or scientifically justified EAC available, nor is there a unified statistical method for determining EAC. One statistically-based EAC is proposed by Liao and Darken (2013) in which the EAC is based on a plausibility interval derived from comparing the RP against itself. To fill this void, the FDA recently used an equivalence margin of $\delta = 1.5\sigma_R$ (FDA, 2015b). Since σ_R is unknown, it was estimated by a sample of RP lots using the sample standard deviation, S_R. As pointed out by Shen et al. (2015), Burdick (2015), and Burdick and Ramírez (2015), there are several good reasons for using this EAC to demonstrate analytical similarity:

1. It provides a criterion in a situation where no scientifically-based EAC is available;
2. The criterion can be applied across all products and QAs;
3. The criterion appropriately considers practical sample sizes for biosimilar lots; and
4. Sponsors are rewarded appropriately for increasing biosimilar lots.

10.2.3 Quality Range Approach for Tier 2 QAs

A quality range approach is used for similarity assessment of Tier 2 QAs. The quality range is defined as

$$\mu_R \pm K \times \sigma_R \tag{10.3}$$

where K should be appropriately justified. Considerations for selecting K are discussed in Yang et al. (2018). As with the Tier 1 attributes, μ_R and σ_R are replaced with sample estimates $\bar{X}_R$ and S_R, respectively. The test product passes Tier 2 if a predefined proportion (e.g., 90%) of the measured assay responses from the test lots falls within the quality range.

10.2.4 Raw Data/Graphical Comparison for Tier 3 QAs

For Tier 3 QAs, similarity assessment is carried out by displaying data with graphical representations. As these QAs have the lowest impact on product safety, efficacy, and quality, it is not necessary to perform more stringent statistical evaluations.

10.3 Alternative Statistical Approaches for Tier 1 QAs

Reference drug product lots may be correlated if sourced from the same drug substance or formulated bulk. As noted by Weese and Burdick (2015), correlation among RP lots can lead to an inflated Type I error rate for the TOST; that is, the probability of falsely declaring analytical similarity when analytical similarity is not obtained is greater than desired. Through a series of simulations, they also demonstrated the power of the test in the alternative space considered by Tsong et al. (2015) is decreased.

Yang et al. (2016) extended the results of Weese and Burdick (2015) and provide a statistical confidence interval approach that achievess the desired Type I error rate when the nature of correlation can be identified. Through both theoretical derivations and simulations, it was demonstrated that when the RP lots are positively correlated, the sample standard deviation S_R under-estimates the true RP standard deviation, σ_R. This, along with the pooling of variances and degrees of freedom, are the root causes of the inflated Type I error rate and decreased power of the TOST mentioned above.

Weese and Burdick (2015) noted that when $\delta = 1.5\sigma_R$, the hypotheses in eq. (10.1) may be rewritten as

$$\begin{aligned} H_0 &: \frac{\mu_R - \mu_T}{\sigma_R} \leq -1.5 \text{ or } \frac{\mu_R - \mu_T}{\sigma_R} \geq 1.5 \\ H_A &: -1.5 < \frac{\mu_R - \mu_T}{\sigma_R} < 1.5 \end{aligned} \tag{10.4}$$

The ratio $(\mu_R - \mu_T)/\sigma_R$ is referred to as the effect size relative to the RP. Similar to the TOST tests described in Section 10.2.2, a 90% confidence interval on $(\mu_R - \mu_T)/\sigma_R$ can be used to reject H_0 if the computed confidence interval falls within the range from −1.5 to +1.5. Yang et al. (2016) derived three such confidence intervals under different assumptions using generalized confidence intervals (GCIs). GCIs are similar to Bayesian credible intervals, but founded on the fiducial inference concept (Weerahandi, 2004; Hanning, 2009).

The GCIs test the hypotheses in eq. (10.4) in the same manner that TOST1 and TOST2 test the hypotheses in eq (10.1). The difference is that the equivalence margin used with GCIs is fixed rather than random.

10.4 Bayesian Approach for Equivalence Testing of Tier 1 QAs

The hypotheses of eq.(10.4) are easily investigated with Bayesian methodology. The data models given by Yang et al. (2016) are provided here as M1, M2, and M3.

M1 (pooled variance):

$$X_{Ri}|\mu_R, \sigma \sim N(\mu_R, \sigma^2), \quad i = 1, ..., N_R \tag{10.5}$$

$$X_{Ti}|\mu_T, \sigma \sim N(\mu_T, \sigma^2), \quad i = 1, ..., N_T \tag{10.6}$$

M2 (unpooled variance):

$$X_{Ri}|\mu_R, \sigma_R \sim N(\mu_R, \sigma_R^2), \quad i = 1, ..., N_R \tag{10.7}$$

$$X_{Ti}|\mu_T, \sigma_T \sim N(\mu_T, \sigma_T^2), \quad i = 1, ..., N_T \tag{10.8}$$

M3 (unpooled variance, partially correlated RP lots):

$$X_{Rij}|\mu_R, L_i, \sigma_E \sim N(\mu_R + L_i, \sigma_E^2), \quad i = 1, ..., n \text{ (DS lots)}, \quad j = 1, ..., r \text{ (DP lots)} \tag{10.9}$$

$$L_i|\sigma_L \sim N(0, \sigma_L^2), \quad i = 1, ..., n \tag{10.10}$$

$$X_{Ti}|\mu_T, \sigma_T \sim N(\mu_T, \sigma_T^2), \quad i = 1, ..., N_T \tag{10.11}$$

The total sample size for RP is $N_R = nr$. The within-lot correlation is $\rho_R = \sigma_L^2/\sigma_R^2$, where $\sigma_R^2 = \sigma_L^2 + \sigma_E^2$. For example, if a sample consists of $N_R = 4$ drug product (DP) lots, where each of $n = 2$ drug substance (DS) lots are used to source $r = 2$ DP lots each, the covariance matrix takes the form

$$\begin{pmatrix} \sigma_L^2 + \sigma_E^2 & \sigma_L^2 & 0 & 0 \\ \sigma_L^2 & \sigma_L^2 + \sigma_E^2 & 0 & 0 \\ 0 & 0 & \sigma_L^2 + \sigma_E^2 & \sigma_L^2 \\ 0 & 0 & \sigma_L^2 & \sigma_L^2 + \sigma_E^2 \end{pmatrix}. \tag{10.12}$$

The total RP standard deviation, $\sigma_R = \sqrt{\sigma_R^2}$, is the denominator in eq. 10.4. If $r = 1$ for M3, the system collapses to M2.

After choosing an appropriate likelihood model (M1, M2, or M3) for the data and appropriate prior distributions for the model parameters, the posterior probability $p = \Pr(-1.5 < (\mu_R - \mu_T)/\sigma_R < 1.5|\text{data})$ may be calculated. If, say, $p \geq p_0$ (e.g., $p_0 = 0.9$), the decision is to accept H_A; otherwise tier 1 biosimilarity cannot be declared. This differs from the frequentist approach proposed by the FDA (2018) and by Yang et al. (2016) in that our proposed posterior probability is a two-sided test and the latter use a two one-sided testing approach.

Because H_0 and H_A are mutually exclusive, $1 - p$ is the posterior probability to declare H_0 and, unlike frequentist testing, one may accept H_0 if $1 - p \geq p_0$. Another popular Bayesian testing approach uses the Bayes factor, given by

$$BF = \frac{\Pr(H_A|\text{data})}{\Pr(H_0|\text{data})} \times \frac{\Pr(H_0)}{\Pr(H_A)} \tag{10.13}$$

to quantify the support for one hypotheis over the other (Kass and Raftery, 1995). If, one assumes, a priori, that $\Pr(H_0) = \Pr(H_A)$, then the Bayes factor is $BF = p/(1-p)$ and, equivalently, $p = BF/(1+BF)$. For this situation, the Bayes factor $BF \geq BF_0$ provides the same decision-making mechanism as $p \geq p_0$.

It is straightforward to evaluate the hypotheses in eq. (10.4) under the three different data models. It is reasonable to assume vaguely-informative priors for mean parameters, such as $\mu_R, \mu_T \sim N(\mu_0, \sigma_0^2)$ so that the distribution covers that the data completely while staying within plausible boundaries. For example, if product specification limits are 50–150 units, then, for most problems, $\mu_0 = 100$ and $\sigma_0 = 20$ will constrain the mean parameters to a reasonable space without adding information to the likelihood. As suggested by Gelman et al. (2013), half Cauchy distributions for the standard deviation parameters are good vague priors.

10.4.1 Illustrations with `brms`

A computer-generated data set will be used to illustrate Bayesian hypothesis testing of eq. (10.4) using the `brm()` function from the `brms` library in R (R Core Team, 2021). The `brms` library provides a simplified interface to the Stan library (Carpenter et al., 2017), a Bayesian computing language, for a large variety of problems.

In the R language, let `d` denote a data.frame constructed as

```
nR = 20
xR = c(88.7, 92.1, 93.5, 93.7, 94.4, 94.6, 95.1, 95.3, 95.9,
       97, 97.8, 97.9, 98.2, 98.8, 99, 100.2, 101.5, 103.5,
       107.6, 109)
nT = 10
xT = c(89.2, 98.5, 100, 100.2, 101.4, 103.6, 104.2, 105.3,
       108.9, 112.8)
d = data.frame(x=c(xR, xT), Source=factor( rep(c("RP", "TP"),
                                          c(nR, nT)) ))
```

Model M1:

It may be reasonable to assume that the RP and TP data share a standard deviation, which is the assumption under M1. The Bayesian model fit and test of eq. (10.4) is given by the following lines of code, which set the priors to $\mu_R, \mu_T \sim N(100, 20^2)$ and $\sigma \sim$ half-Cauchy$(0, 1)$.

```
  ## Set priors
bprior = prior(normal(100, 20), class=b) + prior(cauchy(0, 1),
                                          class = sigma)
  ## Fit model
fit.m1 = brm( x~Source-1, data=d, prior=bprior,
              chains=4, warmup=2000, iter=2000+10000, cores=4)
  ## Extract posterior parameters
post.m1 = as.matrix(fit.m1)
  ## Test eq 6.4
```

```
ratio.m1 = (post.m1[,"b_SourceRP"] -
            post.m1[,"b_SourceTP"])/post.m1[,"sigma"]
p.m1 = mean( ratio.m1 > -1.5 & ratio.m1 < 1.5 )
```

In `fit.m1`, we opted to sample from the posterior distribution with four independent chains (`chains=4`). Sampling from multiple chains permits an evaluation to determine if the MCMC algorithm has reached equilibrium. We also selected 2,000 burn-in samples (warmup) and 10,000 posterior draws (`iter=12000`, which includes the warmup), which, for ANOVA modeling is sufficient. The output shows successful draws from the posterior distribution with Rhat $= 1$ for all parameters, large effective sample sizes (ESS), and an inspection (not shown) of the trace plots and density plots. The output from `fit.m1` is shown below.

```
Family: gaussian
  Links: mu = identity; sigma = identity
Formula: x ~ Source - 1
   Data: d (Number of observations: 30)
  Draws: 4 chains, each with iter = 12000; warmup = 2000; thin = 1;
         total post-warmup draws = 40000

Population-Level Effects:
         Estimate Est.Error l-95% CI u-95% CI Rhat Bulk_ESS Tail_ESS
SourceRP    97.72      1.25    95.26   100.17 1.00    36002    27798
SourceTP   102.40      1.75    98.94   105.87 1.00    32890    26089

Family Specific Parameters:
      Estimate Est.Error l-95% CI u-95% CI Rhat Bulk_ESS Tail_ESS
sigma     5.51      0.76     4.27     7.27 1.00    31970    25271

Draws were sampled using sampling(NUTS). For each parameter, Bulk_ESS
and Tail_ESS are effective sample size measures, and Rhat is the
potential scale reduction factor on split chains (at convergence,
Rhat = 1).
```

The posterior probability p is 0.94, which shows good evidence to declare biosimilarity.

Model M2:
When different standard deviations are assumed for the RP and TP batches, either separate models may be fitted to the RP and TP data or a model term may be added to the `brm()` formula. We prefer the former, but computer code is provided for both approaches. To add a model for the variance as a function of the `Source`(RP or TP), the formula interface `x~Source-1` is extended to `bf( x~Source-1, sigma~Source-1)`. The prior for the standard deviation terms is on the natural logarithm scale so that the prior is set to $\log(\sigma_{\text{source}}) \sim \pi(\cdot)$. If the `bprior` was applied to the M2 model, the prior for σ_R, σ_T are both log-Cauchy$(0, 1)$, which is not a bad choice, but is different from the half-Cauchy$(0, 1)$ previously assigned. To accommodate the model for the log standard deviation, the `bprior` priors are changed to

```
## log-Cauchy prior for sigma[R] and sigma[T]
bprior = prior(normal(100, 20), class=b) +
         prior(cauchy(0, 1), class = b, dpar=sigma)
```

To set the prior for the standard deviation parameters on the original scale, we recommend fitting separate models to the RP and TP data with `brm()`. Because the model only contains an intercept term, the prior `class` is changed from `b` to `Intercept`.

```
  ## Set priors
bprior = prior(normal(100, 20), class=Intercept) +
         prior(cauchy(0, 1), class = sigma)
  ## Fit separate models for RP and TP
fit.m2.R = brm( x~(1), data=subset(d, Source=="RP"),
                prior=bprior,chains=4, warmup=2000,
                iter=2000+10000, cores=4 )
fit.m2.T = brm( x~(1), data=subset(d, Source=="TP"),
                prior=bprior,chains=4, warmup=2000,
                iter=2000+10000, cores=4 )

  ## Extract posterior parameters
post.m2.R = as.matrix(fit.m2.R)
post.m2.T = as.matrix(fit.m2.T)

  ## Test eq 6.4
ratio.m2 = (post.m2.R[,"b_Intercept"] -
              post.m2.T[,"b_Intercept"]) /
              post.m2.R[,"sigma"]
p.m2 = mean( ratio.m2 > -1.5 & ratio.m2 < 1.5 )
```

As before, the output shows successful draws from the posterior distribution with Rhat = 1 for all parameters, large effective sample sizes (ESS), and an inspection (not shown) of the trace plots and density plots shows good agreement across the four chains. The output from `fit.m2.R` and `fit.m2.T` are shown below.

```
> fit.m2.R
 Family: gaussian
  Links: mu = identity; sigma = identity
Formula: x ~ (1)
   Data: subset(d, Source == "RP") (Number of observations: 20)
  Draws: 4 chains, each with iter = 12000; warmup = 2000; thin = 1;
         total post-warmup draws = 40000

Population-Level Effects:
          Estimate Est.Error l-95% CI u-95% CI Rhat Bulk_ESS Tail_ESS
```

```
Intercept    97.70      1.14    95.44    99.94 1.00    27623    23125

Family Specific Parameters:
      Estimate Est.Error l-95% CI u-95% CI Rhat Bulk_ESS Tail_ESS
sigma     5.03      0.84     3.71     6.96 1.00    27522    22703

Draws were sampled using sampling(NUTS). For each parameter, Bulk_ESS
and Tail_ESS are effective sample size measures, and Rhat is the
potential scale reduction factor on split chains (at convergence,
Rhat = 1).

> fit.m2.T
 Family: gaussian
  Links: mu = identity; sigma = identity
Formula: x ~ (1)
   Data: subset(d, Source == "TP") (Number of observations: 10)
  Draws: 4 chains, each with iter = 12000; warmup = 2000; thin = 1;
         total post-warmup draws = 40000

Population-Level Effects:
          Estimate Est.Error l-95% CI u-95% CI Rhat Bulk_ESS Tail_ESS
Intercept   102.38      2.12    98.12   106.64 1.00    21604    18849

Family Specific Parameters:
      Estimate Est.Error l-95% CI u-95% CI Rhat Bulk_ESS Tail_ESS
sigma     6.54      1.65     4.22    10.52 1.00    22486    20318

Draws were sampled using sampling(NUTS). For each parameter, Bulk_ESS
and Tail_ESS are effective sample size measures, and Rhat is the
potential scale reduction factor on split chains (at convergence,
Rhat = 1).
```

Unsurprisingly, because the standard deviation parameter distributions had to be estimated separately, the posterior probability p dropped to 0.87. Because $p < 0.90$ (or the pre-defined cutoff), we would not be able to declare biosimilarity of the test and reference products. The same probability was derived when using the single `brm()` call to model the standard deviations separately for each source.

Model M3:
For model M3, it is assumed that some of the reference DP batches are sourced from the same DS lots so that correlation is induced into the model. A data frame (`d.R`) for the reference data is created with partial correlation $\rho_R = 0.8$ introduced by generating four DP reference batches for each of five DS lots with the following code.

```
set.seed(424)
d.R = data.frame( Lot=factor(rep(1:5, each=4)), x=NA )
sigmaR = 5
rhoR = 0.8
sigmaL = sqrt(rhoR)*sigmaR
sigmaE = sqrt(1-rhoR)*sigmaR
```

```
d.R$x = 100 + rnorm(5, mean=0, sd=sigmaL)[unclass(d.R$Lot)] +
              rnorm(nrow(d.R), mean=0, sd=sigmaE)
ggplot(d.R, aes(Lot, x) ) + geom_jitter(width=0.05) +
      ylab("Value")
```

The data are shown in Figure 10.3.

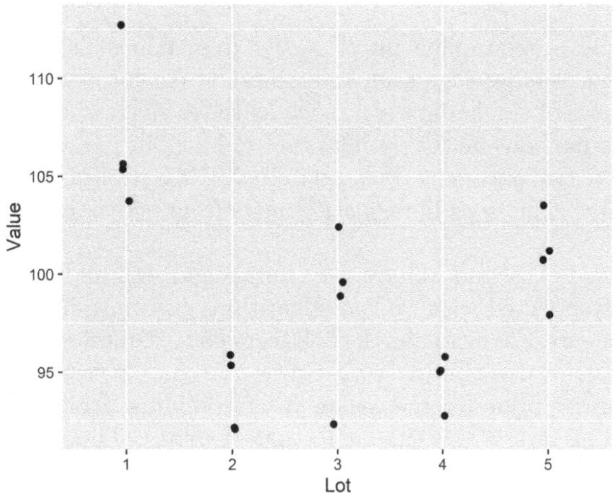

FIGURE 10.3
Reference lots with partial correlation.

For model M3, we add the priors $\sigma_L, \sigma_E \sim$ half-Cauchy$(0, 1)$ and fit the model in `brm()` using the variance-components model. The number of warmups and MCMC iterations were raised to reflect the increased model complexity. The model `fit.m2.T` is retained from the previous code snippet.

```
  ## Set priors
bprior.m3 = prior(normal(100, 20), class=Intercept) +
        prior(cauchy(0, 1), class = sd) + ## prior for sigmaL
        prior(cauchy(0, 1), class=sigma)  ## prior for sigmaE
  ## Fit model
fit.m3.R = brm( x~(1|Lot), data=d.R, prior=bprior.m3,
              chains=4, warmup=10000, iter=10000+25000,
              cores=4 )
  ## Extract posterior parameters
post.m3.R = as.matrix(fit.m3.R)
  ## Get posterior for sigma.R = sqrt( sigmaL^2 + sigmaE^2 )
sigma.R = sqrt( post.m3.R[,"sd_Lot__Intercept"]^2 +
                post.m3.R[,"sigma"]^2 )
  ## Test eq 4
ratio.m3 = (post.m3.R[,"b_Intercept"] -
```

```
                  post.m2.T[,"b_Intercept"])/sigma.R
p.m3 = mean( ratio.m3 > -1.5 & ratio.m3 < 1.5 )
```

With model M3, the posterior probability p is 0.94, which again shows support for a biosimilarity declaration.

10.4.2 Simulation

Because of its simple programming interface, its tremendous flexibility, and its reliance on the well-respected, leading-edge Stan programming platform, we recommend the brms library for the analysis of single data sets, such as those given in this chapter. For simulations, however, brms may not be the optimal choice. Flexibility in brms comes with a price, namely a compilation step and reduced speed in its MCMC procedures compared to certain competitor procedures. The brms library also suffers from occasional stability issues, which may deter users.

Because models M1, M2, and M3 are very simple and well understood, for simulations, the user may be better served with MCMC algorithms custom tailored for linear modeling and variance components. For example, the MCMCregress() function in the MCMCpack library draws from the posterior distribution with Gibbs sampling by constraining the prior into semi-conjugacy (normal prior for the mean, inverse-gamma prior for the variance). The MCMCregress() coding interface is similar to that of brm(). The MCMCregress() function runs a single MCMC chain with default burn in, number of draws, and vague prior that are typically sufficient for most problems. Replacing fit.m1, fit.m2.R, and fit.m2.T from the previous section, the code is given by the following with seed values (replacing the default seed = 12345) provided to ensure that each model starts at a different point in the pseudo-random number generator.

```
fit.m1 = MCMCregress( x~Source-1, data=d, seed=241 )
fit.m2.R = MCMCregress( x~(1), data=subset(d, Source=="RP"),
                       seed=5152 )
fit.m2.T = MCMCregress( x~(1), data=subset(d, Source=="TP"),
                        seed=890 )
```

For model M3, the MCMCpack library does contain the function MCMChregress() for variance components; however, for simulations, we recommend the mature library MCMCglmm with function MCMCglmm(). As with MCMCregress(), its increase in speed over brm() comes with prior constraints, namely a normal prior for the means and inverse-gamma (or inverse-Wishart) for the variance components. MCMCglmm() also runs a single MCMC chain. Replacement code for fit.m3.R using MCMCglmm() is shown below.

```
  ## The priors are sigma[L]^2 ~ inverse-chisquare(df=0.001)
  ##                 sigma[E]^2 ~ inverse-chisquare(df=0.001)
prior.Rcorr = list(R=list(V=1, nu=0.002),
                   G=list(G1=list(V=1, nu=0.002)))
```

```
fit.m3.R = MCMCglmm(fixed=x~(1), random=~Lot, data=d.R,
                    nitt=50000, thin=1, burnin=10000,
                    prior=prior.Rcorr)
```

Using `MCMCregress()` and `MCMCglmm()`, the resulting posterior probabilities given by the R variables `p.m1`, `p.m2`, and `p.m3`, were equivalent to the `brm()` results from the previous section.

We performed simulation testing of the hypotheses in eq. (10.4) using `MCMCregress()` and `MCMCglmm()` in order to gauge the frequentist long-term properties of type I error (i.e., test size) and statistical power. In addition, model misspecification was also examined by fitting models M1 and M2 to data generated under model M3. Test size and power were estimated by Monte Carlo simulation with the posterior probability p. The simulation scenarios, shown in Table 10.1, are a subset of those posed by Yang et al. (2016). The cutoff $p_0 = 0.95$ was applied so that H_A is declared whenever $p = \Pr(-1.5 < (\mu_R - \mu_T)/\sigma_R < 1.5|\text{data}) \geq 0.95$. For each scenario 10,000 Monte Carlo runs were performed to estimate the power, defined here as $\Pr(p \geq 0.95|\text{Scenario})$.

TABLE 10.1
Simulation parameters for Tier 1.

N_R	N_T	$(\mu_R - \mu_T)/\sigma_R$	ρ_R	r	σ_T/σ_R
10, 20	10	1/8, 1.5	0	–	0.5, 1, 2
10, 20	10	1/8, 1.5	0.8	2, 5	0.5, 1, 2

The parameters $(\mu_R - \mu_T)/\sigma_R = 1/8$ represents a scenario that should declare in favor of H_A. The simulated power at $(\mu_R - \mu_T)/\sigma_R = 1/8$ is of interest because it is the point on the power curve evaluated by the FDA in selecting the present equivalence margin of $1.5\sigma_R$. On the other hand, $(\mu_R - \mu_T)/\sigma_R = 1.5$ represents a scenario on the H_0/H_A border, which should result in an H_A declaration about 5% of the time. It is expected that power will be higher whenever $N_R = 20$ (vs $N_R = 10$) and when σ_T/σ_R is smaller.

Results for test size are shown in Figure 10.4, in which a line is drawn at the nominal test size of 0.05. Wherever the data model (M1, M2, M3) assumptions are met with the scenario's data generation, the Bayesian procedure appears to adhere well to frequentist properties, yielding test sizes at or below the 0.05 limit. The reference lots sample size ($N_R = 10, 20$) did not play a role in the long-term test size result. It is clear that pooling the standard deviation (M1) provides the least robust method, leading to false H_A declarations just north of 30% when $(\sigma_R/\sigma_T) = 0.5$, regardless of the value of the number of reference DS batches (r). The pooled standard deviation method also struggles when $r > 1$, except in the case where $(\sigma_R/\sigma_T) = 2$. The unpooled model (M2) resulted in the nominal test size whenever $r = 1$, but type I error starts to rise when $r > 1$. Finally, when $r > 1$, the unpooled + corr (M3) model performed well for all cases. In terms of test size, models M2 and M3 are recommended, respectively, for the cases $r = 1$ and $r > 1$.

Results for statistical power are shown in Figure 10.5, showing cases from Figure 10.4 for which the Monte Carlo test size < 0.07. A line is drawn at 0.80 to guide the eye. A quick look at Figure 10.5 unsurprisingly shows higher statistical power whenever the larger number of reference lots are generated ($N_R = 20$). In all cases for which $(\sigma_R/\sigma_T) = 0.5$, statistical power is appropriately low, reflecting the fact that the test lot data are twice as noisy as the

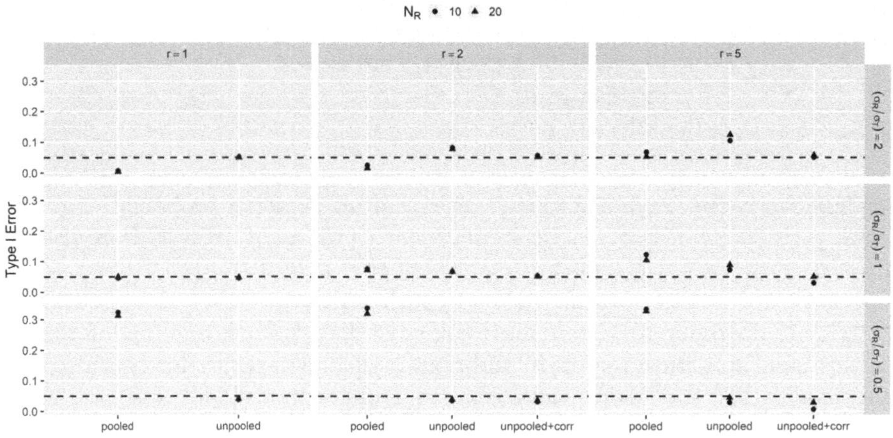

FIGURE 10.4
Long-term Monte Carlo type I error (test size) to decalre H_A in eq. (10.4) for Tier 1 acceptance criteria with line drawn at 0.05.

reference lots. For the cases $r = 1$ and $(\sigma_R/\sigma_T) \geq 1$, statistical power is near to or above 0.80. As noted in Yang et al. (2016), when reference lots are partially correlated, statistical power drops considerably, even when model M3 is fitted to the data. The relatively small size of the reference data results in a less confident posterior distribution when σ_R comprises two variance components instead of one.

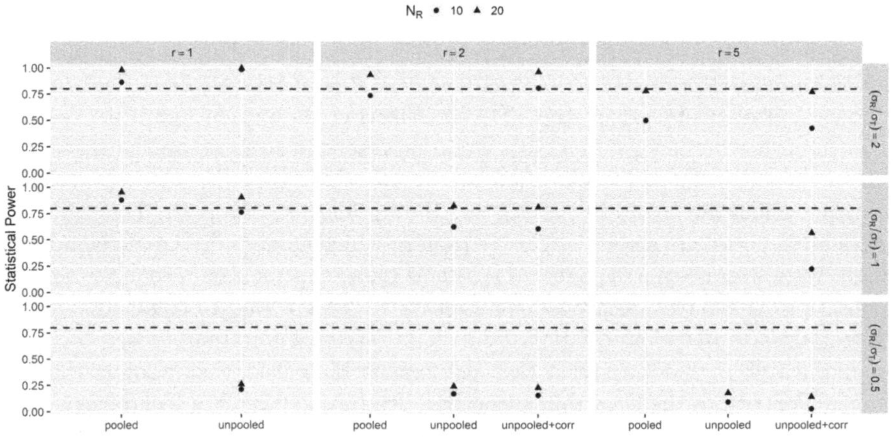

FIGURE 10.5
Long-term Monte Carlo type I error (test size) to decalre H_A in eq. (10.4) for Tier 1 acceptance criteria with line drawn at 0.8.

10.5 Bayesian Approach for Equivalence Testing of Tier 2 QAs

In Tier 2 testing, the test product is declared similar to the reference if a large proportion, q, of measured test-lot values are contained in the interval $(-\Delta_K, \Delta_K)$, where $\Delta_K = \bar{X}_R + KS_R$ and $\bar{X}_R$ and S_R are the sample mean and standard deviation from the reference lots. Yang et al. (2016) propose a two one-sided parametric tolerance interval (Krishnamoorthy and Mathew, 2009) test to compare

$$\begin{aligned} H_0 &: \text{Fewer than } 100 \times q\% \text{ of test lots lie between } -\Delta_K \text{ and } \Delta_K \\ H_A &: \text{At least } 100 \times q\% \text{ of test lots lie between } -\Delta_K \text{ and } \Delta_K \end{aligned} \tag{10.14}$$

Yang et al. (2016) construct the parametric tolerance intervals via GCIs with $q = 0.9$. Instead, we propose testing eq. (10.14) with the Bayesian posterior probability

$$p_q = \Pr\left(\Phi\left(\frac{\Delta_K - \mu_T}{\sigma_T}\right) - \Phi\left(\frac{-\Delta_K - \mu_T}{\sigma_T}\right) > q \middle| \text{data}\right), \tag{10.15}$$

where $\Phi(\cdot)$ is the standard normal cumulative distribution function. A decision can be made to accept H_A if, say, $p_q \geq 0.95$. As with our suggested test method for eq. (10.4), the posterior probability is a two-sided test.

To demonstrate the method, we conducted a simulation with parameters shown in Table 10.2. Reference and test lots are generated with $\mu_R = \mu_T$ and $\sigma_R = \sigma_T$. For the case $\rho_R = 0$, data are generated from model M2 (or M3 with $r = 1$). For the case $\rho_R > 0$, data are generated from model M3 with the number of DP reference batches per DS lot set to $r = 2$. The data were fitted via either `MCMCregress()` or `MCMCglmm()` as in the previous section using the model from which the data were generated (either M2 or M3). The cutoff $p_0 = 0.95$ was applied so that H_A in (10.14) is declared whenever

$$p_q = \Pr\left(\Phi\left(\frac{\Delta_K - \mu_T}{\sigma_T}\right) - \Phi\left(\frac{-\Delta_K - \mu_T}{\sigma_T}\right) > q|\text{data}\right) \geq 0.95. \tag{10.16}$$

For each scenario 10,000 Monte Carlo runs were performed to estimate the power, defined here as $\Pr(p_q \geq 0.95|\text{ Scenario})$.

TABLE 10.2
Simulation parameters for Tier 2.

N_R	N_T	ρ_R	r	K	q
16	8, 10	0 – 0.8	2	2, 3	0.8, 0.9

For model M2, for some positive integer value of K, letting `Y.r` denote a vector of reference product values, Δ_K is computed as

```
xbar.R = mean(Y.r)
sigma.hat.R = sd(Y.r)
delta.K = xbar.R + K*sigma.hat.R
```

For model M3, Δ_K is computed as

```
fit.R = lmer( Y.r~(1|Batch) )
xbar.R = mean(Y.r)
sigma.hat.R = sqrt( VarCorr(fit.R)[["Batch"]][1,1] +
                    sigma(fit.R)^2 )
delta.K = xbar.R + K*sigma.hat.R
```

Letting `Y.t` denote the test product values, the test data are modeled by

```
## For some positive integer zzz
fit.T = MCMCregress(Y.t~(1), seed=zzz)
```

The posterior probability p_q is calculated as

```
pr.q = mean(
          pnorm( (delta.K-fit.T[,"(Intercept)"]) /
                    sqrt(fit.T[,"sigma2"]) ) -
          pnorm( (-delta.K-fit.T[,"(Intercept)"]) /
          sqrt(fit.T[,"sigma2"]) ) >= q )
```

Results of the simulation are shown in Figure 10.6. As expected, and in line with results from Yang et al. (2016), the Tier 2 statistical power is higher for $K = 3$ compared to $K = 2$. Similarly, power is higher for the case $q = 0.8$ compared to $q = 0.9$. Whereas larger partial correlation in the reference lots (ρ_R) appeared detrimental to statistical power in Yang et al. (2016) (see Yang et al. (2016), Figure 8), it did appear to have an appreciable impact on statistical power with the Bayesian procedure.

10.6 Concluding Remarks

Analytical characterizations are the most sensitive measures for assessing similarity between a biosimilar and reference product. The FDA draft guidance recommends a tiered approach and use of statistical methods for assessing analytical similarity. When appropriately applied, statistical methods can provide a high degree of confidence for demonstration of analytical similarity. However, development of such statistical methods can be challenging due to the limited number of reference lots and lack of knowledge concerning their sourcing information. Further compounding the issue is the fact that Tier 1 and Tier 2 acceptance criteria must be established using RP lots. The uncertainties in these acceptance criteria have been shown to inflate the type I error rate and reduce statistical power. For Tier 1 evaluations, these issues can be mitigated by reformulating the analytical similarity hypotheses

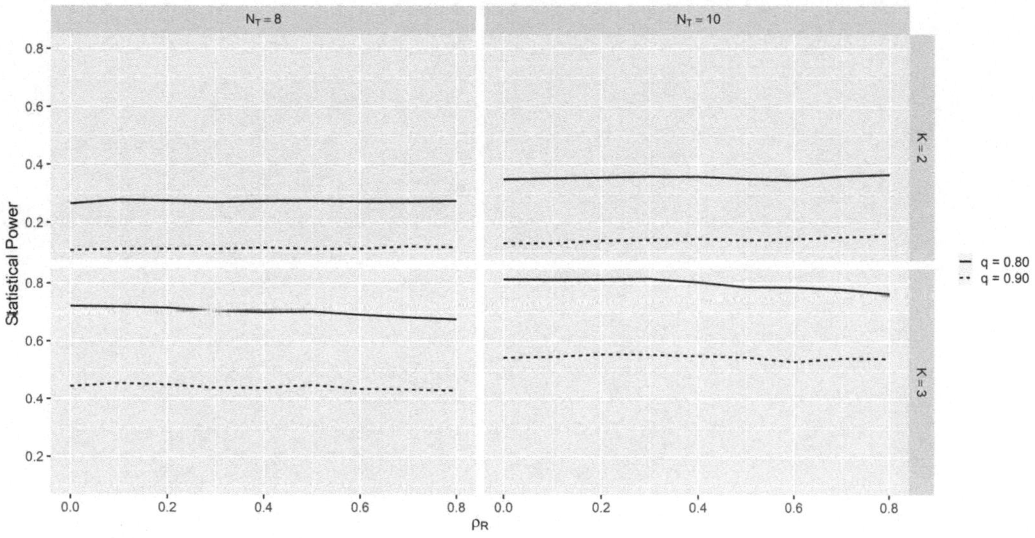

FIGURE 10.6
Long-term Monte Carlo probability to decalre H_A in eq. (10.14) for Tier 2 acceptance criteria.

in terms of the effect size. To test the new hypotheses, generalized confidence intervals can be used if product variances are not equal, or if an existing correlation structure in either the RP or TP lots can be identified. In this chapter, we propose three alternate Bayesian methods for demonstrating analytical similarity. The performance of these methods was evaluated through a simulation study and practice guide on the use of these methods discussed.

11

Bayesian Evaluation and Monitoring of Process Comparability

Ke Wang and Aili Cheng

Pharmaceutical Sciences and Manufacturing Statistics, Pfizer

CONTENTS

11.1 Introduction

Process change is quite common in the drug development process both during the development and post-approval. A process comparability assessment is needed to ensure the continuity and consistency of the drug quality. Depending on the types of change and stage of the development, the scrutiny level of the process comparability assessment will differ. Comparability testing is generally not as extensive for an approved product as it is for changes in early development phase. However, it should be as comprehensive as for an approved product if the changes occur in the late development stage and no additional clinical studies are planned to support biologics license application (BLA) (ICH Q5E, 2005; Brunelle, 2016). The data required for comparability is driven by the risk assessment of the change. The change associated with higher risk demands more comprehensive data (Lee et al., 2012). In

DOI: 10.1201/9781003255093-11

many cases a comparability protocol is recommended with predefined comparability criteria to allow an objective assessment (ICH Q5E, 2005).

For biological products, ICH Q5E (2005) provides a general guidance on two aspects: 1) comparing pre- and post-change product following the manufacturing changes; 2) assessing the impact of the observed differences as it relates to safety and efficacy. It points out that the goal of the process comparability exercise is to ensure the quality, safety, and efficacy of product produced by a change, through the collection and evaluation of the relevant data. The determination of process comparability is based on the assessment up to three levels: analytical tests, nonclinical, and clinical studies. "If a manufacturer can provide assurance of comparability through analytical studies alone, non-clinical or clinical studies with the post-change product are not warranted" (ICH Q5E, 2005).

Therefore, the demonstration of analytical comparability is a critical step needed to avoid unnecessary resource waste and effort for additional nonclinical/clinical studies. The demonstration of comparability does not necessarily mean that the quality attributes of the pre-change and post-change products are identical. It is not even realistic to demonstrate "sameness" given the natural variability of the process. The goal is to demonstrate that the processes are highly similar, and that the existing knowledge is sufficiently predictive to ensure that any differences in quality attributes have no adverse impact upon safety or efficacy of the product (ICH Q5E, 2005).

An analytical comparability exercise usually includes the assessment of three areas: batch release tests, characterization studies, and stability studies (ICH Q5E, 2005; Brunelle, 2016). In this chapter, we will focus on the statistical assessment for the quantitative batch release tests, which can be conducted at the time of release or in a side-by-side manner (SBS).

Several statistical approaches have been developed and applied for comparing two groups of data. Some commonly used statistical approaches can be summarized into two categories: 1) statistical intervals such as minimum and maximum, confidence intervals, prediction intervals, mean $\pm$ 3SD, and tolerance intervals; 2) hypothesis testing including t-test and equivalence test (see details in pages 331-356 of Burdick et al. (2017), and Chatfield et al. (2011)). The minimum and maximum are frequently used by scientists, but they have little predictive capability, in that the range of the current data does not necessarily represent the range of the future data. Furthermore, the min/max based on a limited sample size is subject to large uncertainty (Dong et al., 2015) and is often narrower than the true range of the data. It is also criticized by the European Medicines Agency (EMA) reflection paper on comparative assessment (EMA, 2017). Therefore, using the min/max is not recommended for comparability assessment. Other statistical intervals are simple to calculate and easy to use in the comparability setting, but require a sufficiently large sample size, specifically for the number of pre-change batches, if a prediction interval is used (See details in the comparability chapter of McCormac et al. (2021)). Even the quality range, in the form of mean$\pm k \times$SD as proposed by the Food and Drug Administration (FDA) similarity guidance (FDA, 2019a), requires at least 10 reference product batches and 6 to 10 proposed biosimilar batches.

The most common hypothesis test for demonstrating comparability in the mean is an equivalence test. However, meaningful equivalence criterion setting is one of the most challenging tasks for an equivalence test. Yu et al. (2017) proposed a Bayesian approach to setting an equivalence criterion that is linked to the allowable out of specification (OOS) rate. This approach not only provides a promising way to set a meaningful criterion, but also allows the proper use of historical data which often results in a reduced sample size required for the equivalence test. However, mean equivalence does not directly translate to process comparability where the comparability of the individual batch values often matters the most. It is worth noting that the available data and data structure vary quite a bit from project to project. It would be ideal if the comparability exercise is properly powered and designed by statistical principles, which often would result in balanced data structure (e.g., equal number of pre- and post-change batches) and a sufficiently large sample size to power the hypothesis test. However, the available data are often driven by operational factors such as the clinical need, the stage of the development, and the time of the comparability exercise. For instance, if it is a post-approval change of a monoclonal antibody, the number of pre-change batches could be relatively large, such as 10 or more. However, the number of post-change batches planned for the comparability exercise could be quite limited, such as 3 or 4. For expected post-approval changes, the comparability criterion needs to be set and documented in the comparability protocol before the post-change batches are produced. For the changes made during the development for gene therapy products, side-by-side tests are often required to reduce the impact of the assay variability on the comparison. However, depending on the indication and dose, only a few batches may be needed clinically, limiting the number of batches available for comparability (McCormac et al., 2021, see the comparability chapter). As a result, sample size imbalance and/or small sample sizes are very common in the process comparability setting. In such situations, the equivalence test may not be appropriate in that the result could be dominated by one of the processes.

Frequentist statistical intervals may not be appropriate either when the sample size, especially the pre-change sample size, is small. In real life applications, researchers' scientific priors and process knowledge plays a big part in driving the determination of the comparability criterion. However, this inevitably creates inconsistent results from project to project, depending on the project team's experience. This motivates us to formulate a simple and intuitive workflow that provides consistent quantification of scientific beliefs and the evaluation of the uncertainty associated with such beliefs. In this chapter, we demonstrate a straightforward method to establish a comparability criterion that could be applicable to all of the above comparability situations, including both balanced and unbalanced data, as well as large and small sample size situations.

Regulatory guidance points out that manufacturing control trends are more suitable to serve as comparability criteria in lieu of the release specification. ICH Q5E (2005) states that "Results within the established acceptance criteria, but outside historical manufacturing **control trends**, might suggest product differences that warrant additional study or analysis." All release test results are expected to meet the release specification. However, the release specifications themselves are not considered sufficient to serve as the comparability criteria. Therefore, the term "comparability criteria" is used for comparability assessment instead of the typical term "acceptance criteria". Acceptance criteria are used to determine if a batch is acceptable to be used in patients or healthy subjects. Generally speaking, a batch is acceptable if it meets specification limits. Comparability criteria might be tighter than specifications in that not meeting comparability criteria does not necessarily mean that a batch is out of specification.

Similar points have been expressed in an EMA (2021) and FDA (2016). Therefore defining "control trends" or comparability criteria based on historical manufacturing experience is a critical step for comparability assessment. Facing the limited sample size, Bayesian methodology permits the leveraging of similar manufacturing experience and scientific beliefs in the process comparability exercises.

We propose using the Bayesian highest density interval (HDI) based on the pre-change batches and relevant prior information to form the comparability criteria. Bayesian HDI has potential applicability to all of the above comparability situations, including balanced and unbalanced designs as well as large and small sample size situations. Moreover, it is straightforward and flexible enough to be adapted to multiple situations or quality attributes (for instance, quality attributes that may follow distributions other than the normal distribution).

The Bayesian approach is consistent with multiple guidelines. For instance, the FDA guidance for approval application recommended the use of prior knowledge sources such as related principles, literature, and manufacturing experience when assessing the impact of a change (FDA, 2021). The idea of developing a CMC database which gathers information from similar molecules and processes to be the prior knowledge was also discussed in the comparability workshop for the expedited development program for biological products (Schrieber et al., 1998). These guidelines together with ICH Q5E (2005) provide practical guidance on where to seek prior information, but no details on how.

For the rest of the chapter, we will describe the setup of the Bayesian framework for process comparability assessments. Since prior justification is the most challenging step in Bayesian application, a strategy on how to construct a prior and further assess the chosen prior in the context of process comparability is provided in a separate section, followed by a case study, summary and discussions.

11.2 Bayesian Setup for the Process Comparability Criteria

To establish the Bayesian version of the comparability criteria, i.e., HDI, two distributions need to be defined: the distribution for the quality attribute (i.e., the likelihood of the data), and the prior distribution for the related parameters.

11.2.1 Choice of the Distribution for the Quality Attribute

The underlying distribution of a quality attribute is determined by the data generating process, its scientific nature, and the available data collected so far. From a process control point of view, a quantity of interest from a well-controlled process is often described by a normal distribution centered at the expected value and variance equal to the process and analytical variances. However, the normal distribution is sensitive to "abnormal" values which can impact the estimation of the distribution parameters. The impact is more significant with small sample sizes. To reduce the influence of potentially unusual batches on the estimation of population distribution parameters, we proposed using a Student-t distribution to fit the batch data from the pre-change process.

Let y_i,$i = 1, ..., n$, be an observed pre-change process quality attribute value from the i-th batch, assuming it follows a Student-t distribution with mean μ_y, standard deviation σ_y, and degrees of freedom ν, i.e.,

$$y_i \sim t(\nu, \mu_y, \sigma_y) \tag{11.1}$$

To model this practically, the Stan density functional form of a Student-t distribution will be used, where the three parameters ν, μ_y, σ_y characterize the tails, the center, and the scale of a Student-t distribution (Stan Development Team, 2021b). Bayesian estimation of the parameters of the Student-t distribution was performed using the `rstan` package (Stan Development Team, 2021a) and R (R Core Team, 2021).

11.2.2 Choice of Prior Distribution

The following prior distributions are assigned to the parameters ν, μ_y, σ_y in the Student-t distribution

$$\mu_y \sim N(\mu_\mu, \sigma_\mu) \tag{11.2}$$

$$\sigma_y \sim \text{Half-Normal}(0, H) \tag{11.3}$$

$$\nu \sim \text{Gamma}(\alpha, \beta) \quad \text{with } \nu \geq 1 \tag{11.4}$$

Here, μ_y has a normal distribution with mean μ_μ, and standard deviation σ_μ. The parameter σ_y follows a half-normal distribution with mean 0 and standard deviation H. The degrees of freedom, ν, follows a Gamma distribution with shape parameter α and rate parameter β. For small sample size, a reasonable distribution for degrees of freedom is Gamma(2,0.1) (Juárez and Steel, 2010). As shown in the density plot in Figure 11.1, the Gamma(2,0.1) distribution is spread over a wide range of values but majority of its mass is placed on smaller values (< 50) and it has a mode at 10.

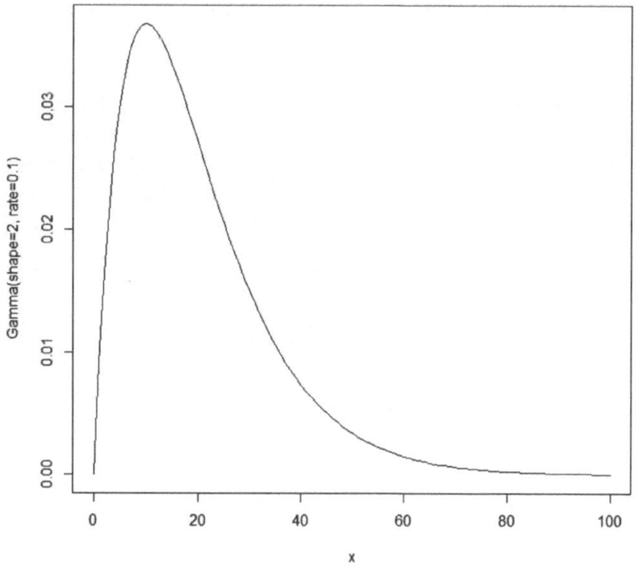

FIGURE 11.1
Density plot of a Gamma(2, 0.1) distribution.

We put a lower bound $\nu \geq 1$ on the degrees of freedom in the t-distribution to ensure that the Student-t distribution has a finite mean. The lower bounded scalar in Stan can be specified by adding `<lower=1>` in the parameter specification. The following Stan code specifies $\nu \geq 1$, $\sigma_y \geq 0$ and no constraints on μ_y.

```
parameters {
  real<lower=1> nu;
  real mu;
  real<lower=0> sigma;
}
```

The hyperparameters μ_μ, σ_μ and H are often specified based on expert opinion, historical information, and scientific knowledge of the quantity of interest. For example, a typical bioassay is centered at 100 and usually ranges from 50 to 150. Therefore, μ_μ can be set at 100. The parameter σ_μ can be set at 20, and H can be set at 50, for example. This can serve as an initial prior. Before using this prior for Bayesian inference, it is critical to understand the impact of the prior on the posterior distribution. This can be achieved via a prior sensitivity analysis (Kruschke, 2015; Depaoli and van de Schoot, 2017). In a prior sensitivity analysis, competing priors are set to examine the impact. The competing priors could be different forms of distributions or the same type of prior distributions but with different hyperparameter settings. The latter was used in our prior sensitivity analysis which is described in Section 11.3. The chosen prior is deemed sensitive if a small change in the prior results in significant changes in posterior distribution. In such a case, it is critical to justify using this sensitive prior. Alternatively, a less sensitive prior could be considered based on the sensitivity evaluation.

Values of σ_μ and H determine the degree of informativeness of the priors, where large values (e.g., $\sigma_\mu = 500$, $H = 500$) introduce diffuse priors, and smaller values (e.g., $\sigma_\mu = 5$, $H = 5$) represent informative priors. Both σ_μ and H result from historical total variability, including process and method variability. Since estimates of process variability are usually difficult to obtain, especially in the early development, method variability is proposed as a convenient way to formulate priors. The method variability, e.g., intermediate precision (IP), is often available from the corresponding qualification or validation study of the same or similar compounds. To build method variability into the prior in a structured way, we reformulate the variance hyperparameters as $\sigma_\mu = \text{multiple.mu} \times \text{IP}$ and $H = \text{multiple.sigma} \times \text{IP}$. Varying multiple.mu and multiple.sigma in the prior sensitivity analysis is equivalent to varying values of σ_μ and H. As a result, priors with smaller values of multiple.mu and multiple.sigma are informative, while priors with larger values of multiple.mu and multiple.sigma can be very diffuse. Using a very diffuse prior as a default is not practical in comparability assessment as it does not bring additional information to help define the distribution of the pre-change process.

11.2.3 Bayesian Inference with Posterior Predictive Intervals

Once the prior and likelihood distributions are set and pre-change batch release data are available, the posterior samples of parameters ν, μ_y, σ_y and the quantity of interest y are generated via a Markov chain Monte Carlo (MCMC) sampling algorithm. Stan samples from the posterior distribution are obtained using either Hamiltonian Monte Carlo or its variant, No-U-turn sampler (NUTS). The latter was used in our simulation. For more details on Stan MCMC algorithms, see Stan Development Team (2021b).

Bayesian inference can be conducted by obtaining a sufficient number of posterior samples to summarize the unknown parameters and their uncertainty. One common approach is to calculate some sort of Bayesian interval. The Bayesian $p\%$ credible interval of a parameter has a similar goal as the frequentist confidence interval but would be interpreted as a range that the parameter of interest lies in with a $p\%$ probability. As shown by Kruschke (2015), the highest density interval (HDI) is the narrowest interval with the same $p\%$ of the distribution for a unimodal probability distribution. "All the values inside the HDI have higher probability density (i.e., credibility) than any value outside the HDI. The HDI therefore includes the most credible values." (Kruschke, 2015). Thus, it makes more sense to use the HDI for decision making rather than an equal-tailed interval. Note, although a Bayesian HDI is usually used for the posterior distribution, we use it for the posterior predictive distribution as well in our study. The Bayesian approach can return a full distribution for the unobserved quantity of interest (i.e., the posterior predictive distribution) and so the HDI can be calculated for this distribution. The calculated HDI from the posterior predictive distribution of the pre-change process batches will guide the setup of a "comparability criterion" in the process comparability exercise. If a process change brings no or little impact to the process attribute, there is a high probability that the post-change batches will fall within the HDI. Therefore, the HDI can serve as the comparability criterion.

11.2.4 Comparability Assessment and Update

If all the post-change batches fall within the HDI as determined above, we can claim that the comparability between the pre- and post-change process is established, or at least that no evidence of non-comparability is found. Then we can update the posterior predictive distribution (distribution A) with the post-change batch data which is considered comparable so far. In other words, using distribution A as the new prior distribution and the post-change data as the new data, a new posterior predictive distribution (distribution B) can be obtained. The HDI from distribution B can then be used as the comparability criterion for the next round of process changes. Such an approach to quantify and update learning is one of key benefits of a Bayesian approach.

If one or two post-change batches fall outside the HDI, it is suggested to conduct an investigation before proceeding to the next step. If the post-change batch or batches fall outside HDI by a small margin, the study owner may decide to either collect more post-change batches or assess the impact of the difference on safety and efficacy as recommended by ICH Q5E (2005). If no adverse impact on safety and efficacy is expected from the difference, then comparability may still be claimed. On the other hand, if a possible adverse impact cannot be excluded, additional nonclinical or clinical studies should be considered. If the difference between pre- and post-change processes is deemed significant enough, then the conclusion of "not comparable" should be reached (Figure 11.2).

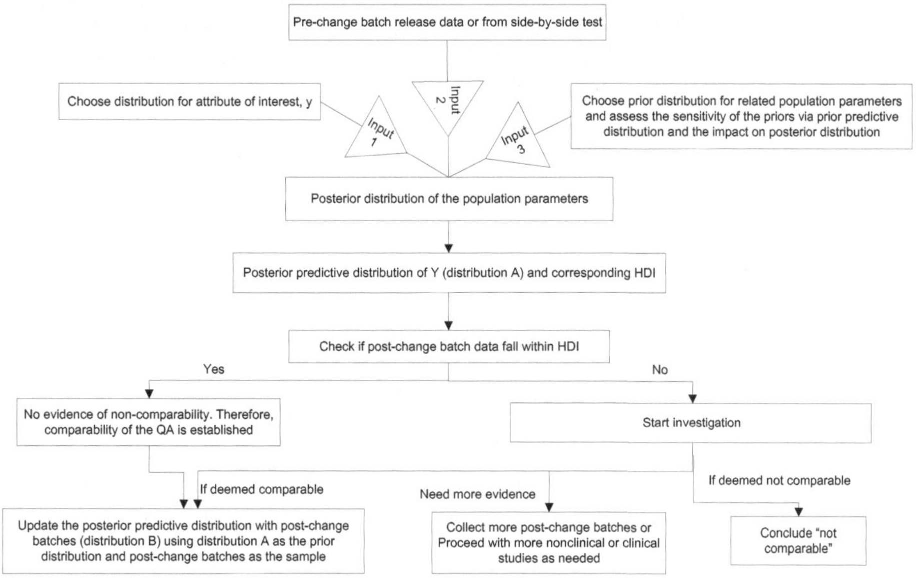

FIGURE 11.2
Bayesian framework for process comparability assessment.

11.2.5 Choice of the Coverage Level of HDI

As a pre-defined criterion, the width of HDI is critical. HDI with higher probability is wider and has higher probability to cover the post-change lots, leading to higher chance to claim comparability. In the context of the process comparability exercise, the HDI serves as the "control trend" in ICH Q5E (2005). The control trend is usually set as mean $\pm$ 3SD range (i.e. 99.73% coverage) in an ideal situation. Therefore, 99.73% would be the ideal coverage for comparability criteria setting as well. However, several practical factors also need to be taken into consideration.

- A HDI with higher coverage requires a larger effective sample size (ESS) to be stable. ESS can be determined by evaluating the Monte Carlo simulation error as a function of the length of the Markov chains (MC). This is also demonstrated in the case study below.
- Unlike specification limits, comparability criteria are not used to accept or reject batches. The role of comparability criteria (i.e., HDI in this case) is to signal if the difference between the pre- and post-change processes is significant. Therefore, the HDI could be more stringent or narrower than specification limit.
- HDI is also affected by the number of pre-change batches and the informativeness of the priors. A small sample size and less informative priors could lead to an HDI that is subject to high uncertainty. In such case, the coverage level needs to be lower to reflect the fact that we do not have high confidence in the interval due to the limited input information.
- Like any interval-based criterion, the more post-change batches to compare against this interval, the higher chance that at least one post-change batch will fall outside the interval. This leads to a disincentive to generate more data points for the comparability exercise. One way to deal with this problem is to choose the coverage level of the HDI based on the anticipated sample size of the post-change batches, e.g., gradually increase the coverage level with increasing sample size, m. For instance, choose 0.97 for $m = 3$ post-change batches, and gradually increase to 0.99 or higher as m increases (Figure 11.3) to ensure the simultaneous coverage level (i.e., the probability that all the post-change batches fall within HDI simultaneously) remains at the same or at a similar level.

Based on the above considerations, the HDI with coverage level of 90% of higher is recommended.

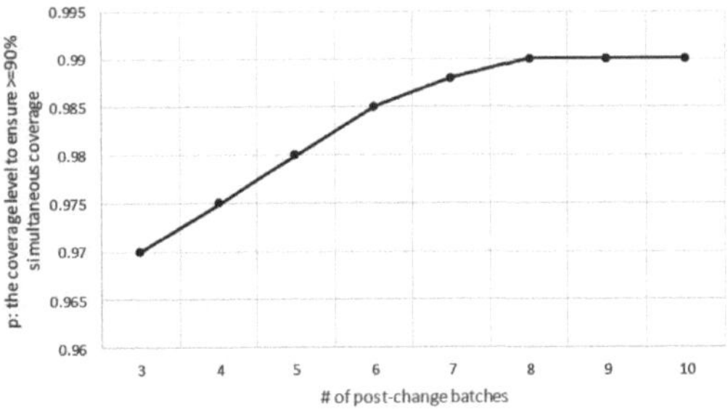

m (number of post-change batches)	p	Prob (all in HDI)
3	0.97	0.913
4	0.975	0.904
5	0.98	0.904
6	0.985	0.913
7	0.988	0.919
8	0.99	0.923
9	0.99	0.914
10	0.99	0.904

FIGURE 11.3
Coverage level, p, of HDI to ensure the simultaneous coverage $\geq$ 90% with different number of post-change batches.

11.3 Prior Sensitivity Assessment

It is critical to understand how the choice of priors impacts the posterior distributions. We recommend two assessments of prior sensitivity: 1) the prior predictive distribution;

2) the impact of the prior on the posterior and posterior predictive distributions. The prior predictive distribution checks the degree of informativeness by comparison to scientific expectation, while the assessment of the posterior distribution evaluates how robust the posterior results are when the priors are altered. A step-by-step illustration on how to conduct the assessment and interpret the results through plotting is provided in this section to emphasize the importance of conducting prior sensitivity analysis in Bayesian estimation.

11.3.1 Prior Predictive Distribution Check

The prior predictive distribution of a quantity of interest can be simulated before collecting data to evaluate whether the chosen prior aligns with subject matter expert's (SME) scientific beliefs. Comparing the prior predictive distribution to the expected scientific ranges of the attribute also helps categorize the degree of prior informativeness.

We demonstrate the prior predictive distribution check via a set of simulated bioassay results from a monoclonal antibody. The scientific belief is that the total variability (including both process and method variability) is larger than method variability alone. In this case, let IP = 5% represent the method variability quantified in an early qualification study. The scientific priors can be introduced to Bayesian estimation through hyperparameters H = multiple.sigma $\times$ IP and σ_μ = multiple.mu $\times$ IP. Based on the expert opinion, $\mu_y \sim N(100, H = 3 \times \text{IP})$ and $\sigma_y \sim \text{Half-Normal}(0, \sigma_\mu = 5 \times \text{IP})$ are chosen as the initial priors. To assess the sensitivity of the initial priors, we first produce prior predictive distributions in Figure 11.4 with varying levels of the two multipliers for H and σ_μ.

```
IP.sim <- 5
a1 <- c(3,5, 10,20) #  levels of multiple.mu
a2 <- c(5,10,20, 50) # levels of multiple.sigma
a.m <- expand.grid(a1, a2)  # a matrix for all
                            # 16 prior settings
```

The following function `priorpredcode` defines a Stan model of the above Student-t distribution with priors for the model parameters and a quantity of interest (i.e., `y_sim` is the product assay).

```
priorpredcode = "
  data {
    real IP;
    real  multiplier.mu;
    real  multiplier.sigma;
  }
  transformed data {
    real H;
    real musigma;
    H = multiplier.sigma *IP;
    musigma = multiplier.mu *IP;
  }
  parameters {
```

```
    real<lower=1> nu;
    real mu;
    real<lower=0> sigma;
  }
  model {
    nu ~ gamma(2, 0.1);
    mu ~ normal(100, musigma);
    sigma ~ normal(0, H);
   }
  generated quantities{
    real  y_sim;
    y_sim = student_t_rng(nu, mu, sigma);
}
"
```

Next pass the specified IP value and levels of multipliers as data to the Stan model to generate the prior predictive samples for all 16 prior settings. The samples are saved and reformatted into a data frame, `ysim`, for further evaluation. For more details about the options in the sampling function for a Stan model, refer to Stan Development Team (2021b).

```
library(rstan) # load library rstan
for (i in 1:nrow(a.m)) {
    datasim.list <- list(
       IP=IP.sim, multiplier.mu=a.m[i,1],
          multiplier.sigma= a.m[i,2])
# fit model
    standmodel <- stan_model(model_code=priorpredcode)

    stanfit.sim <- sampling(standmodel,
                            data=datasim.list,
                            algorithm="NUTS",
                            control=list(adapt_delta=0.85),
                            iter=3000,
                            warmup=500,
                            chains=4,
                            cores=2,
                            seed=9182567)

# convert standfit object to matrix
    y_sim <- round(as.matrix(stanfit.sim),2)
    ysim <- data.frame(multiplier.mu = rep(a.m[i,1],
            nrow(y_sim)),multiplier.sigma = rep(a.m[i,2],
            nrow(y_sim)), y_sim[,"y_sim"])
}
```

With all the generated samples, R package ggplot2 (Wickham, 2016) was used to overlay the prior predictive distributions (Figure 11.4).

```
library(ggplot2)
ysim$multiple.mu <- as.factor(ysim$multiple.mu )
ysim$multiple.sigma <- as.factor(ysim$multiple.sigma)
p = ggplot(data= ysim.plot, aes(x=y_sim,
                              color=multiple.sigma)) +
  facet_wrap(~ multiple.mu, nrow=2, labeller=label_both) +
  geom_density()+  xlim(c(0,200))+
  stat_function(fun=dnorm,n=101, args=list(mean=100, sd=25),
                colour="black", linetype=2,lwd=1, alpha=0.8) +
  xlim(c(0,200))+ylab("")+theme(legend.position="right")
p+scale_color_grey(start = 0.1, end = .8)+  theme_classic()
```

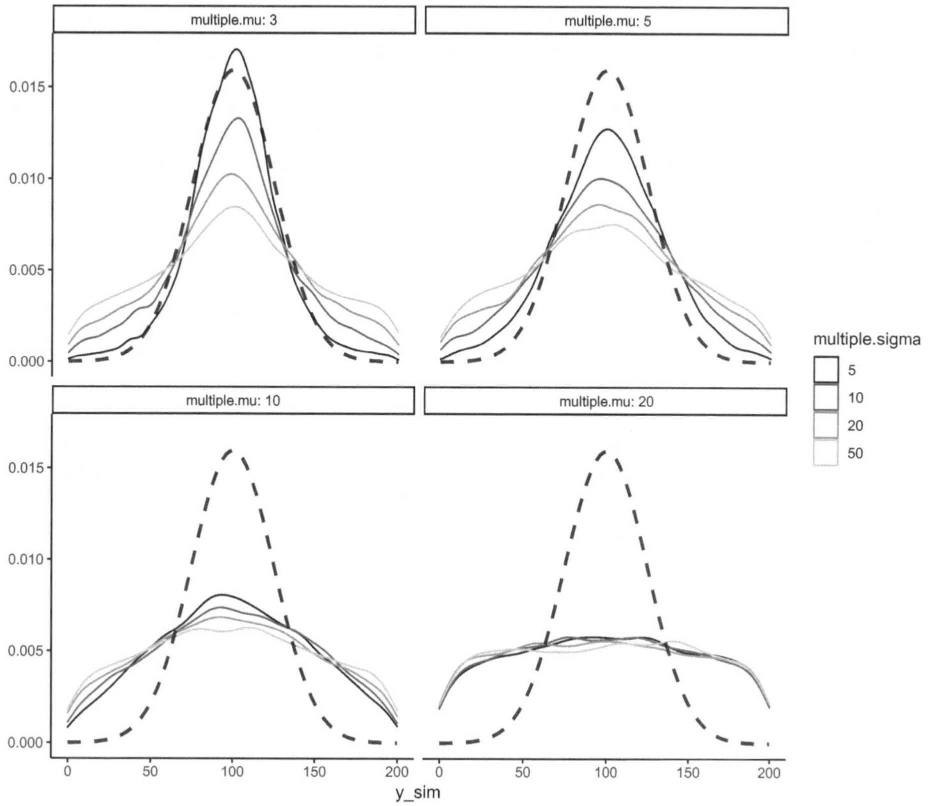

FIGURE 11.4
Simulated prior predictive distributions of product quality attribute values under different prior settings with levels of multiple.mu and multiple.sigma. The dashed black line is the density curve of a $N(100, 5 \times \text{IP})$ to mimic expected assay distribution based on the scientific beliefs that the total variability is five times the method variability.

Historical range for a typical potency assay of a monoclonal antibody is usually within [50%, 150%] in the early stage of development, and within [70%, 130%] in the later stage of development. If a prior predictive distribution is spread far beyond the scientifically meaningful area, its priors are diffuse or noninformative. As shown in the bottom right panel in Figure 11.4, the prior $\mu_y \sim N(100, 20 \times \text{IP})$ is diffuse because all the prior predictive distributions are flat over [0, 200] and their 95% HDIs are unreasonably wide, from -1000 to 1000. On the other hand, the priors $\mu_y \sim N(100, 3 \times \text{IP})$ and $\sigma_y \sim \text{Half-Normal}(0, 5 \times \text{IP})$ in top the left panel in Figure 11.4 are relatively informative priors. Its prior predictive distribution shows a large probability mass over a tight range of attribute values. The dashed black line is the density curve of a $N(100, 5 \times \text{IP})$ to mimic scientific belief that the total variability is five times the method variability. As the multiple.mu and multiple.sigma increase, the prior becomes less informative.

11.3.2 The Impact of Prior on Posterior and Posterior Predictive Distributions

The same set of priors were used to evaluate their impact on the posterior and posterior predictive distributions when the priors are altered for different number of pre-change process batches.

11.3.2.1 Simulation Process

The simulation process is described as follows:

1. Simulate a set of 24 assay values from normal distribution $N(100, 10)$. Take the first 3, 6, 12, and all 24 values to form four data sets for pre-change batches. The mean and sample standard deviation for each data set are summarized in Table 11.1.
2. Let IP $=$ 5%, σ_μ $=$ multiple.mu $\times$ IP, and H $=$ multiple.sigma $\times$ IP, where multiple.mu varies over four values 3, 5, 10, 20 and multiple.sigma varies over a different set of four values 5, 10, 20, 50. The resulting 16 conditions have prior variances from small to large.
3. For each of the 64 different conditions (16 prior settings $\times$ 4 different sample sizes), draw MCMC samples using RStan with four Markov chains, 1000 iterations per chain and remove the first half of the sequence as burn-in length.
4. Check the MCMC convergence for each condition using Rhat and ESS.
5. Summarize the posterior means of model parameters and the predicted assay values.

TABLE 11.1
The sample mean and standard deviation of the four simulated data sets.

Data Set	sample.size	sample.mean	sample.sd
1	3	103	13.5
2	6	100.8	9.6
3	12	100.3	9.7
4	24	99.3	9.8

The following script of `postpredcode` defines a Stan model of a Student-t distribution, the input data, parameters, and quantity of interest:

```
postpredcode = "
  data {
    int<lower=1> n;
    real<lower=0> y[n];
    real IP;
    real  multiplier.mu;
    real  multiplier.sigma;
  }
  transformed data {
    real H;
    real musigma;
    H = multiplier.sigma *IP;
    musigma = multiplier.mu *IP;
  }
  parameters {
    real<lower=1> nu;
    real mu;
    real<lower=0> sigma;
  }
  model {
    nu ~ gamma(2, 0.1);
    mu ~ normal(100, musigma);
    sigma ~ normal(0, H);
     y ~ student_t(nu, mu, sigma);
  }
  generated quantities{
    real  y_pred;
    y_pred = student_t_rng(nu, mu, sigma);
  }
"
```

The posterior samples for each of the 64 conditions are generated by executing the following script. Rstan function `monitor()` summarizes MCMC draws. The summary results of the 64 conditions were consolidated into one data frame for the overall convergence diagnoses and posterior analysis.

```
for (j in 1:4) {   # index for four levels of sample size
  for (i in 1:nrow(a.m)) {  # index for prior settings
    N.sim <- c(N.m[[j]])
    y.sim <- c(y.m[[j]])
    datasim.list <- list(
      n=N.sim, y=y.sim, meanY=100, IP=IP.sim,
      multiplier.mu = a.m[i,1], multiplier.sigma = a.m[i,2])
    standmodel <- stan_model(model_code=postpredcode)
```

```
    stanfit.sim <- sampling(standmodel,
                            data=datasim.list,
                            algorithm="NUTS",
                            control=list(adapt_delta=0.85),
                            iter=1000,
                            warmup=500,
                            chains=4,
                           seed=9182567)

# MCMC posterior sample summary statistics
    summary.post <- monitor(stanfit.sim, permute=FALSE,
                       inc_warmup=FALSE,digits_summary = 2)
    summary.m <- data.frame(param=rownames(summary.post),
                        size=rep(N.sim,nrow(summary.post)),
                        mean.y=rep(mean(y.sim),
                                   nrow(summary.post)),
                        sd.y=rep(sd(y.sim),
                                   nrow(summary.post)),
                          multiplier.mu = rep(a.mu,
                                       nrow(summary.post)),
                        multiplier.sigma = rep(a.y,
                        nrow(summary.post)), summary.post)
   write.table(summary.m,file="postsummary-potency-mu100.csv",
               sep = ",", row.names=FALSE, append = T)
  }
}
```

11.3.2.2 Posterior Analysis

Rhat ($\hat{R}$) value and ESS are commonly used as convergence and efficiency diagnostic tools for Markov Chains. The original $\hat{R}$ refers to potential scale reduction statistics from Gelman and Rubin (1992), and compares the within-chain and the between-chain variance for model parameter estimates. If the chains converge to a common distribution, $\hat{R}$ will be one. Due to the flaws associated with the traditional Rhat in diagnosing convergence of thick tailed chains, rstan produces an improved rank-based Rhat, as proposed by Vehtari et al. (2021), to measure chain convergence for model parameter estimates and other univariate quantities of interest. On the rstan webpage (`https://mc-stan.org/rstan/reference/Rhat.html`), it is recommended to run "at least four chains by default and only using the sample if R-hat is less than 1.05". If convergence is not achieved, increasing chain length and thinning can be considered.

Violin plots are used to visualize the 64 Rhat values for the convergence of the five model parameter estimates, lp_(the unnormalized log posterior density $\log p(\mu_y, \sigma_y|y)$), mu (Student-t center location parameter: μ_y), nu (Student-t degrees of freedom: ν), sigma (Student-t scale parameter: σ_y), and y_pred (the predicted quantity of interest: assay value y). This was done by loading the summary statistics of MC samples into R, and then using `ggplot()` to create the violin plot in the top panel in Figure 11.5. Almost all Rhat values are less than 1.01, with a few between 1.01-1.03, indicating that the four chains of posterior samples mixed well and converged to a common distribution.

```
# load posterior sample summary statistics
mc.m <-  read.csv("postsummary-potency-mu100.csv",header=TRUE)
mc.m$multiplier.mu <- as.factor(mc.m$multiplier.mu)
mc.m$multiplier.sigma <- as.factor(mc.m$multiplier.sigma)
mc.m$size <- factor(mc.m$size,levels=c("3", "6","12","24"),
                    labels=c("3", "6","12","24"))

ggplot(mc.m, aes(x=param, y=Rhat)) +
  geom_violin(trim=TRUE)+
  geom_boxplot(width=0.1)+
  ylim(c(0.995, 1.03))+  xlab("")+  theme_minimal()
```

Similarly, replacing the Rhat in the y-axis in the above code with Bulk_ESS and Tail_ESS will produce the violin plots for the ESS. Bulk_ESS and Tail_ESS are also the improved version for measuring MC sampling efficiency in the bulk (e.g., mean) and tails (5% and 95% quantiles) of the distribution using rank normalized draws (for more details, see Vehtari et al. (2021)). The recommended minimum ESS for achieving reliable estimates of the posterior quantiles is 100 per MC, and so a minimum ESS of 400 is desired with four chains. As shown in Figure 11.5, majority Bulk and tail ESS of all five quantities are greater than 400, indicating the adequate sampling efficiency in the bulk and tails of the distribution, producing reliable estimates of respective posterior quantiles.

Looking more closely at the Rhat and Tail_ESS values allows us to further analyze the impact of prior and sample size on the convergence and sampling efficiency. For illustration purposes, Figure 11.6 displays the Rhat and Tail_ESS of the predicted quantity of interest (y) at 64 unique conditions using `varPlot()` in the R `VCA` package (Schuetzenmeister and Dufey, 2020). Tail_ESS plot was produced by replacing Rhat with Tail_ESS in the code below.

```
library(VCA)  # load library VCA for varPlot

# only look at y_pred as an example
rhat.m <- mc.m %>%  filter(param=="y_pred")
varPlot(Rhat~multiplier.mu/multiplier.sigma, rhat.m,
        VCnam=list(text=c("multiplier.mu","multiplier.sigma"),
                          cex=0.9, col="black"),
        VarLab = list(cex = 0.9, adj = c(0.5, 0.5)),
        YLabel = list(text ="y_pred: Rhat", side = 2,
                      line =3.5, cex = 1.0),
        mar=c(0.1,6,0.5,1), htab = 0.2,
        Points = list(pch = list(var="size", pch=1:4),
                      cex = 1, col = "black"),
        Mean = NULL,  ylim=c(0.995, 1.02))
legend( x = 0, y = 1.02, pch=1:4, pt.cex=c(1,1,1,1),
        legend=c("size=3", "size=6", "size=12", "size=24"),
                 cex=0.9)
```

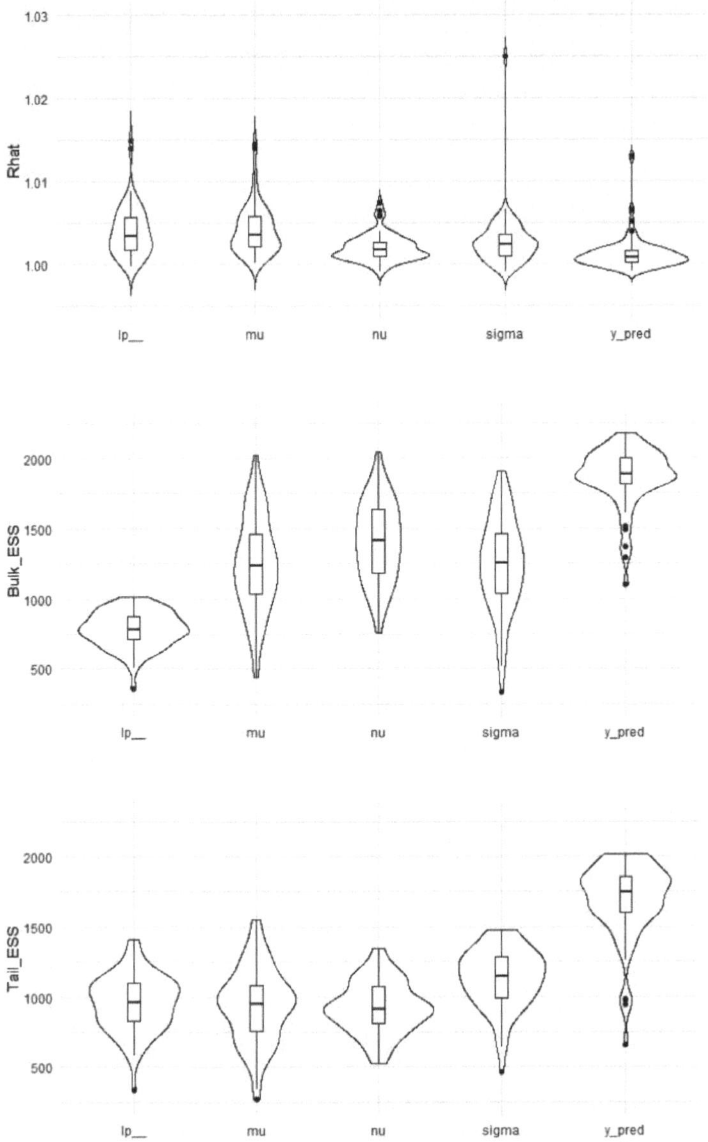

FIGURE 11.5
Rhat, Bulk, and Tail ESS estimates for parameters nu(ν), sigma(σ_y), lp_(the log posterior density), and y_pred(the predicted quantity of interest, assay values) for all 64 conditions.

As shown in Figure 11.6, the conditions with higher values of Rhat (> 1.01) and smaller tail ESS (< 1000) have the smallest sample size of 3 and diffuse priors ($\sigma_\mu = 20 \times \text{IP}$ and $\sigma_y = 50 \times \text{IP}$). Note that from the prior predictive check, $\mu_y \sim N(100, 20 \times \text{IP})$ and/or $\sigma_y \sim \text{Half-Normal}(0, 50 \times \text{IP})$ are very diffuse priors based on the scientific expectation of the attribute. Increasing the MC iterations might help improve mixing and stabilize the posterior estimates. However, only increasing the MC chain does not guarantee the convergence of the MC. Other approaches such as model reparameterization could be considered as well. This section only provides first level evaluation of the recommended minimum ESS. Minimum ESS, however, will need to be further investigated by checking the Monte Carlo

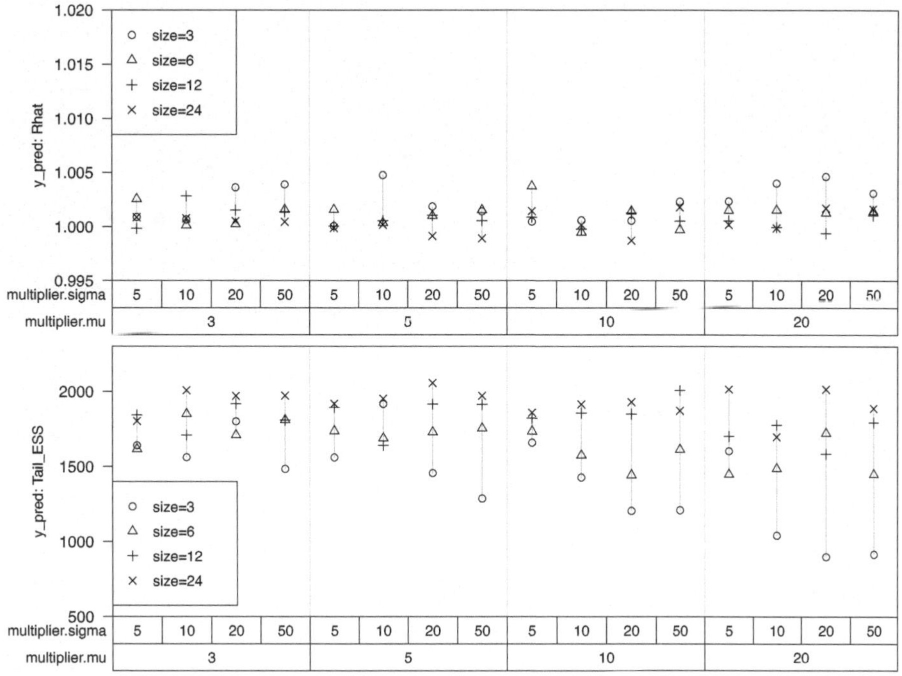

FIGURE 11.6
Rhat and tail effective sample size estimates for y_pred, the predicted quantity of interest at the 64 unique conditions.

standard errors (MCSE) with different lengths of Markov Chains. The investigation of the MCSE vs ESS is demonstrated in our case study in later sections.

Here we have demonstrated convergence of all the conditions. Next, we move to the evaluation of prior impact on the posterior estimates. The sensitivity analysis will show how much the posterior estimates change when priors are altered. Plots of the posterior mean estimates of μ_y, σ_y, and y in Figure 11.7 are generated to visualize the impact of the priors and sample sizes. At a sample size of 6 or above, the posterior mean estimates are insensitive to the current prior settings. The posterior mean estimate is robust with the chosen informative priors, where $\mu_y \sim N(100, 3 \times \text{IP})$ and $\sigma_y \sim$ Half-Normal$(0, 5 \times \text{IP})$. At a sample size of 3, the mean estimates of quantities of interests are not as robust as those with relatively larger sample sizes, especially with respect to the variance estimates. This is expected when sample size is small. In such a case, it is even more critical to justify the choice of priors. An informative prior that is sensitive does not suggest "bad" results. As a good practice, we recommend that practitioners always address the choice of priors, document the sensitivity results, and have a clear understanding of the impact of these choices on posterior inference.

11.4 A Case Study Based on a Simulated Data Set

To demonstrate the implementation of the proposed Bayesian approach in a real-life application, a subset of six values and a subset of three values are selected out of the above simulated 24 values to represent the relative potency of the pre-change (process 1) and

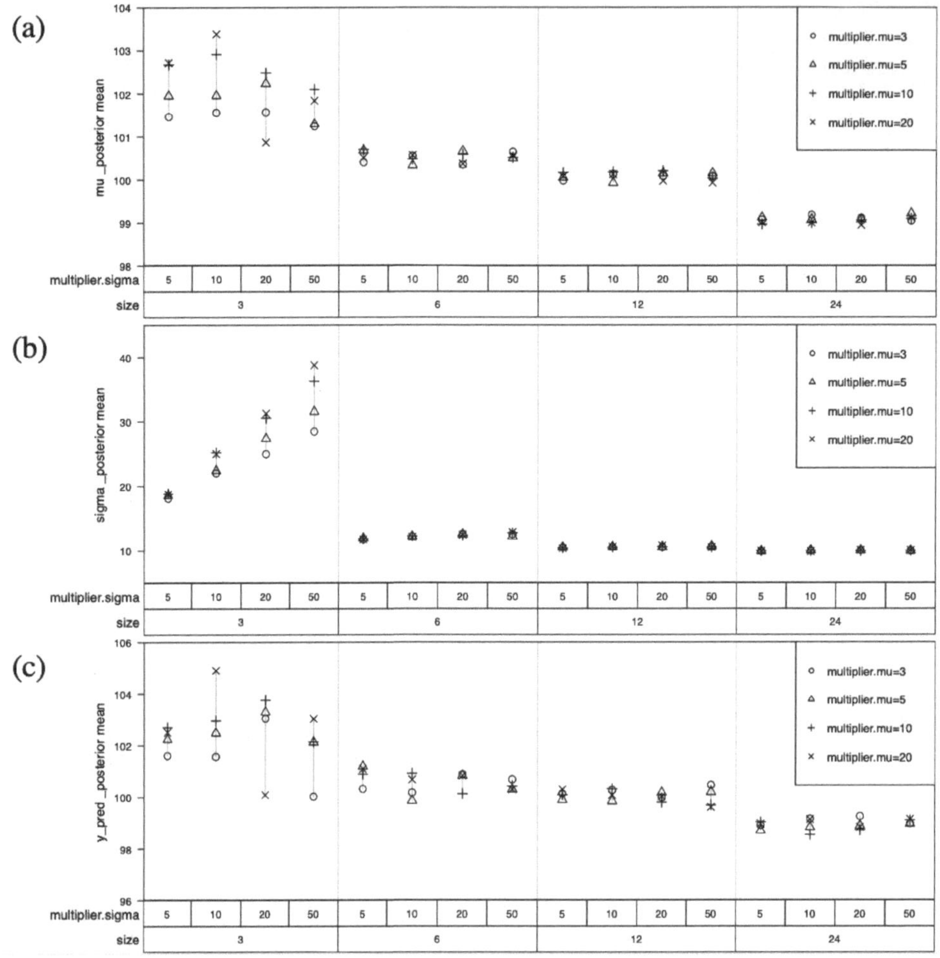

FIGURE 11.7
Posterior mean estimates for (a) mu(μ_y), (b) sigma(σ_y), and (c) y_pred (the predicted quantity of interest) at the 64 unique conditions.

post-change (process 2) process drug product batches at the time of release, from a monoclonal antibody compound. We created a data frame for the simulated data and the associated processes:

```
myData0 <- round(c(81.38162,95.55772,98.71117,94.61979,
                    101.02236,104.56085,116.30879,103.16120,
                    98.71117 ),2)
process <- c(rep("Process_1", 6), rep("Process_2", 3))
breaks <- round(c(mean(myData0[1:6]),
                   mean(myData0[1:6])+3*sd(myData0[1:6]),
                   mean(myData0[1:6])-3*sd(myData0[1:6])),1)
example <- data.frame(lot=factor(1:length(myData0)),
                       process=process, Assay=myData0)
```

The batch release values are displayed in Figure 11.8 with the batch number on the x-axis. The black dashed line represents the sample mean of 96. The two gray dashed lines represent the sample mean $\pm\, 3 \times$ sample standard deviation (SD) limits of (72, 120) based on the six pre-change batch values.

```
example %>%
ggplot(aes(x=lot, y=Assay, shape=process)) +
  scale_y_continuous(limits = c(70, 130),breaks=breaks )+
  geom_point(size=3) +
  geom_hline(yintercept= breaks[1], lty=2, col="black") +
  geom_hline(yintercept= breaks[2:3], lty=2, col="darkgray") +
  theme_classic()+
  theme(legend.position="top",
        axis.text = element_text(size = 12),
        axis.title = element_text(size = 12))
```

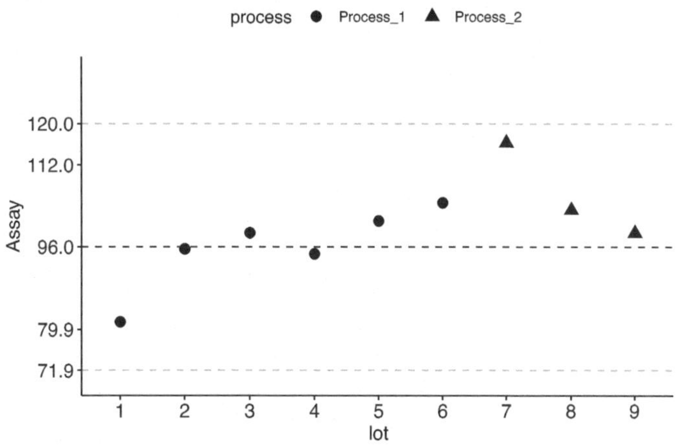

FIGURE 11.8
Simulated potency assay data from pre-change process (process 1) and post-change process (process 2). The gray dashed lines are mean $\pm\, 3 \times$ SD based on six pre-change batch assay values. The middle black dashed line represents the sample mean of the six pre-change batches.

A 10% method variability was obtained from an early qualification study. The total variability is believed to be at most two to three times the method variability based on expert opinions and historical manufacturing experience of similar products. Assume that the potency values follow a Student-t distribution with an expected mean at 100. The priors $\mu_y \sim N(100, \sigma_\mu = 2 \times \text{IP} = 20)$ and $\sigma_y \sim \text{Half-Normal}(0, H = 5 \times \text{IP} = 50)$ were chosen as the initial priors. Note that σ_μ represents the spread of the process mean and is expected to be smaller than the variability of the batch release data. However, we intentionally chose σ_μ to be larger than the scientific belief to ensure the resulting prior predictive distribution covers, and even extends a little beyond, the expected values. The same logic applies to the choice of H. Prior sensitivity analysis is carried out based on these choices. As shown in the prior sensitivity section above, these priors result in a prior predictive distribution that covers well the possible potency data range. These priors are quite robust in terms of their impact on the posterior distribution compared to other less informative priors. Therefore, $\mu_y \sim N(100, \sigma_\mu = 2 \times \text{IP} = 20)$ and $\sigma_y \sim \text{Half-Normal}(0, H = 5 \times \text{IP} = 50)$ were chosen as the priors for the following Bayesian HDI calculation.

The pre-change batch data and prior settings were passed to the previous defined Stan model, `postpredcode`. Five different post burn-in posterior samples of different sizes were collected, 2000, 6000, 10000, 20000 and 30000, and were saved for model diagnosis and HDI calculation. The results are shown in the following subsections.

```
IP.sim <- 10 #
multiplier.mu <- 2
multiplier.sigma <- 5
nchain <- 4
datasim.list <- list(n=n, y=y, meanY=100, IP=IP.sim,
                     a_mu=a.mu, a_y=a.y)
standmodel <- stan_model(model_code=postpredcode)

#vary iteration and warmup numbers to change the chain size
stanfit.sim <- sampling(standmodel,
                        data=datasim.list,
                        algorithm="NUTS",
                        iter=1000,
                        warmup=500,
                        chains=nchain,
                        cores=2,
                        seed=182567)
y_sim <- round(as.matrix(stanfit.sim),2)
write.csv(y_sim, file="mcsamples_example2000.csv")
summary.post <- round(monitor(stanfit.sim,
                     permute=FALSE, inc_warmup=FALSE),4)
write.csv(summary.post, file=" mcmcdiag_n2000.csv")
```

11.4.1 MCMC Convergence

Table 11.2 lists the summary statistics of 2000 posterior samples. All Rhat values are less than 1.01, both bulk and tail ESS are about 50% of the total posterior samples, suggesting good sampling efficiency and that the four chains have mixed well.

TABLE 11.2
Summary statistics of the posterior sample estimates of three model parameters.

Parameters	mean	median	se_mean	sd	Rhat	Bulk_ESS	Tail_ESS
nu	20.82	17.18	0.35	14.22	1.0022	1194	915
mu	96.53	96.47	0.14	4.27	1.0017	990	923
sigma	10.01	9.03	0.14	4.49	1.0019	1118	1062

Common MCMC diagnostic plots, such as the trace plots in Figure 11.9 (A), autocorrelation plots in Figure 11.9 (B) and bivariate plots in Figure 11.9 (C), are produced using R package `bayesplot` (Gabry and Mahr, 2021) to visualize MCMC convergence. In addition, NUTS-specific divergence transition plots are provided to check if the parameter space has been sufficiently explored. Two types of violin plots were produced by `mcmc_nuts_divergence` function to display the distribution of the log-posterior and acceptance probabilities for iterations that encountered divergent transition and those that did not. The divergence plots are unique to Hamiltonian Monte Carlo and its variant NUT sampler which are implemented in Stan to explore the target distribution. How far the exploration moves each time is controlled by a step size. If a step size is too big, it can miss local features in the target distribution, resulting in a divergence. Divergences indicate some part of the posterior is not being explored. Figure 11.9 (D) reports zero leapfrog transitions with diverging error, which is why no divergence violin plots are displayed. Therefore, all diagnostic plots have demonstrated that the four chains have converged to a common distribution and have efficiently explored the parameter space.

```
library(bayesplot)
lp_cp <- log_posterior(stanfit.sim)
np_cp <- nuts_params(stanfit.sim)

#(A) trace plot
color_scheme_set("gray")
mcmc_trace(stanfit.sim, pars = c("mu","sigma","nu"),
facet_args = list(ncol = 1, strip.position = "left"))+
                   xlab("Post-warmup iteration")

# (B) Autocorrelation function (ACF)
mcmc_acf(stanfit.sim, pars = c("mu","sigma","nu"), lags = 10)

# (C) parameter scatter plot
mcmc_pairs((stanfit.sim), pars = c("mu", "sigma", "nu"),
            np = np_cp, off_diag_args = list(size = 0.75))

# (D) NUT divergence plot
mcmc_nuts_divergence(np_cp, lp_cp)
```

11.4.2 Posterior Accuracy

The saved MCMC samples with five different post burn-in sample sizes of 2000, 6000, 10000, 20000 and 30000 are loaded into R and combined for estimate accuracy evaluation.

```
# load the files with different post buin-in MCMC samples
setwd("C:\\home\\Research\\processcomparability\\simulation")
mcse.n2000 <- read.csv("mcmcdiag_n2000.csv", header=TRUE)
mcse.n6000 <- read.csv("mcmcdiag_n6000.csv", header=TRUE)
mcse.n10000 <- read.csv("mcmcdiag_n10000.csv", header=TRUE)
```

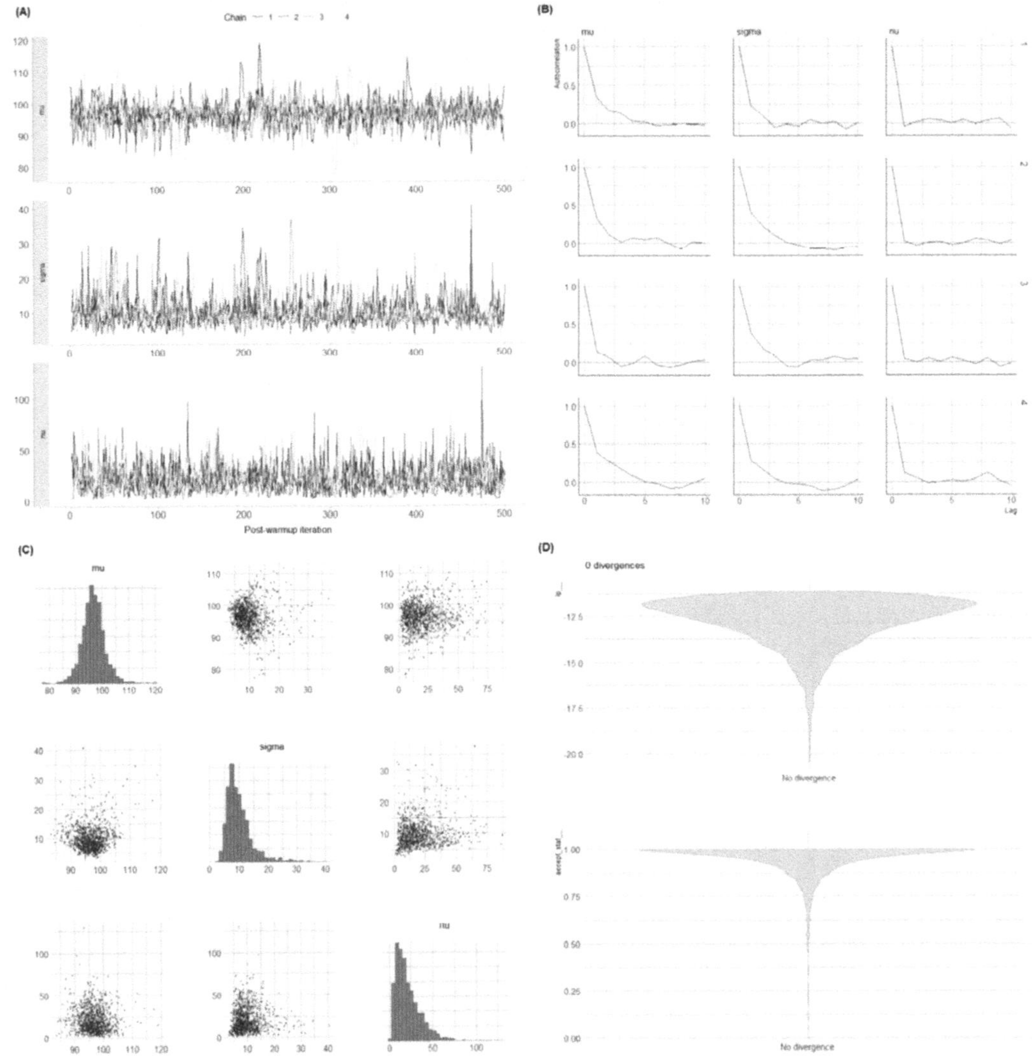

FIGURE 11.9
General MCMC diagnostic plots: (A) Parameter posterior sample trace plots do not show any stuck chains, or chain not being mixed. (B) Autocorrelation function (ACF) plots with lag=10 indicate sample correlation quickly drops to zero within 5 lags. (C) Bivariate scatter plot does not show collinearity among parameters. All parameters have unimodal posterior distributions as shown in the diagonal histograms. (D) NUTS divergence plot (note, no divergent plots are produced), the diagnostic plot does not identify divergence error in any part of the distributions of the log-posterior or NUTS acceptance statistics, meaning that the parameter space has been well explored.

```
mcse.n20000 <- read.csv("mcmcdiag_n20000.csv", header=TRUE)
mcse.n30000 <- read.csv("mcmcdiag_n30000.csv", header=TRUE)

mcse.n <- data.frame(size=rep(c(2000, 6000, 10000,
                                20000, 30000), each=5),
rbind(mcse.n2000,mcse.n6000, mcse.n10000,mcse.n20000,
      mcse.n30000)) %>%
    filter(X %in% c( "mu", "sigma", "nu", "y_pred"))
```

Posterior accuracy was first evaluated with the median estimates of all three parameters via plots of MCSE as a function of chain length. As shown in the top of Figure 11.10, the number of post burn-in iterations is the x-axis and the median estimate of parameters $\pm 1 \times$ MCSE is the y-axis. Substituting "mu" with either "sigma" or "nu" in the code below will produce all three plots in Figure 11.10. Only slight differences were observed with median estimates, suggesting that a post burn-in sample size of 2000 is sufficient for the posterior median estimates.

```
mcse.n %>%
  filter(X=="mu") %>%
  ggplot(aes(x=factor(size), y=Q50))+
  geom_point()+  geom_line()+
  geom_errorbar(aes(ymin=Q50-MCSE_Q50,ymax=Q50+MCSE_Q50),
                width=.3,position="dodge")+
  ylab("mean")+  xlab("iterations")+  theme_bw()
```

Next we compare the posterior accuracy for the 50%, 75%, and 97.5% quantile estimates of the posterior distributions of the model parameters and the posterior predictive distribution of relative potency values via evaluating the ratio of MCSE to the posterior sample standard deviation (MCSE/sd ratio). The following code produces the MCSE/sd ratio plot for the 50% quantile estimates, substituting "MCSE_Q50/sd" in the `ggplot yaxis` with "MCSE_Q75/sd" and "MCSE_Q97.5/sd" produces three plots in the bottom of Figure 11.10. The MCSE/sd ratio is less than 5% for the 50% and 75% estimates for all quantities of interest. However, an accurate estimate of the tails in the distribution such as 97.5% would require minimum 20,000 posterior samples.

```
mcse.n %>%
  ggplot(aes(x=factor(size), y=MCSE_Q50/sd, shape=X,group=X))+
  geom_point()+  geom_line()+    ylab("MCSE_Q50/sd")+
  xlab("iterations")+  ylim(c(0,0.05))+  theme_classic2()
```

Putting this all together, Figure 11.10 plots the median estimates and $\pm 1 \times$ MCSE interval estimates for the three parameters with varying post burn-in chain length from 2,000 to 30,000 iterations. The centroid estimates (i.e., median) are stable with 2000 samples (note that the scale of the centroid differences across different chain lengths is practically small), while the MCSE/sd ratio plots of the quantiles in Figure 11.10 suggest at least 20,000 samples are required to stabilize the estimation of tail quantile 97.5%. Based on this finding, the MCMC samples with post burn-in chain length of 20,000 will be used in later sections when comparing prior and posterior distributions and making inference with 95% HDIs.

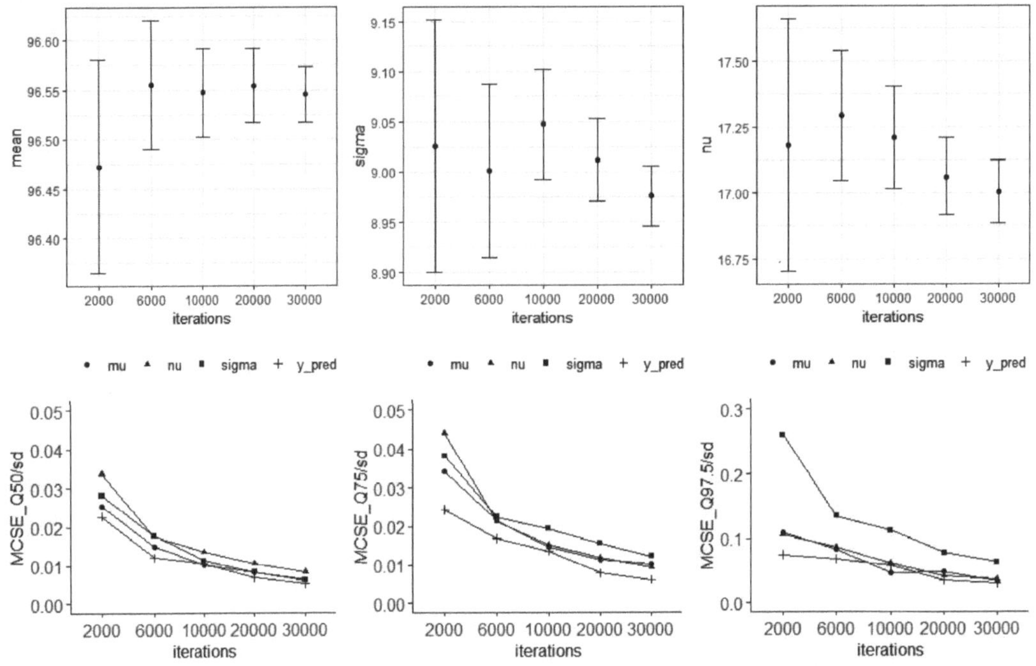

FIGURE 11.10
The plot on top is a plot of post burn-in samples with posterior median $\pm 1 \times$ MCSE interval estimates of mu(μ_y), sigma(σ_y), and nu(ν). The bottom plot is the MCSE/sd ratio plot of the 50%, 75%, and 97.5% quantile estimates of mu(μ_y), sigma(σ_y), nu(ν), and y_pred as function of post burn-in sample sizes.

11.4.3 Prior to Posterior Comparison

A simple way to demonstrate how priors are updated with the new information (pre-change batch release data in this case) is to overlay the prior and posterior distributions in a plot. Here we generate 20,000 samples from the prior predictive distributions and the posterior predictive distributions, load the saved MCMC sample .csv files into R, and consolidate the two sets into one data frame:

```
y_pred <- read.csv("mcsamples_example20000.csv", header=TRUE)
y_sim <- read.csv("priorpredmcsamples_example20000.csv",
                  header=TRUE)
vardistr <- data.frame(bayes=rep(c("posterior","prior"),
            c(length(y_pred[,"mu"]),length(y_sim[,"mu"]))),
            mu=c(y_pred[,"mu"],y_sim[,"mu"]),
```

```
                    sigma=c(y_pred[,"sigma"],y_sim[,"sigma"]),
                    nu=c(y_pred[,"nu"],y_sim[,"nu"]),
                    y=c(y_pred[,"y_pred"],y_sim[,"y_pred"]))
```

Next we use a flexible R package **ggh4x** (van den Brand, 2021) for the superposed distributions over selected ranges of each quantity of interest to produce Figure 11.11.

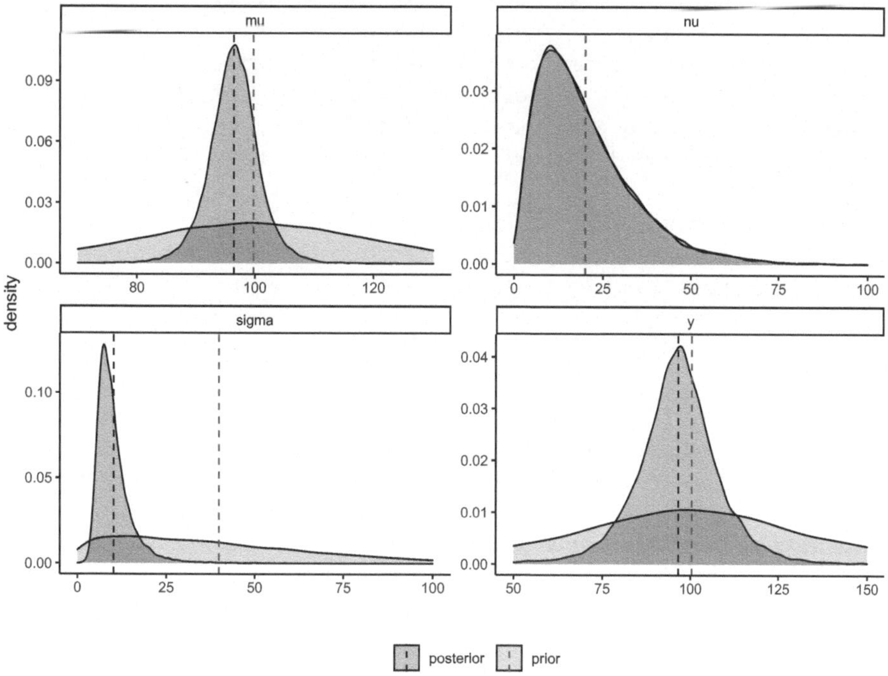

FIGURE 11.11
Overlaid prior and posterior distributions of mu(μ_y), sigma(σ_y), nu(ν), and y_pred.

```
library(ggh4x)
scales <- list(
  scale_x_continuous(minor_breaks = c(80,90, 100, 110,120),
                                    limits=c(70, 130)),
  scale_x_continuous(minor_breaks = c(10, 30, 50, 80),
                                    limits=c(0,100)),
  scale_x_continuous(minor_breaks = c(10, 30, 50, 80),
                                    limits=c(0,100)),
scale_x_continuous(minor_breaks = c(70,80,90,100,110,120,130),
                                    limits=c(50, 150))
)
vardistr %>%
  pivot_longer(cols=c("mu", "sigma", "nu", "y"),
```

```
                 names_to="parameters",
                 values_to="values") %>%
  dplyr::select("parameters", "values", "bayes") -> plot11

p <- ggplot(data=plot11, aes(x = values, fill=bayes)) +
  geom_density(alpha=0.3) +  xlab("") +
  facet_wrap(~ factor(parameters), scales = "free", nrow = 2)+
  facetted_pos_scales(x = scales) +
  geom_vline(data=group.mean, aes(xintercept = values,
             color=bayes), linetype="dashed")+
    theme_classic()+   theme(legend.position="bottom",
                             legend.title=element_blank())+
   theme(strip.text.x=element_text(size=16, colour="black"),
        strip.background = element_rect(fill="white",
                                       colour="gray",size=2))
p+scale_color_grey(start = 0.1, end = .5)+
scale_fill_grey(start = 0.1, end = .5)+ theme_classic() +
  theme(legend.position="bottom",legend.title=element_blank())
```

As shown in Figure 11.11, the priors are relatively vague for the location of the center and the spread of the distribution. The posterior and prior distributions of ν are almost identical, suggesting the pre-change batch data is not able to accurately estimate the degrees of freedom in the Student-t distribution. As discussed in Gelman et al. (2013) and Kruschke (2015), accurate estimation of a small value ν requires values from the extreme tails of the distribution, which are rare in the drug manufacturing process. The degree of freedom is included in the model estimation to cope with any potential outliers.

11.4.4 Bayesian Inference on Process Comparability

The `plotPost` function in `bayesboot` (Bäth, 2018) can be used to generate the posterior distributions of model parameters and the posterior predictive distribution of the predicted values. Moreover, this function also calculates the probability mass within a pre-specified interval. The following one-line code produces the posterior predictive distribution of the predicted relative potency values in the bottom left panel in Figure 11.12. The 95% HDI is [70%, 123%].

```
library(bayesboot)
plotPost(as.numeric(na.omit(y_sim[,"y_pred "])), col='gray',
         credMass = 0.95, HDItextPlace =0.95, xlab="values")
```

One of the greatest benefits of the Bayesian method is that we can acquire the posterior predictive distribution not only for the quantity of interest itself, but also for the functions of the quantity of interest. Figure 11.12 shows the density plots for the three model parameters and a predicted quantity y, as well as the density plots of a normalized process mean, $(\mu_y - 100)/\sigma_y$, and a normalized y, $(y - 100)/\sigma_y$, both as functions of the target center 100 and process variability. Similar inference can be made with the full predictive distributions.

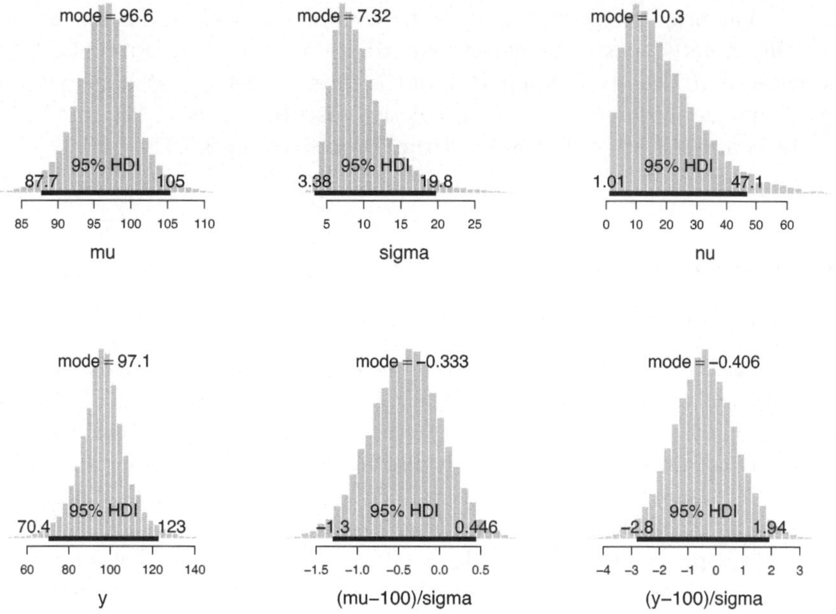

FIGURE 11.12
Posterior distributions of quantities of interest. The horizontal solid black lines represent the 95% HDI.

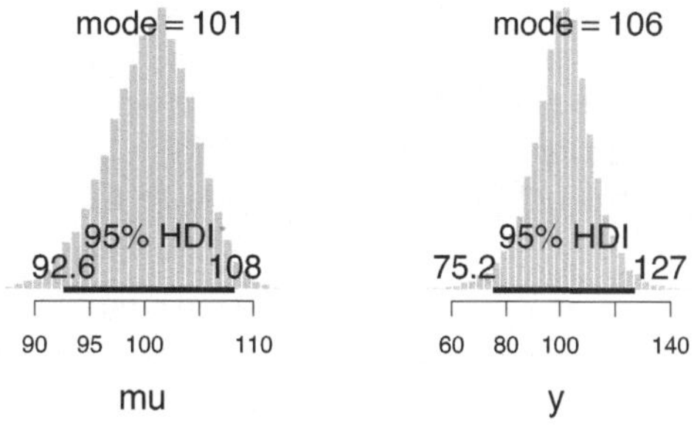

FIGURE 11.13
The updated posterior density distributions of mu(μ_y) (left panel) and predicted assay y (right panel) with three post-change batches using the pre-change posterior density as informative priors. The horizontal solid black lines are the updated 95% HDI.

The 95% HDI of the posterior predictive distribution, 70%-123%, is used as the comparability criterion. All three post-change batch values fall within the range. Process comparability is established.

Following the flowchart (Figure 11.2), the Bayesian framework can be easily used for process updating. In this case, the pre-change process posteriors could be taken as the new priors, i.e., $\mu_y \sim N(96.6, 5)$ and $\sigma_y \sim$ Half-Normal$(0, 10)$, and they can be updated with the post-change process data. Even though process comparability is established, we highly recommend that prior sensitivity analysis be conducted when updating the priors. As an example, the updated posterior density distribution of μ_y in Figure 11.13 indicates the process center at 101%, which resulted from the three higher post-change batch values. The 95% HDI from the updated posterior predictive distribution is 75.2% to 127%, which can serve as the comparability criterion for future process changes.

11.5 Summary and Discussion

Process comparability at the analytical level is a critical step to ensure consistency of drug quality, safety, and efficacy. Like most of the comparative studies in the CMC field, a limited sample size is one of the most challenging factors. Making a comparability decision based on limited data is not only difficult, but it is also impractical. Leveraging scientific knowledge into such decision-making is highly recommended by multiple guidelines. To encourage consistent usage of historical manufacturing experience and scientific beliefs, a Bayesian HDI approach is proposed that provides a structured way to build prior information into the comparability assessment framework (Figure 11.2), that is easy to implement.

To ensure successful implementation of this approach, it is critical to understand the roles that different factors play in this framework. Some of the key factors, such as prior and sample size, are further summarized and discussed below.

1. **Prior Selection**
   A Student-*t* distribution was used as an example to describe the data likelihood. Users may adopt other distributions depending on the property of their data. A weakly informative prior was selected in the simulation study based on prior sensitivity analysis, which includes a prior predictive check and an assessment on the impact to the posterior estimates. The prior predictive check provides information to categorize the priors from informative, weakly informative, to noninformative. Then the impact of prior on posterior estimates needs to be assessed, reviewed, and discussed with the subject matter experts to finalize the prior selection.
2. **Multiples of IP**
   Multiples of the method variability (i.e., IP) are introduced to set up the hyperparameters and to vary the degree of prior informativeness. We chose to use the IP because it is generally available and easy to obtain during the process development. Prior knowledge often varies from person to person, which could lead to inconsistent use of prior information. The introduction of multiples of the IP provides a structured and consistent way for scientists to quantify the priors with associated uncertainty.
3. **Limited Sample Size**
   Although increasing sample size provides more confidence in the process comparability exercise, the sample size of both pre- and post-change batches is often determined by practical restrictions like the supply need for clinical development and commercial production. For an early comparability exercise, sample sizes of 1 or 2 batches are quite common (Brunelle, 2016). Any frequentist approach could be meaningless with such a small sample size. However, the Bayesian framework as proposed here would still be useful. The Bayesian approach allows users to

visualize the prior predictive distribution and to see how the prior predictive distribution gets updated even with 1 or 2 batches. The ability to visualize the prior predictive distribution even without any pre- and post-change data is still helpful in increasing quantitative understanding.

4. **Process Update and Monitoring**
   As demonstrated in the example, a Bayesian approach has the flexibility to update the posterior distribution as new information becomes available. In the case of very limited batches, such as one or two lots for gene therapy product, the process comparability exercise strongly depends on scientific knowledge and similar assay methods. In the Bayesian framework, we can turn the strong scientific prior knowledge into an simulated prior predictive distribution. The variability in the prior can be varied from small to high in order to improve understanding of process risk and to determine how tight the process variability needs to be controlled to ensure the same quality level. The posterior distribution becomes the new prior for the next process comparability exercise. Using the posterior predictive distribution of the pre-change batches, an HDI or other type of credible interval can be considered as the "control trend" or the process comparability criterion for the post-change process. The post-change posterior distributions can be updated multiple times as the process evolves.

5. **Prior Information**
   This chapter used method intermediate precision as an example to build the prior. Besides IP, which is relatively easy to obtain, there are many other potential inputs that could be used for prior building, including established chemical and biological engineering principles, related literature and manufacturing experience (FDA, 2021), process development studies, small scale evaluation/validation studies, experience with earlier process changes, experience with equipment in similar operations, changes in similar manufacturing processes with similar products, and literature (ICH Q5E, 2005). However, how to systematically use different sources of information in addition to IP is still a big challenge. Our plan is to use IP as the starting point. As we gain more experience in applying Bayesian HDI to process comparability studies, we hope to develop a better understanding of how to convert the above sources into quantitative priors.

6. **Assessment vs Conclusion/Decision**
   The Bayesian HDI does not impose any requirement on the sample size of the post-change batches. However, the knowledge about the post-change process is often limited by the number of post-change batches. The fact that all the post-change batches fall within HDI does not necessarily guarantee that the pre-change and post-change process are the same. It simply means that there is no clear evidence, or signal, to claim that the post-change process is not comparable to the pre-change process. On the other hand, if one or more of the post-change batches fall outside HDI, it is a signal to raise the alert and an investigation should be considered. If no assignable cause is identified and the number of post-change batches are as limited as 2 or 3, more batches may need to be collected before drawing the conclusion. Although Bayesian HDI is an important input to the decision-making process, the comparability decision should not be based solely on statistical analysis results. Not all prior knowledge is incorporated into the construction of prior distribution building and so a holistic assessment is still needed. However, the assessment will be much easier if it starts with HDI.

12

Bayesian Alternatives to Traditional Methods for Estimating Product Shelf-Life and Internal Release Limits

Perceval Sondag

Novo Nordisk Inc.

Ji Young Kim

Merck & Co. Inc.

Laurent Natalis

PharmaLex Belgium SA

Tara Scherder

SynoloStats LLC

CONTENTS

DOI: 10.1201/9781003255093-12

12.1 Introduction

Every commercialized pharmaceutical product, including small molecules drugs, large molecules biologics, and vaccines, must have an expiration date and storage instructions (FDA, 2015a). To obtain these two crucial pieces of information, companies are required to perform rigorous stability studies. Stability studies are conducted to assess the quality of a drug substance (DS) or a drug product (DP) through time, under specific storage conditions (specifically, temperature and relative humidity). Shelf-life is defined as the time period during which a pharmaceutical product is expected to remain within the approved specifications for each of its quality attributes (ICH Q1A(R2), 2003) and defines the expiration date.

The most commonly referenced regulatory guidance for the calculation of shelf-life is the International Conference on Harmonisation (ICH) Q1E: Evaluation for Stability Data (ICH Q1E, 2003). The main purpose of stability studies as described in this guidance is to establish confidence that a future batch will remain within specification throughout its shelf-life. However, the proposed statistical methodology in the guidance has been shown not to be fit for this purpose (Kiermeier et al., 2004; Quinlan et al., 2013; Capen et al., 2018). From ICH Q1E:
"An appropriate approach to [...] shelf-life estimation is to analyze a quantitative attribute (e.g., assay, degradation products) by determining the earliest time at which the 95 percent confidence limit for the mean intersects the proposed acceptance criterion."

While the statement seems appropriate, ICH Q1E suggests that the confidence interval of the mean be calculated separately for a minimum of three batches – using a fixed batch analysis – and to consider the shortest estimated shelf-life to be the product shelf-life. Results using this approach can be deficient considering: (1) the worst of three observed batches is highly unlikely to be the worst of all future batches, and (2) it can encourage manufacturers to base results on a strict minimum of batches as increasing study size can decrease the estimated shelf-life.

While the guidance proposes poolability tests to potentially combine batches, a fixed batch analysis is inappropriate when the objective is to predict the shelf-life of future batches. Instead, hierarchical modeling (Chen et al., 1995) is more suitable for prediction. By treating batches as random, it becomes possible to determine shelf-life using the model projection for a future batch instead of a worst-case estimate from existing batches.

When a sufficient number of stability batches (6 or more) are available, Burdick et al. (2017) recommend treating batch as a random effect. The sensitivity of the fixed batch method recommended in ICH Q1E may preclude pooling the batches due to the increased batch-to-batch variability, and the worst-case philosophy can underestimate the shelf-life for the population of future batches.

Confidence intervals for linear mixed effects hierarchical models rely on substantial approximation of the degrees of freedom. The extent of approximation increases when the model becomes more complex (inclusion of various effects accounting for storage conditions, packaging types, or other factors). To address this limitation, Burdick et al. (2017) strongly recommend a Bayesian approach, which does not require the degrees of freedom calculations needed for a frequentist mixed model. The Bayesian approach also permits the use of prior information when available, which can be highly beneficial in the early stages of manufacturing when limited knowledge on the product stability is available. Moreover, the posterior distribution can be derived for any function of the parameters and so it provides a solution for quantifying challenging probabilistic statements not possible with a frequentist approach.

Once a specific shelf-life is approved (or claimed), ongoing assurance that future batches will meet the desired shelf-life is required. This can be achieved with a release range that accounts for expected change across the shelf-life. These internal release limits (IRLs) can assure, with a defined level of confidence, that the product will remain within specifications throughout the entire shelf-life, while stored at the labeled storage conditions. Use of IRL's is discretionary, and no guidance related to IRL's is included in ICH Q1E. Allen et al. (1991) first proposed a method to derive IRLs that is similar to ICH Q1E's shelf-life determination, while other authors have proposed different approaches, including using mixed effect models (Egan and Schofield, 2009; Altan et al., 2018). Whether using fixed or mixed effect models, deriving IRLs based on frequentist models poses the same challenges as estimating shelf-life.

In contrast, Bayesian approaches allow for a risk-based approach for both cases. In Section 12.2 of this chapter, we provide computational details for estimation of shelf-life and IRLs for various pharmaceutical products, illustrating how Bayesian statistics can address the multiple challenges that are posed by product stability requirements. In Section 12.3, we present case studies, including results.

12.2 Methodology

12.2.1 Shelf-Life Calculation

In this section, we first present the traditional ICH Q1E method, followed by the mixed effect model alternative using both Bayesian and Frequentist approaches.

12.2.2 The ICH Q1E Method: Fixed Batches Model

The World Health Organization's guidelines on stability evaluation of vaccines (WHO, 2011) and the FDA Guidance for Industry Q1A(R2) Stability Testing of New Drug Substances and Products (ICH Q1A(R2), 2003) both suggest calculating statistical confidence intervals on the regression of stability study measurements to determine the maximum time a batch is likely to conform to acceptance criteria for all critical quality attributes.

Following the ICH Q1E guideline, a minimum of three full scale batches are studied, and three models are usually considered as described in Figure 12.1.

$$\text{MI}: y_{ijk} = \beta_0 + (\text{Time}_k \times \beta_1) + (\text{Batch}_j \times \beta_{2_j}) + (\text{Time}_k \times \text{Batch}_j \times \beta_{3_j}) + \varepsilon_{ijk} \quad (12.1)$$
$$\text{MII}: y_{ijk} = \beta_0 + (\text{Time}_k \times \beta_1) + (\text{Batch}_j \times \beta_{2_j}) + \varepsilon_{ijk} \quad (12.2)$$
$$\text{MIII}: y_{ik} = \beta_0 + (\text{Time}_k \times \beta_1) + \varepsilon_{ik} \quad (12.3)$$

where:

- y_{ijk} is the results, possibly transformed to ensure normality of residuals, for the ith replicate of the jth batch for a specific critical quality attribute (CQA) in the studied conditions at the kth time point;
- Batch_j is a set of j dummy variables (for all batches but a reference batch);
- β_0 is the coefficient for the intercept;
- β_1 is the coefficient for the slope;

- β_{2_j} is the effect of batch j on the intercept;
- β_{3_j} is the effect of batch j on the slope (i.e. the interaction between batch and time);
- Time_k is the kth storage time point, and ICH Q1E typically recommends 0, 3, 6, 9, 12, 18, 24, and 36 month measurements (for a three years study);
- $\varepsilon_{ijk} \sim N(0, \sigma_e^2)$ is the residual error, with σ_e^2 the residual variability.

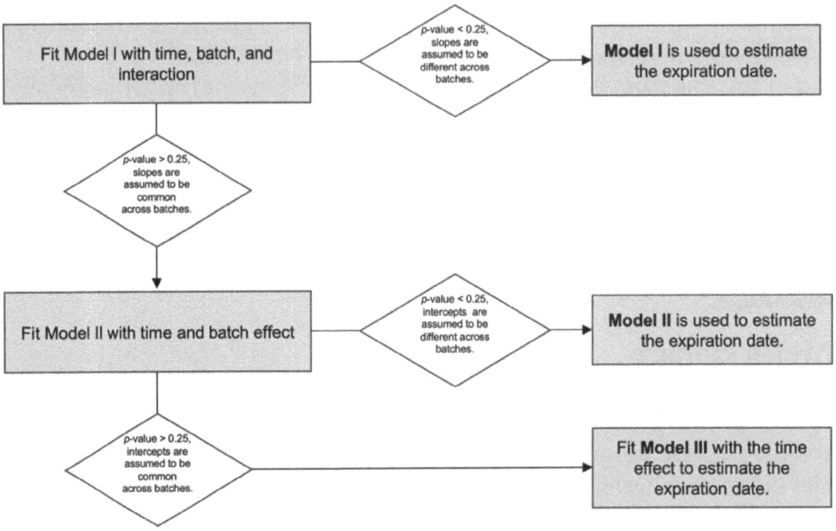

FIGURE 12.1
ICH Q1E guideline for the batch poolability and model definition. By default, model I, which includes distinct slopes and intercepts for each batch, is used. According to ICH Q1E, if the p-value associated with β_3 is not statistically significant at the 0.25 level, model II, which include a common slope and different intercepts, can be used. If the p-value associated with β_2 from model II is not statistically significant at the 0.25 level, model III, which include a common slope and intercept, can then be used. The 0.25 significance level was proposed by Bancroft (1964) to increase statistical power.

Using the selected model, the estimated product shelf-life for a specific CQA is the shortest time that the confidence interval crosses either the lower or the upper specification limit. Shelf-life can be extrapolated beyond the latest observed data point by up to double the observed data or 12 months, whichever is earlier.

12.2.3 Alternative: Random Batch Model

The approach described in Section 12.2.2 has the advantage of simplicity as well as being directly implemented in commercial statistical software such as JMP (JMP, 2022), Minitab (Minitab, LLC, 2022), or Stab-e-Lity (Stab-e-Lity, 2022), as well as some open-source libraries (Lee et al., 2010). Although relatively simple, this approach is flawed for multiple reasons, primarily because a fixed effects model only applies to the observed batches. Assuming the worst of (as little as) three batches is representative of the worst possibility for all future manufactured batches is risky. Burdick et al. (2017) therefore state such a model cannot be used to make inferences about the shelf-life of a future batch.

Although these methods described in the ICH Q1E guideline are widely recommended by regulatory authorities across the globe, we recommend a mixed model. Fortunately, the guidance allows for the use of other statistical approaches, as long as such approach is justified.

Unlike the fixed effect model, mixed-models, or hierarchical models, make predictions and inference possible for future batches. An example of such a model is:

$$y_{ij} = (\beta_0 + \gamma_{0_j}) + (\beta_1 + \gamma_{1_j}) \times \text{Time}_{ij} + \varepsilon_{ij}, \tag{12.4}$$

where:

- y_{ij} is the ith observation of the jth batch, possibly transformed to ensure normality of residuals, for a specific CQA in the studied conditions;
- $\gamma_{0_j} \sim N(0, \sigma_{bI}^2)$ is the effect of batch j on the intercept, with σ_{bI}^2 the batch-to-batch variability for the intercept and β_0 the overall intercept;
- $\gamma_{1_j} \sim N(0, \sigma_{bS}^2)$ is the effect of batch j on the slope, with σ_{bS}^2 the batch-to-batch variability for the slope and β_1 the overall slope;
- Time is the storage time;
- $\varepsilon_{ij} \sim N(0, \sigma_e^2)$ is the residual error, with σ_e^2 the residual variability.

In some cases, this model can be simplified by assuming a common slope among the batches. In other cases, γ_{0_j} and γ_{1_j} should be considered correlated, resulting in a more complex model. While some published methods exist to aid selection of the best hierarchical model (Peng and Lu, 2012; Kuznetsova et al., 2017), we recommend using scientific judgement by reviewing the data and residuals with a subject matter expert, rather than relying on statistical significance.

Using frequentist methods to apply this model presents two main challenges. First, substantial approximation may be required to estimate the degrees of freedom associated with each variance component, which is required to predict future batches accounting for the uncertainty of the model parameters and variance components estimates. This can result in a highly inaccurate shelf-life estimate. Second, while the fixed-effect method highly discourages companies to study more than the minimum required number of batches, mixed models require a larger number of study batches. Companies may revert to the fixed-effect approach simply to avoid additional study batches, as each additional batch incurs substantial resources.

Bayesian statistics can address both challenges discussed above. First, the use of Markov Chain Monte Carlo (MCMC) simulation makes prediction possible without the approximation of the degrees of freedom, as the uncertainty of each parameter and variance component is already accounted for in their respective posterior distributions. Second, using an informative prior distribution may reduce the number of batches needed for a reliable estimation of the product shelf-life.

12.2.3.1 Fit Hierarchical Models Using Stan

Many Bayesian software packages exist, with some of the most popular being JAGS (Depaoli et al., 2016), Stan (Carpenter et al., 2017), and SAS (Chen, 2011). The first two can be applied with an R interface (Plummer, 2003; Stan Development Team, 2021b). Additional R libraries, such as `MCMCglmm` (Hadfield, 2010), `coda` (Plummer et al., 2006), `MCMCpack` (Martin et al., 2011), `brms` (Bürkner, 2017), and more, also provide Bayesian algorithms. In this chapter we focus on Rstan and other packages that run Stan in the background. Several

R packages (e.g., brms, rstanarm (Goodrich et al., 2020)) have been developed to allow convenient fitting of the regression models (both for continuous or categorical responses) based on pre-written stan functions. The R syntax needed to execute Bayesian model fitting is very similar to the standard frequentist models in R (lm, lmer, glm, glmer, etc). Therefore, practitioners unfamiliar with Bayesian theory can easily apply Bayesian modeling as a quick start to exploration of Bayesian approaches. For example, a simplification of the model described in (12.4). with a common slope for each batch, can be fit in R using the following scripts.

```
# Using brms package:
fit <- brm( Y ~ 1 + Time + (1 |Batch), data = your.data.set)

# Using rstanarm package:
fit <- stan_lmer(Y ~ 1 + Time + (1 |Batch),
                                          data = your.data.set)
```

The number of chains, number of iterations, warm-up periods, thinning, number of cores, seeds, or any other simulation configurations can be additionally specified as desired. The posterior draws can be extracted using data.frame(fit) or as.matrix(fit).

```
post <- data.frame(fit)
post <- as.matrix(fit)
```

Additionally, the brms package provides Stan code for those who want to manually modify the underlying script and run the code in rstan. This may be particularly useful for the choice of prior distributions. Further details on prior derivation is provided in Section 12.2.3.3.

As with any MCMC application, we highly recommend performing model diagnostics, such as assessing the effective sample size for every parameter as well as observing trace plots to assess convergence. Details for proper Bayesian model diagnostics can be found in Seaman Jr. et al. (2020) and Chapter 3 of this book.

12.2.3.2 Making Predictions and Estimating the Shelf-Life

Once the joint posterior distribution of each model parameter and variance component is derived and the model is properly evaluated, posterior distribution draws can be used to estimate the shelf-life of future batches. The posterior distribution of the intercept γ_0 of a future batch is simply obtained by drawing from a random normal distribution with the marginal posterior distribution of the model β_0 as the mean, and the marginal posterior distribution of σ^2_{bI} as the variance. The posterior distribution of the slope γ_1 of a future batch is then obtained by drawing from a random normal distribution with the marginal posterior distribution of the model β_1 as the mean, and the marginal posterior distribution of σ^2_{bS} as the variance.

For example, using M posterior draws obtained from MCMC, the posterior distribution of an intercept of a future batch can be generated as follows:

```
rnorm(nrow(post), post$alpha, sqrt(post$sigma2_batch_int))
```

This will generate an M-vector of posterior draws of the batch intercept, drawn from each set of posterior draws of the associated regression parameters (`alpha` and `sigma2_batch_int`).

Similarly, a posterior distribution of a slope of a future batch can be obtained as follows:

```
rnorm(nrow(post), post$beta, sqrt(post$sigma2_batch_slope))
```

While the above scripts are assuming the model will contain both the random intercept and random slope by batch, one may choose to omit either of the random effects based on the data or historical information, in which case the above script would be reduced. For example, if the model contains only a random intercept but not a random slope, the posterior distribution of a future batch would just be the posterior distribution of the overall slope β_1:

```
post$beta
```

A complete stability analysis is illustrated in Section 12.3.1.2 using a case-study, where R scripts at all steps are provided.

When the slope is assumed to be the same for all batches, the marginal posterior distribution of β_1 can simply be used for the future batch slopes. In cases where the batch intercept and slope are correlated, γ_0 and γ_1 should be drawn from a multivariate normal distribution.

Using each mth posterior draw of the intercept and the slope of a future batch, the mth shelf-life is identified by the value of `Time` when the regression line crosses the specification limit, i.e.,:

$$\text{Shelf-Life}_m = \frac{\text{Limit} - \gamma_{0_m}}{\gamma_{1_m}}, \quad m = 1, ..., M, \tag{12.5}$$

where the "Limit" is either lower or upper specification limit, depending on the slope (lower limit when $\gamma_{1_m} < 0$ and upper limit when $\gamma_{1_m} > 0$. When $\gamma_{1_m} = 0$, the regression line is flat, and $\text{Shelf-Life}_m = \infty$. As suggested in Burdick et al. (2017), the shelf-life of a future batch is determined by taking the 5th percentile of the M draws from the posterior predictive distribution described above, often rounded down to the whole month.

Note: The random seed for generation of random numbers should be specified so that results can be reproduced.

12.2.3.3 Prior Distribution Derivation

Use of prior information in a shelf-life estimate can substantially improve accuracy particularly when data are limited to results for a few batches collected over a short time frame. It is not uncommon to have relevant data that can be justified as appropriate prior information. For instance, stability data for development batches across a longer time frame may be available. Use of prior information in this case reduces uncertainty in a way similar to pooling batches. However, a Bayesian approach increases the opportunity to reduce uncertainty. Specifically, historical stability performance from similar products might also be leveraged. In each case, the expected similarity of the stability profile of the full-scale-stability (FSS) batches to the historical "prior information batches" must be described to justify the method.

The amount of prior information that is applicable depends on relative stability performance of the FSS and the historical batches. In cases where the FSS and historical batches appear to have both the same intercept and slope, prior distributions can be elicited using the historical batches.

When just the intercept of the FSS batches appear different from the historical batches, estimates and standard errors for all model parameters excluding the overall intercept are used as prior information. If both intercept and slope of the historical stability profile are different from the FSS batches, prior information is limited to estimates and standard error of the historical profile variance components.

Our proposed method to derive the prior distributions from historical data is to first fit Equation 1 on the historical batches. In general, the output from statistical software should provide the estimate and standard error of each model parameter and variance component. The parameters β_0 and β_1 can each be assumed to follow a normal distribution and therefore the common way to exploit this knowledge is to use

$$\beta_0 \sim N\left(\hat{\beta}_{0_h}, \mathrm{SE}^2_{\hat{\beta}_{0_h}}\right) \tag{12.6}$$

$$\beta_1 \sim N\left(\hat{\beta}_{1_h}, \mathrm{SE}^2_{\hat{\beta}_{1_h}}\right) \tag{12.7}$$

where $\hat{\beta}_{j_h}$ and $\mathrm{SE}^2_{\hat{\beta}_{j_h}}$ are respectively the restricted maximum likelihood estimate and standard error of β_j ($j = 1, 2$) based on historical batches. If the historical batches differ from the FSS batches and should not be used to provide prior knowledge on β_0 and/or β_1, a noninformative normal prior, such as $N(0, 10^6)$, should be used.

Obtaining priors for the random effect variances is more complex. The first step is to find the Chi-square degrees of freedom associated with each variance component estimate $\hat{\sigma}^2_h$. The Chi-square degrees of freedom associated with a variance estimate from the linear mixed effects model can be computed using the Satterthwaite approach (Van Den Heuvel, E. R., 2010):

$$df = \begin{cases} 2\left(\frac{\hat{\sigma}^2_h}{\mathrm{SE}(\hat{\sigma}^2_h)}\right)^2 & \text{if } 1 \leq 2\left(\frac{\hat{\sigma}^2_h}{\mathrm{SE}(\hat{\sigma}^2_h)}\right)^2 \leq n \\ 1 & \text{if } 2\left(\frac{\hat{\sigma}^2_h}{\mathrm{SE}(\hat{\sigma}^2_h)}\right)^2 < 1 \\ n & \text{if } 2\left(\frac{\hat{\sigma}^2_h}{\mathrm{SE}(\hat{\sigma}^2_h)}\right)^2 > n \end{cases} \tag{12.8}$$

where n is the total number of observations. Then, inverse-gamma priors for the random effect variances can be derived as follows:

$$X = \frac{df \times \hat{\sigma}^2}{\sigma^2} \sim \chi^2(df) = \mathrm{Gamma}\left(\frac{df}{2}, \frac{1}{2}\right), \tag{12.9}$$

where the gamma distribution is parameterized using shape and rate parameters.

Now transitioning to the Bayesian framework, assume σ^2 is a random parameter, and $\hat{\sigma}^2$ is a realized estimate (a constant),

$$\frac{1}{\sigma^2} = \frac{X}{df \times \hat{\sigma}^2} \sim \text{Gamma}\left(\frac{df}{2}, \frac{df \times \hat{\sigma}^2}{2}\right). \tag{12.10}$$

This is equivalent to

$$\sigma^2 \sim \text{Inverse-Gamma}\left(\frac{df}{2}, \frac{df \times \hat{\sigma}^2}{2}\right), \tag{12.11}$$

where the inverse-gamma distribution is using the shape and scale parameterization.

The case study in Section 12.3 presents details and codes for specific variance components.

12.2.4 Internal Release Limits Derivation

IRLs provide assurance with some probability (typically 95%) that the released batch will remain within specification during the expiry period. Typically, the release range is narrower than the filed product specification ranges because it accounts for degradation over time, the uncertainty in the slope estimate, and the measurement method error.

For CQAs that do not change over time, the specification range need only be adjusted by the width of the measurement uncertainty, with measurement uncertainty being calculated by:

$$u(Y^2) = S^2IP + u(\hat{\delta})^2, \tag{12.12}$$

where

- $u(Y^2)$ is the measurement uncertainty,
- S^2IP is the assay intermediate precision,
- $u(\hat{\delta})^2$ is the uncertainty (sampling variability) of the assay accuracy.

Thus, in this case:

$$\text{LRL} = \text{LSL} + u(Y)^2 \tag{12.13}$$

$$\text{URL} = \text{USL} - u(Y)^2 \tag{12.14}$$

where LRL and URL are respectively the lower and upper release limits, and LSL and USL are respectively the lower and upper specification limits.

For CQAs that do change over time, the IRL must account for the model slope, as well as the uncertainty of the model slope. Thus, for CQAs that decrease over time:

$$\text{LRL} = \text{LSL} + \text{expected decline} + \text{measurement uncertainty} + \text{decline uncertainty} \tag{12.15}$$

$$\text{URL} = \text{USL} - \text{measurement uncertainty} \tag{12.16}$$

And for CQAs that increase over time:

$$\text{LRL} = \text{LSL} + \text{measurement uncertainty} \tag{12.17}$$

$$\text{URL} = \text{USL} - \text{expected decline} - \text{measurement uncertainty} - \text{decline uncertainty} \tag{12.18}$$

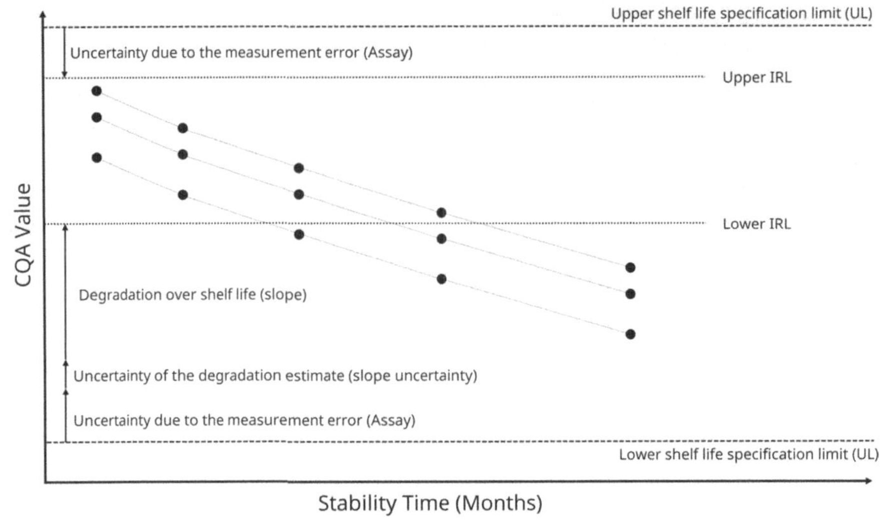

FIGURE 12.2
Graphical display of IRL calculation for an attribute which exhibits degradation over time. Individual batch profiles are represented with linked dots. The horizontal dashed lines are the upper and lower shelf-life specification limits (UL and LL), and the dotted lines represent the calculated lower and upper IRLs for the product's desired shelf-life (dSL). The diminution from the specification range to the release range due to the product degradation over shelf-life (slope), slope uncertainty, and measurement error, are illustrated by vertical arrows.

These relationships are shown graphically for an attribute that decreases over time in Figure 12.2.

12.2.4.1 Traditional Method

Allen et al. (1991) proposed the following formula to estimate LRL and USL, shown here for decreasing CQAs:

$$\text{LRL} = \text{LSL} - \hat{\beta}_1 \times x_{SL} + t_{df_L,\alpha/2}\sqrt{\hat{\sigma}^2_{\beta_1} \times x^2_{SL} + \frac{\hat{\sigma}^2_Y}{n_R}} \tag{12.19}$$

$$\text{URL} = \text{USL} + t_{df_U,\alpha/2}\hat{\sigma}^2_Y \tag{12.20}$$

where

- $\hat{\beta}_1$ is the model slope;
- x_{SL} is the desired shelf-life;
- $t_{df_L,\alpha/2}$ is the $(\alpha/2)^{th}$ quantile for a t distribution with df_L degrees of freedom;
- $t_{df_U,\alpha/2}$ is the $(\alpha/2)^{th}$ quantile for a t distribution with df_U degrees of freedom;
- $\hat{\sigma}^2_{\beta_1}$ is the uncertainty in the slope estimation;

- $\hat{\sigma}_Y^2$ is the assay variability;
- n_R is the number of sample that will be measured for each batch release testing.

Allen et al. (1991) propose that df_L be estimated using Satterthwaite's method although other methods exist (Egan and Schofield, 2009):

$$df_L = \frac{\left(\hat{\sigma}_{\beta_1}^2 + \hat{\sigma}_Y^2\right)^2}{\frac{\hat{\sigma}_{\beta_1}^4}{df_{\beta_1}} + \frac{\hat{\sigma}_Y^4}{df_y}} \tag{12.21}$$

where $\hat{\sigma}_{\beta_1}^2$, $\hat{\sigma}_Y^2$ and their respective associated degrees of freedom df_{β_1} and df_Y may be obtained from the selected model described in Section 12.2.2. If the slopes can be pooled (model I and II), the overall slope can be used, and if the slopes cannot be pooled (model III), the steepest slope should be used (Yang, 2018). While Allen et al. (1991) believe that URL is not useful, we suggest calculating it, because a single measurement within specifications does not guarantee that the true batch release value also meets the specifications.

12.2.4.2 Bayesian Alternative

The limitations of ICH Q1E's proposed method for shelf-life estimation also exist for the Allen et al. (1991) method for IRL derivation. Mixed effect models are a better alternative (Montes et al., 2019), though they present the same challenges as described for shelf-life determination. These challenges can again be addressed with a Bayesian approach, which uses the same model for shelf-life estimation and IRL derivation.

The first step is prior derivation and model fitting. See Sections 12.2.3.1 and 12.2.3.3 for details. Once the joint posterior distribution of each model parameter and variance component is derived and the model is properly evaluated, posterior distribution chains are used to estimate the probability that a batch will meet specification throughout the product desired shelf-life, for a specific *measured* release value. Note that a batch will be accepted or rejected based on its *measured* value, but whether that same batch falls (or not) within specifications at shelf-life depends on the *true* release value.

Next, generate a grid of K release values across the specification range. The larger K is, the more precise the IRL range will be. The release values k represent the average of n_R measured samples at release. For each release value k:

1. Draw M samples from $N(k, \ddot{\sigma}_Y^2/n_R)$, where $\ddot{\sigma}_Y^2$ is distributed as the marginal posterior distribution of σ_Y^2;
2. Obtain the posterior distribution of γ_1 as described in Section 12.2.3.3.
3. Derive the posterior predictive distribution of Y_{SL}, where Y_{SL} is the true value of Y at shelf-life: $Y_{SL} = Y_R + \gamma_1 \times x_{SL}$, where Y_R is the chain of true release values obtained in Step 1;
4. Calculate $\pi = \Pr(\text{LSL} \leq Y_{SL} \leq \text{USL}|\text{Data}, I, k)$, the probability that the true value of Y at shelf-life falls within the specification limits (where I represents the available information).

IRLs are then defined as the widest range of measured release values for which π reaches the desired confidence (probability). As IRLs are usually for internal use only, and not part of a regulatory submission, they can be updated as study data become available.

12.3 Case Study

In this section, an example dataset is analyzed to demonstrate

- how to estimate a shelf-life using ICH Q1E approach (ICH Q1E, 2003) and Bayesian random batch model;
- how to derive IRLs using the Allen et al. (1991) approach and a Bayesian approach.

The data are shown in Table 12.1 and in Figure 12.3. The dataset contains stability data for 6 batches. Batches 1, 2, and 3 have stability data only up to 24 months, while the batches 4, 5, and 6 have data up to 12 months. In this example, batches 4, 5, and 6 are the Process Performance Qualification (PPQ) batches used for the full-scale stability study, while batches 1, 2, and 3 are historical batches that can only be used to derive the prior. A Bayesian mixed effects model was fit to batches 4, 5, and 6 with noninformative and informative priors, where the informative priors were derived from the data for batches 1, 2, and 3.

TABLE 12.1
Example data.

Time (Month)	Y	Batch	Time (Month)	Y	Batch
0	107.21	1	12	104.78	3
3	106.38	1	18	106.02	3
6	103.86	1	24	102.98	3
9	103.75	1	0	100.89	4
12	101.69	1	3	102.69	4
18	104.41	1	6	100.55	4
24	100.66	1	9	101.91	4
0	107.66	2	12	98.93	4
3	105.92	2	0	104.93	5
6	106.03	2	3	103.62	5
9	104.66	2	6	101.46	5
12	102.58	2	9	102.85	5
18	103.8	2	12	99.7	5
24	101.29	2	0	105.84	6
0	109.21	3	3	107.59	6
3	106.93	3	6	104.65	6
6	106.61	3	9	104.88	6
9	106.82	3	12	103.99	6

12.3.1 Shelf-Life Estimation

12.3.1.1 Fixed Batch Approach Using ICH Q1E

In this section, the frequentists' method as suggested by ICH was used to estimate the shelf-life based on the worst-batch case. The significance level of 0.25 was used to determine the statistical significance of the interaction effect between `Time` and `Batch`, as well as the statistical significance of the `Batch` effect. According to the ICH Q1E guideline, the following three linear models are considered:

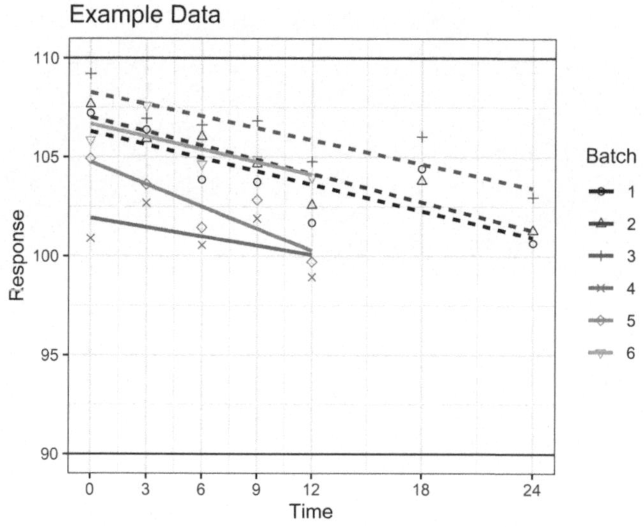

FIGURE 12.3
Stability data from 6 batches. Batches 1, 2, and 3 are historical batches.

- MI: Model with different slopes and different intercepts across batches
- MII: Model with a common slope and different intercepts across batches
- MIII: Model with a common slope and a common slope across batches

Among these 3 models, the best model for the shelf-life estimation is determined based on sequential tests: By default, MI (a different slope and a different intercept for each batch) is fitted and the interaction term is selected. If the p-value for the interaction term is ≥ 0.25, then MII (a common slope and different intercepts) will be selected. If the p-value for the batch effect in MII is ≥ 0.25, then MIII (a common slope and a common intercept) will be selected.

Analysis can be performed with the following script in R, which was written with the `tidyverse` and `car` libraries loaded.

```
library(tidyverse)
library(car) # for Anova function
```

First, create a new data frame keeping only the FSS batches (Batches 4, 5, 6):

```
d1 <- d %>% filter(as.numeric(Batch) > 3)
```

Fit the model M1:

```
> fit.f1 <- lm(Y ~ Time*Batch, data=d1)
> Anova(fit.f1)
```

```
Anova Table (Type II tests)

Response: Y
            Sum Sq Df F value    Pr(>F)
Time        16.684  1 11.3366 0.0082966 **
Batch       49.834  2 16.9311 0.0008908 ***
Time:Batch   2.302  2  0.7823 0.4861434
Residuals   13.245  9
```

P-value for the interaction term was found to be $0.486 > 0.25$, indicating that the interaction effect is not statistically significant at a 25% level of significance. Therefore, MII was fitted by dropping the interaction term.

```
> fit.f2 <- lm(Y ~ Time + Batch, data=d1)
> Anova(fit.f2)
Anova Table (Type II tests)

Response: Y
          Sum Sq Df F value    Pr(>F)
Time      16.684  1  11.804 0.0055670 **
Batch     49.834  2  17.629 0.0003708 ***
Residuals 15.548 11
```

The p-value for the batch effect in MII is 0.0004, indicating that the Batch effect is statistically significant. Therefore, MII is selected to be the final model (the model with a common slope and different intercepts across batches). The regression summary for the final model MII is shown below.

```
fit.f <- fit.f2 # Final model

> summary(fit.f)

Call:
lm(formula = Y ~ Time + Batch, data = d1)

Residuals:
     Min       1Q   Median       3Q      Max
-1.59397 -0.89054  0.08751  0.93820  1.65789

Coefficients:
             Estimate Std. Error t value Pr(>|t|)
(Intercept) 102.48674    0.68640 149.312  < 2e-16 ***
Time         -0.24858    0.07235  -3.436 0.005567 **
Batch5        1.51533    0.75191   2.015 0.068969 .
Batch6        4.39470    0.75191   5.845 0.000112 ***
```

```
Residual standard error: 1.189 on 11 degrees of freedom
Multiple R-squared:  0.8105,Adjusted R-squared:  0.7589
F-statistic: 15.69 on 3 and 11 DF,  p-value: 0.0002747
```

Next, the predicted values and the associated 95% confidence bands were obtained:

```
Newdata = expand.grid(Batch = unique(d1$Batch),
                      Time = seq(0,40, by = 0.01))
Pred <- predict(fit.f, Newdata, interval = "confidence")
Predicted <- data.frame(Newdata, Pred) %>%
             mutate(within.spec = lwr >= LSL & upr <= USL)
```

The shelf-life is the earliest time point that any of the confidence intervals goes out of specification limits.

```
SL.f = Predicted %>% filter(within.spec == F) %>%
       select(Time) %>% min()

> SL.f
[1] 32.58
```

Figure 12.4 shows the prediction lines and 95% bands, created with the following script:

```
ggplot(data = Predicted, aes(x = Time, y = fit)) +
  theme_bw() +
  scale_shape_manual(values = 1:length(unique(d1$Batch))) +
  scale_colour_grey(start = 0.1, end = 0.4,
               na.value = "black", aesthetics = "colour") +
  scale_colour_grey(start = 0.1, end = 0.4,
               na.value = "black", aesthetics = "fill") +
  scale_linetype_manual(values = c("dotdash", "dashed",
                                   "longdash")) +

  geom_ribbon(aes(ymin = lwr, ymax = upr, fill = Batch),
               alpha = 0.3) +
  geom_line(aes(color=Batch, linetype = Batch)) +

  geom_hline(yintercept = LSL, col = 1, linetype = 1) +
  geom_hline(yintercept = USL, col = 1, linetype = 1) +

  scale_x_continuous(breaks = seq(0, 40, by=5)) +
```

```
labs(x = "Time", y = "Response",
     title = "95% Confidence Bands by Batch")
```

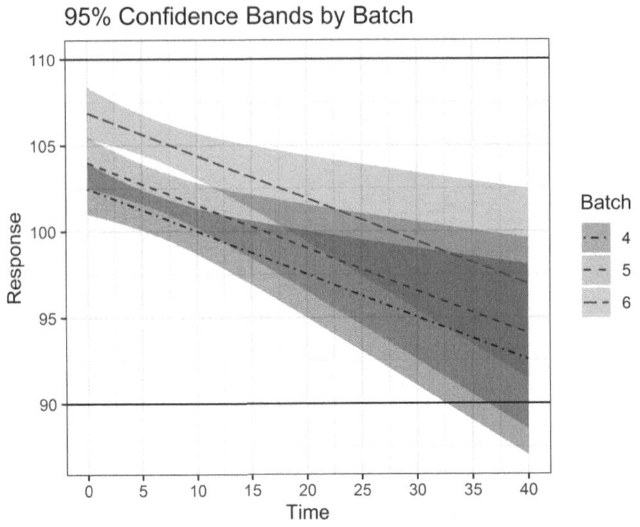

FIGURE 12.4
95% confidence bands by batch extrapolated up to time 40 months.

Figure 12.4 shows the 95% confidence bands extrapolated up to 40 months. The confidence band of Batch 1 hits the specification the earliest, at Time = 32.58 months. By taking the floor of the value, the shelf-life estimate would be 32 months.

As noted in Section 12.1, this estimate is unlikely to be the worst of all future batches. Hierarchical modeling is more suitable for prediction of the future batches, and a Bayesian approach is strongly recommended for the various benefits relative to the frequentist mixed model. In the next section, we will present a Bayesian methodology for analysis of the data in Table 12.1, with and without prior information.

12.3.1.2 Random Batch Approach Using Bayesian Estimation

In this section, the data for batches 4, 5, and 6 were analyzed using Bayesian approach with and without using prior information. A Bayesian linear mixed effect model was fitted with Y as the response, Time as a fixed effect, and a random intercept by batch. Since the slopes in Figure 12.4 appear to be similar across batches, a random slope was not included in the model.

The ith observation of the jth batch was expressed as follows:

$$y_{ij} = \beta_0 + \delta_{0_j} + \beta_1 \times \text{Time}_{ij} + \varepsilon_{ij} \tag{12.22}$$

where $\delta_{0_j} \sim N(0, \sigma^2_{\text{batch intercept}})$ and $\varepsilon_{ij} \sim N(0, \sigma^2_e)$.

The Bayesian analyses have been performed using various platforms and packages that require manual coding. We illustrate the analyses using R and rstan. The following is an example of manual coding for rstan (with noninformative priors).
Using the rstan package:

```
standata = list(

  N = nrow(d1),
  N_Batch = length(unique(d1$Batch)),
  Batch = as.numeric(as.factor(d1$Batch)),
  Y = d1$Y,
  Time = d1$Time
)

stanmodel_no_priors ="

  data{

    int N ;
    int N_Batch;
    vector[N] Y;
    vector[N] Time;
    int Batch[N];
  }

  parameters{

  real alpha;
  real beta;
  real<lower=0> sigma2_batch_int;
  real<lower=0> sigma2_resid;

  // generated values for random effects
  vector[N_Batch] u_batch_int; // random intercept by batch
}
  model {
  vector[N] mu; // mean vector

// noninformative Priors
    alpha ~ normal(0, 1e3);
    beta ~ normal(0, 1e3);
    sigma2_resid ~ inv_gamma(0.0001, 0.0001);
    sigma2_batch_int ~ inv_gamma(0.0001, 0.0001);

// Random effects distributions
u_batch_int ~ normal(0, sqrt(sigma2_batch_int));

// Mean vector
for (i in 1:N){
mu[i] = alpha +  u_batch_int[Batch[i]] + beta * Time[i] ;
}

// Distribution of Y
Y ~ normal(mu, sqrt(sigma2_resid)); // vector of length N
```

```
}
"
fit_rstan <- stan(model_code = stanmodel_no_priors,
                  data = standata)
```

The posterior from rstan can be extracted using

```
post <- data.frame(extract(fit))
```

For illustration, the first 10 rows of the posterior draws from rstan are shown in Table 12.2, where

- alpha represents the fixed intercept
- beta represents the fixed slope
- sigma2_batch_int represents the variance of the random intercept by batch
- sigma2_resid represents the residual variance
- u_batch_int.1 ~ u_batch_int.3 represent the differences between each batch intercept and the overall (fixed) intercept.

The intercept and the slope of a future batch are defined as follows based on the model:

- Intercept of a future batch = fixed intercept + intercept of a future batch
- Slope of a future batch = fixed slope (since no random effect was assumed)

TABLE 12.2
Chain of the joint posterior distribution.

alpha	beta	sigma2_batch_int	sigma2_resid	u_batch_int.1	u_batch_int.2	u_batch_int.3	lp__
106.041	−0.36	10.369	1.161	−2.397	−1.015	1.599	−14.027
103.497	−0.082	17.192	2.499	−3.244	−1.034	1.158	−19.457
106.099	−0.534	1.45	4.205	−1.531	0.538	1.631	−18.653
102.515	−0.298	92.911	1.823	0.756	1.568	5.107	−16.57
101.701	−0.16	25.778	1.275	1.163	1.514	5.244	−16.678
104.08	−0.16	4.435	6.698	−0.795	−0.077	1.912	−19.117
106.094	−0.259	4.295	2.008	−3.02	−1.974	1.383	−13.743
105.376	−0.243	6.484	1.77	−2.573	−0.758	1.09	−13.113
105.292	−0.246	5.399	1.608	−2.092	−1.772	1.956	−13.374
103.732	−0.262	2.526	1.873	−0.659	0.72	3.146	−12.949

The posterior draws of the random intercept can be generated from $N(0, \sigma^2_{\text{batch intercept}})$ using each set of posterior draws of $\sigma^2_{\text{batch intercept}}$.

```
int.fut <- rnorm(nrow(post), post$alpha,
                 sqrt(post$sigma2_batch_int))
slope.fut <- post$beta
```

As an optional feature, the fitted object in `rstanarm` additionally provides posterior draws of the random effect of a future batch (labeled as `NEW` in the output) as well as for the current batches, which can be directly used to obtain the posterior distributions of the intercept and slope of a future batch.

```
int.fut <- post[, "(Intercept)"] +
           post[,"b[(Intercept) Batch:_NEW_Batch]"]
slope.fut <- post[, "Time"]
```

Using each mth posterior draw of the intercept and the slope of a future batch, i.e., $\text{Intercept}^{[m]}_{\text{future}}$ and $\text{Slope}^{[m]}_{\text{future}}$, where $m = 1, ..., M$, the mth shelf-life is calculated by finding a value of Time, where the regression line hits the specification limit:

$$\text{Shelf-life}^{[m]} = \frac{\text{Limit} - \text{Intercept}^{[m]}_{\text{future}}}{\text{Slope}^{[m]}_{\text{future}}}, \tag{12.23}$$

for $m = 1, ..., M$, where the Limit is either lower or upper stability limit depending on the slope. (Lower limit when $\text{Slope}^{[m]}_{\text{future}} < 0$ and upper limit when $\text{Slope}^{[m]}_{\text{future}} > 0$. When $\text{Slope}^{[m]}_{\text{future}} = 0$, then $\text{Shelf-life}^{[m]} = \infty$, as the regression line will be flat. R scripts to calculate the shelf-life are shown below.

```
SLs <- data.frame(int.fut, slope.fut) %>%
   mutate(sl =
        case_when(slope.fut < 0 ~ (LSL - int.fut)/slope.fut,
                  slope.fut > 0 ~ (USL - int.fut)/slope.fut,
                  slope.fut == 0 ~ Inf))
```

As suggested in Burdick et al. (2017), the shelf-life of a future batch is determined by taking the 5th percentile of the M draws from the posterior predictive distribution described above. (Often the floor of the value is taken as the final shelf-life.)

```
SL.fut.batch <- data.frame(Batch = "Future",
                           SL = quantile(SLs$sl,
                                         0.05, na.rm=T))
print(SL.fut.batch)
floor(SL.fut.batch$SL)
```

It should be emphasized that it is important to set a random seed where random numbers are generated in order to reproduce the results. Below are the results from the Bayesian estimation using rstan using 4 chains, with each chain having 130000 iterations, a warm-up period of 30000, and thinning of 10. The random seeds used to generate these results are shown in the full script we are sharing at `https://github.com/BayesCMC/Book`.

12.3.1.3 Results with Noninformative Prior

The following noninformative priors were used.

- $\beta_0 \sim N(0, 1000^2)$
- $\beta_1 \sim N(0, 1000^2)$
- $\sigma^2_{\text{bath intercept}} \sim \text{Inverse-Gamma}(0.0001, 0.0001)$
- $\sigma^2_e \sim \text{Inverse-Gamma}(0.0001, 0.0001)$

The fit is shown in Figure 12.5, while Figure 12.6 shows trace plots of 4 Markov chains for each regression parameter to inspect sampling behavior and assess mixing across chains and convergence.
To print the summary of the fit:

```
print(fit)
```

```
Inference for Stan model: 94cb7f413f562284ecf62cd786e92964.
4 chains, each with iter=130000; warmup=30000; thin=10;
post-warmup draws per chain=10000, total post-warmup draws=40000.

                   mean se_mean     sd   2.5%    25%    50%    75%  97.5% n_eff Rhat
alpha            104.48    0.03   3.76  98.99 103.37 104.46 105.54 109.82 16245    1
beta              -0.25    0.00   0.08  -0.41  -0.30  -0.25  -0.20  -0.09 37744    1
sigma2_batch_int  49.72    5.27 898.35   0.74   2.90   6.22  15.52 189.91 29094    1
sigma2_resid       1.79    0.01   1.04   0.71   1.15   1.53   2.12   4.50 35750    1
u_batch_int[1]    -1.83    0.03   3.75  -7.28  -2.84  -1.74  -0.71   3.44 16138    1
u_batch_int[2]    -0.44    0.03   3.74  -5.83  -1.45  -0.40   0.62   5.00 16082    1
u_batch_int[3]     2.20    0.03   3.75  -2.87   1.10   2.15   3.25   7.87 16158    1
lp__             -15.49    0.01   2.43 -21.34 -16.80 -15.07 -13.71 -12.06 31618    1
```

FIGURE 12.5
Fit summary based on noninformative priors.

To look at trace plots:

```
stan_trace(fit)
```

Figure 12.7 shows an example of the posterior distributions of the intercept and slope of a future batch using noninformative priors, generated by the following scripts:

```
ggplot(data=data.frame(int.fut), aes(x=int.fut)) +
    theme_bw() + xlim(90, 120) +
    labs(x = "Intercept of a Future Batch") +
    geom_density()
```

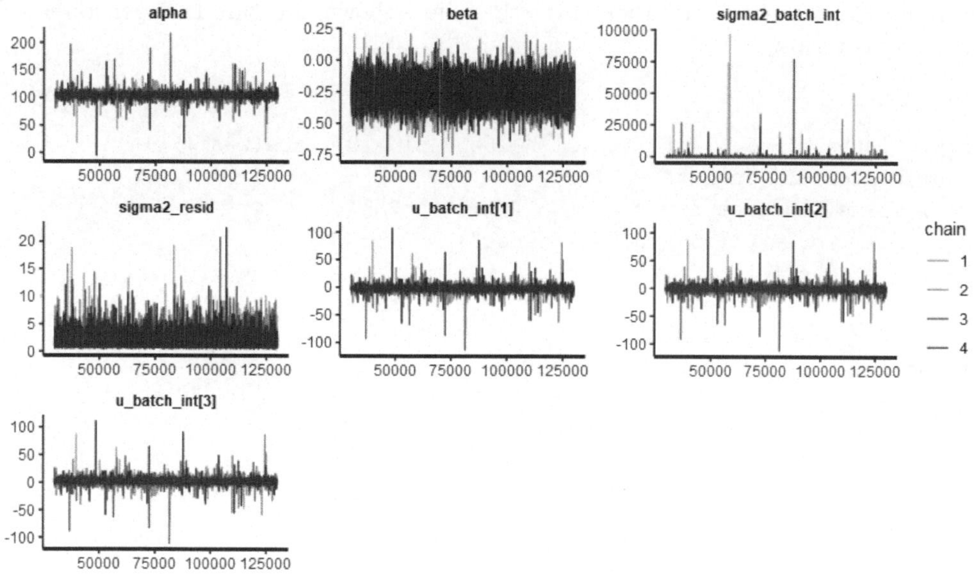

FIGURE 12.6
Trace plots of 4 Markov chains based on noninformative priors.

```
ggplot(data=data.frame(slope.fut), aes(x=slope.fut)) +
    theme_bw() + xlim(-0.75, 0.25) +
    labs(x = "Slope of a Future Batch") +
    geom_density()
```

Note that the histograms are showing partial ranges of intercept and slope to make the high-density areas more visible.

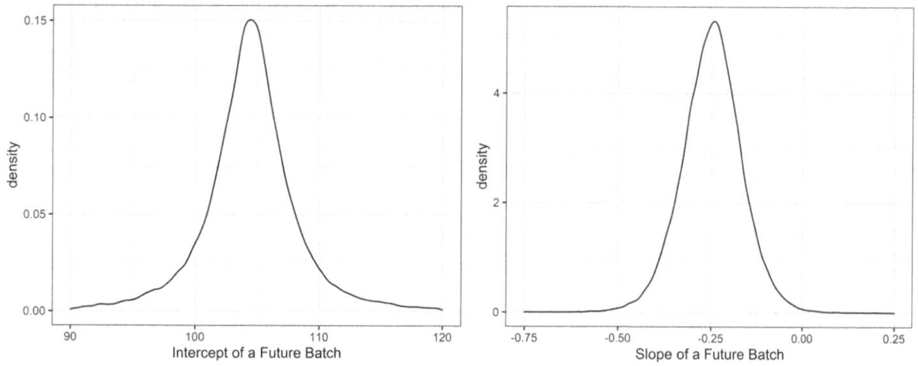

FIGURE 12.7
Distributions of the intercept and slope of a future batch (using noninformative priors).

The resulting posterior distribution of the shelf-life is shown in Figure 12.8, generated using the following script:

```
ggplot(data = SLs %>% filter(sl < 250 & sl > 0), aes(x=sl)) +
geom_histogram(binwidth = 2) +
geom_vline(xintercept = round(SL.fut.batch$SL),
           col=2, linetype = "dashed") +
labs(x = "Shelf-Life", title = "Posterior distribution of
          shelf-life between 0 and 250 months",
          y = "Response") +
theme_bw()
```

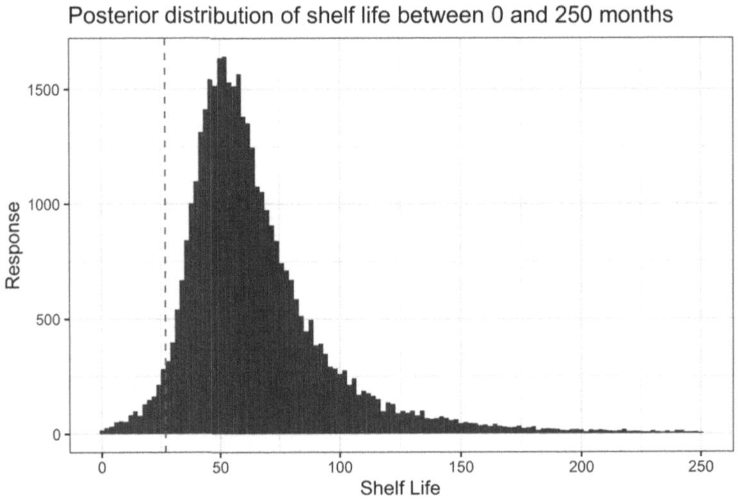

FIGURE 12.8
Posterior distribution of the shelf-life of a future batch between 0 and 250 months for visibility.

The resulting shelf-life for a future batch was estimated to be only 27.18 months (27 months as the nearest lower integer).

Gelman (2006) discussed potential issues in the use of Inverse-Gamma (IG) distribution as a noninformative prior. The paper illustrated that the choice of Inverse-Gamma parameters for group-level variance could have a big impact on the inferences, especially when the group level variance is near 0. We performed a sensitivity analysis (not presented) and observed that the results were consistent regardless of the scale and shape of the noninformative IG. However, when using Half-Normal or Half-Cauchy distributions, the results were highly sensitive to the scale parameter chosen for the prior. Therefore, it seemed that the Inverse-Gamma was an appropriate choice.

12.3.1.4 Results with Informative Prior

The following noninformative prior was used for the fixed intercept:

- $\beta_0 \sim N(0, 1000^2)$

For the fixed slope and variance parameters, the following informative priors were used:

- $\beta_1 \sim N(-0.22134, 0.03093^2)$
- $\sigma^2_{\text{bath intercept}} \sim \text{Inverse-Gamma}(0.75, 0.95)$
- $\sigma^2_e \sim \text{Inverse-Gamma}(8.5, 12.9)$

This was based on the prior information derived from the batches 4, 5, and 6, which had data from longer stability time periods. While there are many ways to obtain prior information, we present one approach to determine priors, based on a regression fitted to the prior data (assuming prior data are available).

Determination of priors for regression parameters based on prior data
The same linear mixed model that is to be fitted on the FSS batches was fit on the historical batches (1 to 3). The following is the regression output from the prior data (batches 1-3):

```
lmr <- lmer(Y ~ Time + (1 |Batch), data = d %>%
          filter(Batch %in% 1:3))
summary(lmr)
Linear mixed model fit by REML. t-tests use
       Satterthwaite's method ['lmerModLmerTest']
Formula: Y ~ Time + (1 | Batch)
   Data: d %>% filter(Batch %in% 1:3)

REML criterion at convergence: 72.1

Scaled residuals:
    Min      1Q  Median      3Q     Max
-1.8477 -0.5875 -0.2106  0.6976  1.8037

Random effects:
 Groups   Name        Variance Std.Dev.
 Batch    (Intercept) 1.127    1.062
 Residual             1.232    1.110
Number of obs: 21, groups:  Batch, 3

Fixed effects:
             Estimate Std. Error        df t value Pr(>|t|)
(Intercept) 107.19354    0.73179   3.02107 146.480 6.44e-07 ***
Time         -0.22134    0.03093  17.00000  -7.157 1.61e-06 ***
```

The fitted object contains estimates and standard errors (SEs) of the estimates both for the fixed and random effect parameters. The SEs for the estimators of batch-to-batch variance and residual variance are not shown in the default summary output, but can be obtained as follows:

```
# Standard error of random effects variances
se_vars <- vcov(lmr, full = TRUE); se_vars
```

TABLE 12.3
A 4 by 4 variance-covariance matrix of the estimators. The 3rd and 4th diagonal elements are the squared SEs of the batch-to-batch and residual variance estimators.

	Intercept	Time	Batch Intercept	Residual
Intercept	0.536	−0.010	0.000	0.000
Time	−0.010	0.001	0.000	0.000
Batch Intercept	0.000	0.000	1.702	−0.026
Residual	0.000	0.000	−0.026	0.179

The priors for the population intercept and slope can be assumed to be N(`Estimate`, `Std.Error`), where `Estimate` and `Std.Error` are taken from the summary output. In our example, we used an informative prior only for the population slope, and still used a non-informative prior for the intercept:

- $\beta_0 \sim N(0, 1000^2)$
- $\beta_1 \sim N(-0.22134, 0.03093^2)$.

Note that the mean and SD of the slope are from the regression output. On the other hand, obtaining priors for the random effect variances is relatively more complex. We followed the method described in Section 12.2.3.3. The informative priors for the batch-to-batch variance (σ_b^2) and residual variance (σ_r^2) were assumed to be the following inverse-gamma (IG) distributions:

$$\sigma_b^2 \sim \text{Inverse-Gamma}\left(\frac{df_b}{2}, \frac{df_b\hat{\sigma}_b^2}{2}\right) \quad (12.24)$$

$$\sigma_r^2 \sim \text{Inverse-Gamma}\left(\frac{df_r}{2}, \frac{df_r\hat{\sigma}_r^2}{2}\right) \quad (12.25)$$

where $\hat{\sigma}_b^2$ and $\hat{\sigma}_r^2$ are the estimates obtained from the above `lmer` output, and df_b and df_r are the degrees of freedom for the variance components calculated using Satterthwaite approach and the standard errors provided in Table 12.3. Below shows the computation process, taking variance estimates their associated standard errors from the fitted object, and computing the degrees of freedom for each variance:

```
# Estimates of random effects variances
> vars_re <- data.frame(summary(lmr)$varcor)
> sigma2_b <- vars_re$vcov[1]; sigma2_b
[1] 1.127008
> sigma2_r <- vars_re$vcov[2]; sigma2_r
[1] 1.2321

> se.sigma2_b <- sqrt(diag(se_vars)[3]); se.sigma2_b
[1] 1.30442
> se.sigma2_r <- sqrt(diag(se_vars)[4]); se.sigma2_r
[1] 0.4226068
```

```
> df_b <- 2 * (sigma2_b / se.sigma2_b)^2; df_b
[1] 1.492963
> df_r <- 2 * (sigma2_r / se.sigma2_r)^2; df_r
[1] 17

> df_b/2
[1] 0.7464815
> df_b * sigma2_b^2 / 2
[1] 0.9481418

> df_r/2
[1] 8.5
> df_r * sigma2_r^2 / 2
[1] 12.9036
```

The fit is shown in Figure 12.9, while Figure 12.10 shows trace plots of 4 Markov chains for each regression parameter to inspect sampling behavior and assess mixing across chains and convergence.

```
Inference for Stan model: 9ea8e5e9e1d8c445d38f776de9c646e7.
4 chains, each with iter=130000; warmup=30000; thin=10;
post-warmup draws per chain=10000, total post-warmup draws=40000.

                   mean se_mean    sd   2.5%    25%    50%    75%  97.5% n_eff Rhat
alpha            104.32    0.01  1.55 101.30 103.52 104.31 105.11 107.34 33100    1
beta              -0.23    0.00  0.03  -0.28  -0.24  -0.23  -0.21  -0.17 37400    1
sigma2_batch_int   7.31    0.31 60.52   0.84   2.08   3.59   6.76  32.45 38320    1
sigma2_resid       1.56    0.00  0.45   0.92   1.25   1.49   1.79   2.65 40309    1
u_batch_int[1]    -1.78    0.01  1.58  -4.94  -2.58  -1.73  -0.93   1.17 33287    1
u_batch_int[2]    -0.41    0.01  1.57  -3.50  -1.21  -0.40   0.40   2.62 33235    1
u_batch_int[3]     2.19    0.01  1.58  -0.73   1.34   2.15   3.01   5.40 33461    1
lp__             -28.30    0.01  2.09 -33.35 -29.44 -27.92 -26.76 -25.35 38152    1
```

FIGURE 12.9
Fit summary based on informative priors.

Figure 12.11 shows an example of the posterior distributions of the intercept and slope of a future batch using informative priors.
The resulting posterior distribution of the shelf-life between is shown in Figure 12.12.
The shelf-life for a future batch was estimated to be 42.28 months (42 months as the nearest lower integer).

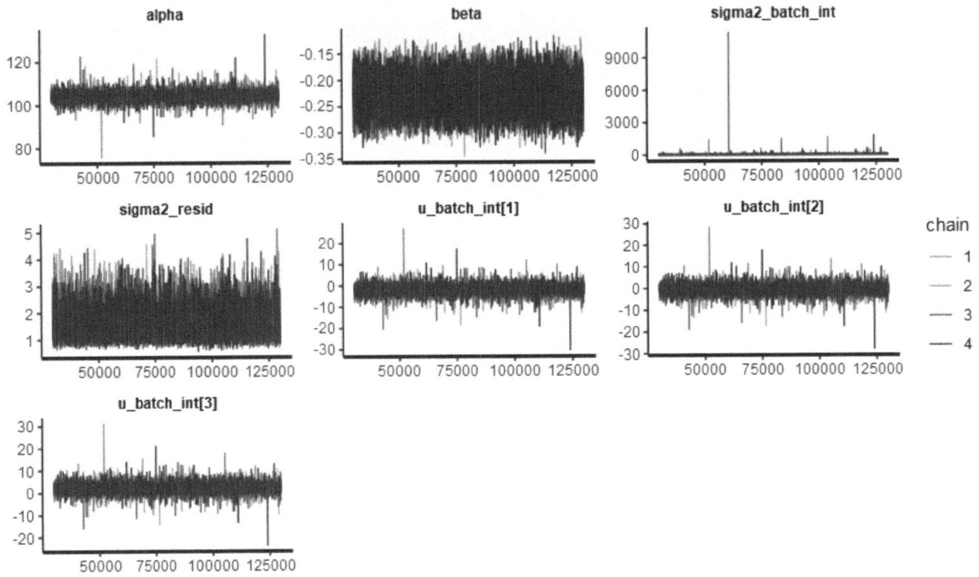

FIGURE 12.10
Trace plots of 4 Markov chains based on informative priors.

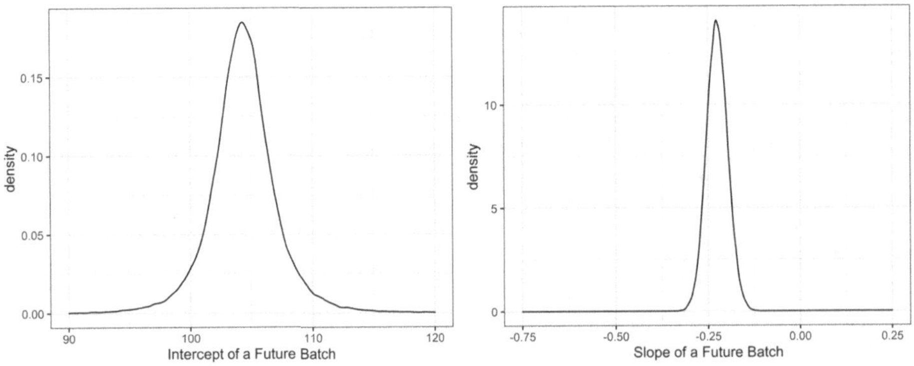

FIGURE 12.11
Distributions of the intercept and slope of a future batch (using informative priors).

12.3.2 Internal Release Limits (IRLs) Estimation

In this section, internal release limits will be computed using a Bayesian approach using the `rstan` package in R.

Internal Release Limit Example

For both the traditional and Bayesian methods, we use $n_R = 1$. Wider release limits can be obtained in both cases by committing to measure more than one sample for each future released batch.

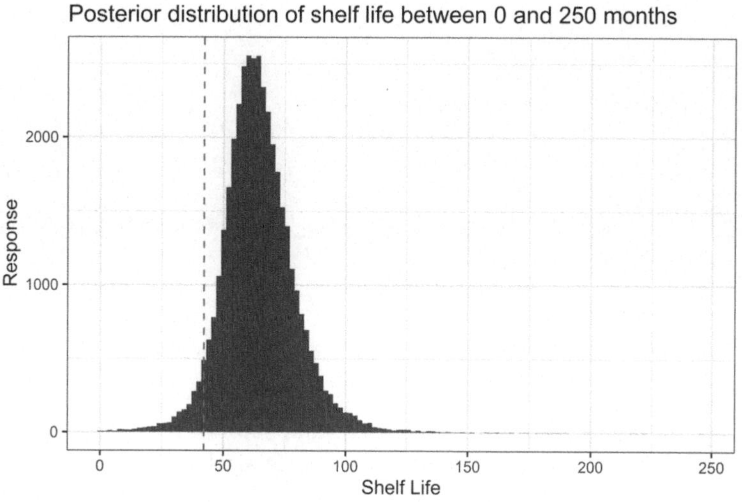

FIGURE 12.12
Posterior distribution of the shelf-life of a future batch using informative priors.

Allen's Method
Allen's method described in Section 12.2.4.1. was implemented as follows in R. The number of replicate assays used for batch release was assumed to be 1 in this example. The slope estimate was obtained from an OLS model with Batch and Time as the fixed effects. The degrees of freedom for residual variance and slope SE were obtained from the fitted model. The shelf-life was set to 36 months for illustration. The resulting internal release limit was 104.1.

```
> n <- 1 # number of replicate assays used for batch release

> lm_d1 <- lm(Y ~ Batch + Time, data = d1)

> assayvar <- sigma(lm_d1)^2

> avg.slope <- summary(lm_d1)$coef["Time", "Estimate"]
> avg.slope
[1] -0.2485797

> se.slope <- summary(lm_d1)$coef["Time", "Std. Error"]
> se.slope
[1] 0.07235241

> df.assayvar <- lm_d1$df.residual
> df.avg.slope <- df.assayvar

> df.t <- (assayvar + se.slope^2)^2 /
  ( (assayvar^2/ df.assayvar)+(se.slope^2^2 / df.avg.slope) )
> df.t
```

```
[1] 11.08148

> tvalue <- qt(0.95, df.t); tvalue
[1] 1.794677

> # with SL of 36
> LSL - avg.slope * 36 + tvalue * sqrt(se.slope^2 * 36^2 +
        (assayvar/n))
[1] 104.0874
```

Bayesian IRL
Using the posterior draws from noninformative and informative priors generated for the shelf-life estimates, internal release limits were calculated for a shelf-life of 36 months. Based on the steps described in Section 12.2.4.2. and the joint posterior distribution of the model parameters extracted in 12.3.1.2, the release limits can be calculated as follows in R:

First, generate K release values within spec range

```
release <- seq(LSL, USL, length=10000)
```

Then compute the probability that the values at the release and at the shelf-life are both within the specification for each release value k:

```
prob_withinspec <- do.call(rbind, lapply(release,function(k){

    # k is each release value
```

Following the steps in Section 12.2.4.2:
1. Draw M Samples from a normal distribution with mean k and variance of $\hat{\sigma}_Y^2/n_R$. $n_R = 1$ in this example and $\hat{\sigma}_Y^2$ is the assay variability, which is represented as a residual variance in this example.

```
Y_R <- rnorm(nrow(post), k, sqrt(post$sigma2_resid))
```

2. Obtain the posterior distribution of γ_1 (slope) – this was already obtained from the shelf-life calculation: `slope.fut`.

3. Derive the posterior predictive distribution of Y_{SL}, where Y_{SL} is the true value of Y at shelf-life: $Y_{SL} = Y_R + \gamma_1 \times x_{SL}$, where Y_R is the chain of true release values obtained in Step 1.

```
Y_SL <- Y_R + slope.fut * 36 # Shelf-life set at 36 months
```

4. Calculate $\pi = \Pr(LSL \leq Y_{SL} \leq USL|\text{Data}, I, k)$, the probability that the true value of Y at shelf-life falls within the specification limits (where I represents the available information).

```
prob_k <- mean(Y_SL >= LSL & Y_SL <= USL &
                   Y_R >= LSL & Y_R <= USL)

    data.frame(k, prob_k)
}))
```

Figures 12.13 and 12.14 show the trajectories of the release values against the computed probabilities. The desired level of within-spec probability is indicated as the blue dashed line (95% was chosen in this example).

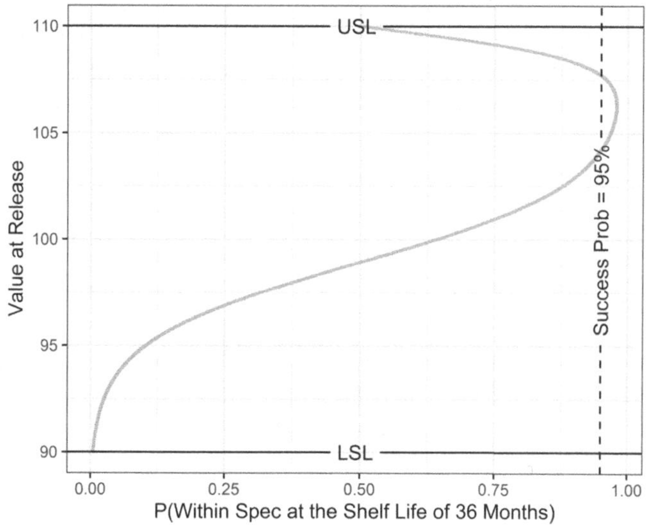

FIGURE 12.13
Plot of the value at release vs the probability of within spec at the shelf-life, using the posterior draws based on noninformative priors.

IRLs are then defined as the window of measured release values for which the probability reaches the desired level.

```
IRL <- prob_withinspec %>%
       filter(prob_k >= 0.95) %>%
       select(k) %>% range()
```

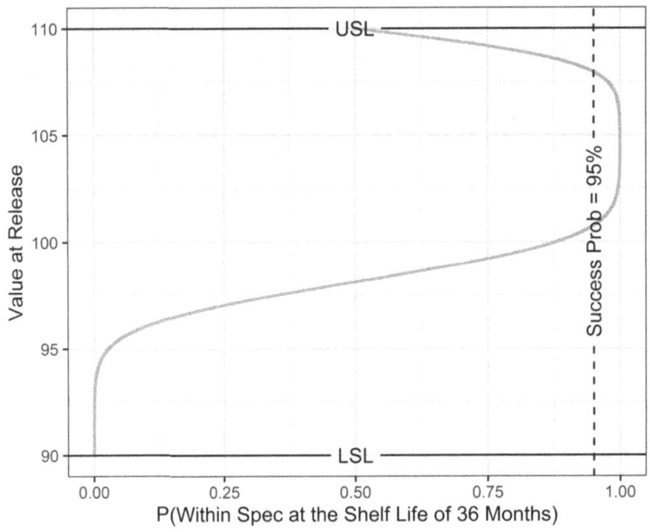

FIGURE 12.14
Plot of the value at release vs the probability of within spec at the shelf-life, using the posterior draws based on informative priors.

The resulting internal release limits that correspond to the success probability $\geq 95\%$ were $(104.17, 107.73)$ for the noninformative prior case, and $(100.76, 107.96)$ for the informative prior case.

12.4 Discussion

The case study results discussed in Section 12.3 highlight two critical justifications to model stability data and obtain shelf-life estimates using a Bayesian approach. First, the difference in shelf-life between the fixed batches model and the mixed effect model with noninformative prior distributions illustrates that the worst of three batches is often not a good representation of the worst possible case. Second, the comparison of the mixed effect model with and without the use of informative prior demonstrates how powerful prior knowledge can be when making predictions based on a small sample size, by leveraging all information to provide more accurate estimation.

In cases of linear mixed models, frequentist methods should give similar results to the Bayesian model with noninformative prior, assuming the frequentist degrees of freedom approximation is reasonable. However, it can be difficult to evaluate the accuracy of this approximation, thereby obscuring the quality of the estimates. There are multiple substantial numeric challenges to fitting a nonlinear model (Jennrich, 1969; Wagner, 1975; Clark and Perry, 1994; Draper and Smith, 1998; Benaroya et al., 2015) that preclude application of frequentist methods for inference and prediction purposes, including the ICH method for shelf-life estimation and Allen et al. (1991) method for IRL derivation for product. Because Bayesian methods are not subject to asymptotic theory and samples are drawn from the exact posterior distributions, they are a better alternative for nonlinear cases (Katz et al.,

1981). While this chapter does not include instructions for fitting nonlinear mixed effect models, the Bayesian methods described are directly applicable to those situations.

In this chapter, we limited discussion to analysis of one CQA at a time. When multiple CQAs are correlated, a closed form for the prediction of a future CQA is not available. Frequentist statistics fall short of providing a practical solution for prediction in the case of generalized linear mixed model, and Bayesian methods are again a viable alternative. See Fong et al. (2010) for details on fitting the model. The posterior distribution manipulation described in this chapter to make predictions can then be used, accounting for the correlation between the response variables of the model.

The main limitation of a Bayesian approach is the lack of user-friendly Bayesian statistical software. All the Bayesian approaches presented in this chapter require access to an experienced Bayesian statistician. Another limitation is the lack of regulatory guidance on the use of Bayesian statistics for CMC (Faya et al., 2021). We hope and believe that increasing awareness of the advantage of Bayesian statistics in stability studies will incentivize solutions to these limitations.

13

Application of Bayesian Methods for Specification Setting

Chris Thompson and Guillermo Miro-Quesada

Data Science and Modeling, BioPharmaceuticals Development, R&D, AstraZeneca, Gaithersburg, Maryland, USA

CONTENTS

13.1 Introduction

Process specifications for therapeutic products must be set considering two factors, the safety and efficacy profile of the product and the capability of the process to consistently produce product within the desired quality range. Determining the process capability requires an understanding of the long term process variability which can be thought of as the expected distribution of the process outputs. Bayesian methods are often useful for determining process capability (Bernardo and Irony, 1996; Wu and Lin, 2009) and therefore determining how tight specifications can be set before the process is not capable of consistently producing releasable product. Results of a Bayesian analysis are typically provided in the form of a distribution of the statistic of interest, rather than an estimate and range which should contain the population statistic with a specified confidence. In addition, the ability to leverage prior information allows the incorporation of platform knowledge and for distributions to be updated when additional data is available. The combination of these pieces make Bayesian approaches closely aligned with how many scientists and engineers think about process development. This eases the integration of these techniques into process development activities, rather than being more of a standalone or gatekeeping exercise to determine whether a particular p-value is achieved. For example, it is still relatively common to determine whether a factor is important to process development based on its significance determined by a p-value, whereas the probability of interest is really the probability that material of acceptable product quality is produced, given the level of process control.

Some important considerations need to be made when working with Bayesian methods. Most notably, the information used for the selection of priors should be clearly stated and justified. Even when vague priors are used, care should be taken to ensure that the choice of prior is not impacting the results. In practice this can be done relatively simply by re-running the model with an alternative choice of prior to confirm that consistent results are obtained (see Chapter 3 for more suggestions) . Other considerations are involved around the Markov

DOI: 10.1201/9781003255093-13

Chain Monte Carlo output to ensure that the solution has converged and is free of undue autocorrelation. For more complex models, consideration should also be given to model formulation and parameterization choices which can significantly impact the computational time taken to run the model.

To construct the process model, Bayesian methods are used to generate a posterior distribution of a product quality attribute (PQA). Per ICH Q11 (2012), the set points and operating ranges of process parameters should be assessed to determine their impact to process reproducibility and critical quality attributes. Typically, this assessment is performed during process characterization using linear regression models that are constructed from statistical Design of Experiments (DoE). The analysis of these models relates the level of the PQA to the controllable process parameters of the unit operation. This approach ensures that any variation in the process parameters within the defined normal operating range (NOR) of the process will result in a consistent process and acceptable product quality. In the Bayesian paradigm, the model estimates the distribution of the parameter estimates (the impact of the process parameters on the model output, PQA) given the available data. From this output a posterior predictive distribution can be obtained for the PQA given the process parameter set point. However, the process parameters over the long term are not expected to always be at the set point. For example, cell culture media and buffer solutions are prepared for each production lot that may vary around their setpoints from lot to lot, yields will vary affecting the loading of the subsequent step in the process and the long term variability due to the level of process control of the process parameters should be included to estimate the range of long term process variability. As the process parameters studied have a defined NOR, the parameters can be considered to vary within this range. The posterior predictive distribution of the PQA is then generated using the expected distribution of the process parameters, rather than the parameters at a fixed set point. These posterior distributions of the PQA could be generated, usually with fairly similar results, using frequentist methods as parameter estimates for linear regression may be similar under both approaches (Christensen et al., 2011). However, estimation of intervals for fixed effects as well as variance components for mixed effect models using a frequentist analysis typically relies on either approximate Wald intervals, asymptotic likelihood profiles or parametric bootstrapping (Bates et al., 2015). In contrast, the Bayesian analysis uses the joint sampling distribution of the model parameters, which makes it relatively simple to assess model and parameter uncertainty. The use of response surface modeling for this purpose has been used in the past (Miro-Quesada et al., 2011) as has been the quantitation of random effects using Bayesian methods (Chen and Ye, 2011). Bayesian models also avoid the frequently encountered issue of negative, or zero, variance components in frequentist models and have also been used as an orthogonal check on the accuracy of intervals calculated from mixed models (Wolfinger, 1998; Montes et al., 2019). Thus, while both frameworks may produce consistent results (in cases where there is minimal contribution from prior information) the Bayesian analysis is often a more robust approach.

The second application presented in this chapter is one where additional data is available to update a previously generated posterior distribution of the PQA. In this case, the previously generated distribution becomes the basis for an informative prior, which is combined with additional data to update our knowledge of the distribution of the PQA and to generate a new posterior. Updating knowledge of a process is intuitively a simple concept, and while this could be challenging to do using frequentist methods, it is exactly what Bayesian methods are designed to do.

Note that process specifications are rarely set using statistical methods alone. While statistical intervals that contain PQA levels for future batches can be obtained (e.g., tolerance intervals) these limits must be assessed in the context of patient safety and product efficacy if they are to be meaningful. The specification must reflect both the available safety and efficacy information as well as process capability. This will ensure that limits are not set so tight that the product cannot be manufactured reliably, or so wide that patient safety cannot be ensured.

13.2 Case Study Part 1: Process Simulation

A frequently encountered problem, especially for late stage projects approaching commercialization, is how to determine the expected long term variability of the manufacturing process. This is complicated by the fact that often there may exist only a small number of previously manufactured clinical batches, and these are typically produced at different scales and with different processes, leaving only the process validation lots as being the most representative of the future process. Additionally, the lots available may only have been run at or close to the target set point and may not have experienced any of the variation in process parameters (intermediate hold times, chromatography loading factors, etc.) that would be expected during extended commercial manufacturing. Fortunately, the factors that might cause this level of variability are explored in process characterization studies of each unit operation. Likewise, the expected levels of variation of these factors, within their control ranges which are generally obtained from the level of control of each factor available in the manufacturing facility. By combining understanding of both the impact of the factors and their respective levels of variation, the expected long term process variability can be estimated.

DoE and the approach of studying unit operations over a design space has become standard for process characterization studies (ICH Q8(R2), 2009). The effect of materials and process parameters on both the process and the product are well studied during process characterization. However, the data collected in these studies are in practice rarely used for more than determining key and critical process parameters. In this case study, the individual unit operation DoE results are combined to simulate the level of the PQA through the process and determine the process capability distribution.

The approach to simulation for each unit operation is to fit a linear regression model and then to simulate the expected variation in the process parameters to predict PQA levels. Figure 13.1 illustrates the relationship between the process inputs and process output described by the linear regression model (typically a response surface design), along with the impact of model parameter uncertainty and assay variation. When combining multiple models, uncertainty in the model parameters is also included at the unit operation level. Importantly, residual variance is not added to simulations of unit operations as this residual variance is mostly a function of assay variation. Instead, an estimate of assay variation is added only once at the end of the process simulation to ensure this variation is not accounted multiple times. Figure 13.2 illustrates the combination of models to simulate the process output. The simulated variability in the process parameters is used to estimate the level and variability of the unit operation output which is the input for the following unit operations.

For simplicity, the dataset used for modeling in this example consists of a bioreactor DoE, an in-process hold study and a chromatography DoE. The bioreactor study is a central composite design with 4 factors with PQA as a response. The study was performed as three blocks and each reactor was sampled on each of three harvest days. The first two blocks contain the corner points at the edge of the normal operating range and a subsequent block contains the axial points outside the normal operating range. A random block variable is included to account for variation in raw materials and media preparation between experimental blocks. To account for variation in scale, 6 pilot scale runs and 3 commercial

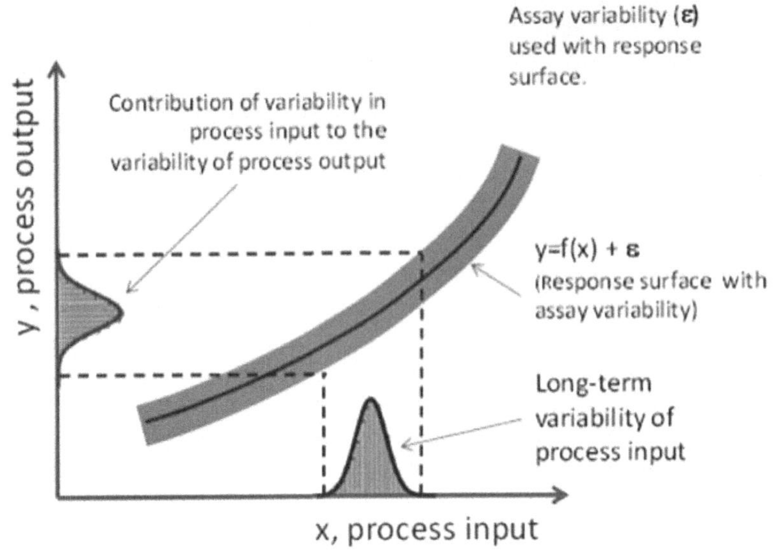

FIGURE 13.1
Prediction of long term process variability due to process inputs plus release assay variability.

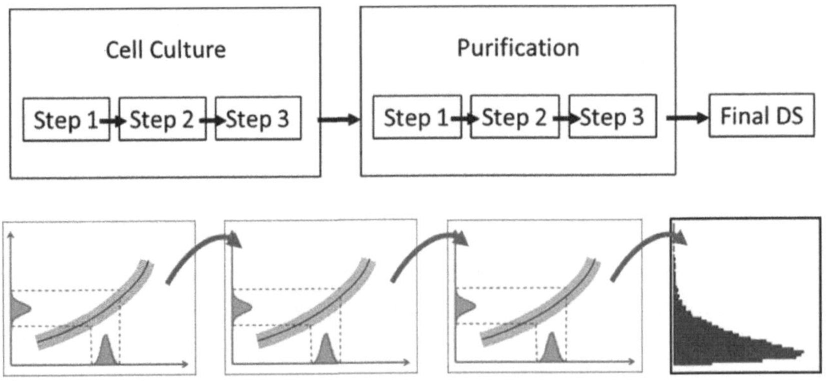

FIGURE 13.2
Combination of process steps to predict overall process variability. Models exist for unit operations within the cell culture and purification process phases. Regression models are constructed for each unit operation and model outputs are generated including expected variability in process parameters. The output of each model is combined to produce a simulated process output at Final DS for each attribute studied.

scale runs are included, giving 3 levels for scale (Lab, Pilot and Commercial). For in-process hold time, lab scale data is generated to determine the change in product quality attributes over time. The chromatography study is a central composite design in a single block with all points within the normal operating range and response of PQA delta (the change in the attribute over the purification step). Figure 13.3 shows the lab scale characterization data and the corresponding pilot and commercial scale process qualification runs. Little variation is observed in the commercial scale runs as few lots have been observed and conditions are expected to have varied little from the target conditions. Interest is in determining how much long term variation in the process outputs is expected based on the level of control of the process inputs at scale and the impact of that variation, which is described by the linear regression model.

Process models would typically consist of multiple hold steps and downstream unit operations to be combined but this reduced example can be easily generalized to a larger process. Care should be taken when modeling to understand the clearance and generation mechanism of product quality species. While small changes are often well approximated by an additive model, larger changes may require a model that considers fold clearance or non-linear changes over steps and so models should be built with consultation from the process subject matter experts.

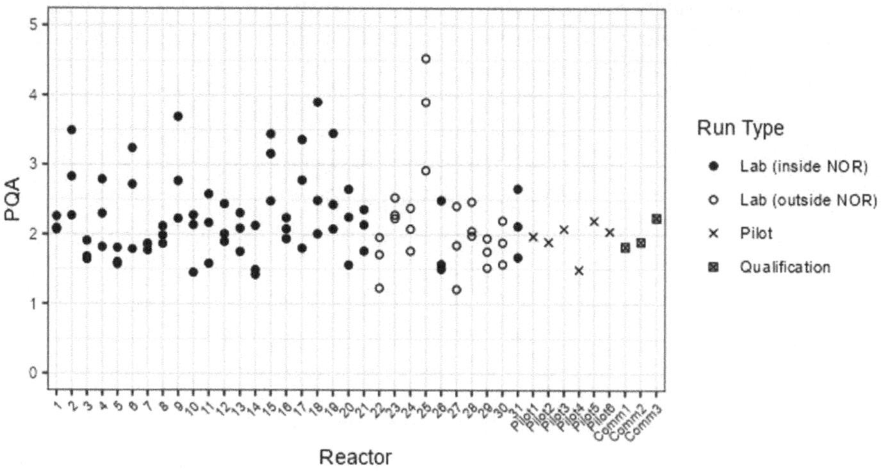

FIGURE 13.3
Bioreactor data illustration.

The model for the bioreactor is shown below, the model consists of a 4 factor response surface fixed effect model including the factors pH, Temperature, Dissolved Oxygen (DO), Seeding Density with each point sampled at multiple times to assess the impact of Harvest Day. An additional fixed effect is included for scale and random effects are added for experimental block and bioreactor:

$$Y_{ijkl} = \beta_1 \mathbf{X}_1 + \beta_2[\mathbf{scale}]_i + \varepsilon_{\text{block},j} + \varepsilon_{\text{bioreactor},k} + \varepsilon_{ijkl}. \tag{13.1}$$

- Y_{ijkl} represents the value of pQA i, for a fixed scale and random block and bioreactor. For this dataset, scale (i) is from 1 to 3 (for the levels: Lab, Pilot and Commercial), block (j) is from 1 to 12, bioreactor (k) is from 1 to 40, and there were 102 total observations.
- β_1, β_2 represent fixed-effects corresponding to the overall intercept and coefficients corresponding to the model matrix and categorical variable scale, respectively. For this dataset β_1 contains the parameters for a 5 factor response surface and so is a vector of length 21, β_2 is a vector of length 3 for the scales.

- $\mathbf{X}_1, [\mathbf{scale}]_i$ represent the response surface model matrix and a fixed effect of scale, respectively. The response surface design space is a 21×102 matrix and the scale design space is a 3×102 matrix.
- $\varepsilon_{\text{block}} \sim N(0, \sigma^2_{\text{block}})$ represent the random effects associated with block.
- $\varepsilon_{\text{bioreactor}} \sim N(0, \sigma^2_{\text{bioreactor}})$ represent the random effects associated with bioreactor.
- $\varepsilon_{\text{block}} \sim N(0, \sigma^2)$ represents the residual variance.

The regression model is fit using the `MCMCglmm` function in R (Hadfield, 2010). `MCMCglmm` by default uses vague priors where the priors are set to be normal for fixed effects and inverse Wishart distributions for variance components. The prior distributions are specified as a list with three components named B, G and R for the fixed effects, random effects and residual variance respectively. For this example, vague priors were selected with unit variance (V) and small degrees of freedom (n) for both random effect and residual variance components in the code below. No prior was specified for the fixed effects and so the default prior was used. The prior specification used is given below:

$$\beta \sim \text{MVN}\left(\mu_\beta, \Sigma_\beta\right) \tag{13.2}$$
$$\text{Scale} \sim \text{MVN}\left(\mu_S, \Sigma_S\right) \tag{13.3}$$
$$\sigma^2_{\text{block}} \sim \text{W}^{-1}\left(V_b, n_b\right) \tag{13.4}$$
$$\sigma^2_{\text{bioreactor}} \sim \text{W}^{-1}\left(V_r, n_r\right) \tag{13.5}$$
$$\sigma^2 \sim \text{W}^{-1}\left(V_{\text{res}}, n_{\text{res}}\right) \tag{13.6}$$

where β is a fixed effect parameter estimate vector (length 21), and Scale fixed effect scale parameter vector (length 3) which are distributed multivariate normal with mean μ and covariance matrix Σ. By default μ is set to a zero vector $[1 \times n]$ and Σ is set to $I_n \times 10^{10}$, (with n set to match the dimension of the fixed effect vectors). $\sigma^2_{\text{block}}, \sigma^2_{\text{bioreactor}}$ and σ^2 are distributed inverse Wishart with scale matrix V and n degrees of freedom. By default V is set to 1 and n is set to zero, which is a flat prior over the range $[0, \infty)$.

The default normal prior with mean zero and variance 10^10 was used for the fixed effects for all models presented. Three alternatives were considered for priors on the variance components. There alternatives were:

1. The default uniform prior over the range of zero to infinity.
2. A vague inverse Wishart prior with scale ($V = 1$) and degrees of freedom ($n = 0.01$).
3. An informative prior with $n = 3$ degrees of freedom and scale set so that the model average of the distribution matched the REML estimate for each variance component.

The latter can be obtained as the modal average of the univariate inverse Wishart distribution used can be determined by the formula below:

$$\text{Mode} = \frac{V \times n}{n + 2} \tag{13.7}$$

As in this case the univariate inverse Wishart is used for the variance components, the priors can be plotted using the inverse gamma function, which is a special case of the inverse

Wishart. Only the priors for the residual variance component are plotted as the same trends can be observed for each component. From the plot in Figure 13.4, the distribution of the three priors over the range of zero to 0.5 can be compared. The REML-based prior has a dense, relatively narrow distribution with a modal average corresponding to the REML estimate of residual variance (0.047). In contrast the vague prior is more skewed but much less dense to allow for a wider range of values, and the uniform prior allows the variance to take any non-negative real number with equal probability.

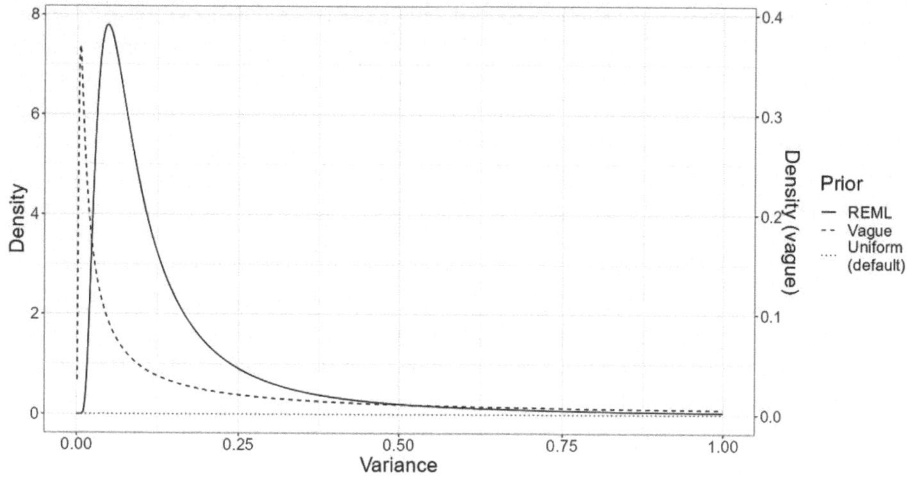

FIGURE 13.4
Plot of prior distributions of the residual variance. The density for the REML prior is plotted against the left axis, the density for the vague prior is plotted on the secondary axis (right) to enable visualization, the uniform prior has a density of zero. More details on the parameterization of the distributions used can be found in the documentation for `MCMCglmm` (Hadfield, 2010) and a density function for the inverse gamma distribution is available in the `MCMCpack` package (Martin et al., 2011).

The `MCMCglmm` function takes a relatively straightforward model specification that does not require a separate model file or a change in scripting language making it more accessible for those less familiar with Markov chain Monte Carlo (MCMC) modeling. The fixed effect formula is specified using standard R formula (abbreviated here for convenience and brevity). The source data file is a regular data frame (and can be downloaded from `https://github.com/BayesCMC/Book`) and the residual variance is specified as Gaussian. Random effects are added as a formula. A simple residual covariance structure is specified (a wide variety of variance structures can be specified and the reader is directed to the package documentation for more information). The list of prior distributions is specified and the MCMC iterations, along with thinning and burn in parameters are specified.

```
fit_brx = MCMCglmm(as.formula(paste("PQA",fix_form_brx,
                                     "+ Scale")),
data=d_brx_s,
       family = "gaussian",
       random=~Reactor+Block, rcov=~units, prior=prior,
       burnin=burn, nitt=burn+thin*iter, thin=thin)
```

The model was run to generate 20,000 samples. After an initial burnin period of 10,000 iterations to allow the chain to stabilize, a sample is taken every 20 iterations until 20,000 samples have been collected, making the total number of iterations $10{,}000 + 20 \times 20{,}000$ (this value is represented by the `nitt=burn+thin*iter` parameter in the code). The model summary outputs effective sample size (ESS) for all parameter estimates along with credible intervals and MCMC derived probabilities for fixed effects that zero is contained within the posterior distribution. The ESS is used to confirm that the MCMC solutions are not autocorrelated and that the samples are well mixed. Ideally, the ESS will be equal to the number of specified samples for the model but this may be reduced due to autocorrelation between samples. Trace and density plots (Figure 13.5) are also useful diagnostics. Trace plots are often described a looking like "fuzzy caterpillars," they should be stable and move around the range of potential solutions without appearing to get stuck at any one point. The equivalent plots for variance components can be harder to look at due to the skew in the distributions. It is suggested that looking at the log traces of the variance components may be easier. Density plots should be smooth and span a range that is narrow enough to be practically useful. Estimates for fixed effect coefficients as well as variance components can be found by obtaining the posterior mode of the resulting distribution and highest posterior density (HPD) intervals describe the smallest span of the support that contains the specified proportion of the distribution of each coefficient. The distribution of the posterior estimate should have moved and tightened from the diffuse prior distribution. Autocorrelation plots may also be used to establish that the thinning of the chain is sufficient that the realizations are approximately independent. This method only generates a single chain, which for designed studies like this one may be sufficient, however the chains may be compared from multiple models using different starting values to confirm that a stable global solution has been reached.

```
#Variance Component Standard Deviation Estimates
sqrt(posterior.mode(fit_brx$VCV))
##      Reactor        Block       units
## 0.08923974  0.07242433  0.21023693
sqrt(HPDinterval(fit_brx$VCV))
##                  lower      upper
## Reactor  0.03484269  0.1924979
## Block    0.02903992  0.2455842
## units    0.17962836  0.2579931
## attr(,"Probability")
## [1] 0.95
```

In this case, the proposed model performed well, other than some minor autocorrelation observed for the Reactor random effect. Comparison between the alternative priors showed comparable performance, although the autocorrelation was higher and ESS was therefore lower for the uniform variance prior model. As illustration, Table 13.1 summarizes the residual variance estimates and highest posterior density intervals as well as the deviance information criteria (DIC) for the model overall. These results illustrate that despite substantial differences in prior specification and some differences observed in model diagnostics, the three models produced consistent estimates and similar overall model fits.

In order to simulate the levels of PQA observed from the bioreactor stage of the process, the fitted model must be combined with the set points of the operating parameters for the process. While the target conditions are defined, many of these will also vary around

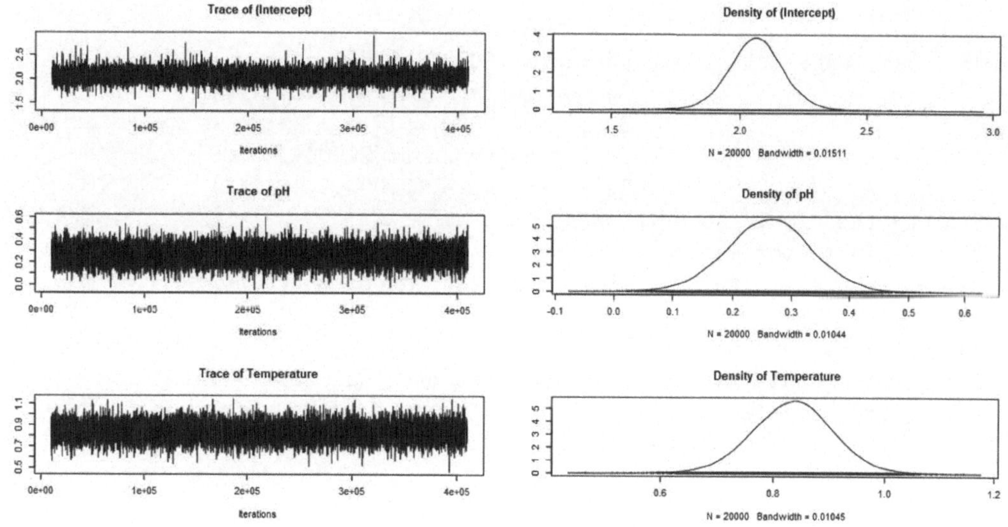

FIGURE 13.5
Plots of trace and density for bioreactor model coefficients.

TABLE 13.1
Summary of residual variance components and DIC across models.

Model Prior Specification	Posterior Mode	Lower 95% HPD CI	Upper 95% HPD CI	DIC
REML	0.0484	0.0334	0.0667	13.35
Vague	0.0462	0.0313	0.0667	13.69
Uniform	0.0459	0.0338	0.0700	15.79

the set point within the NOR of the process. In some cases this is because the level is controlled dynamically in the process, such as the dissolved oxygen (DO) and in some cases this is due to operational variability, such as the ability to harvest the bioreactor on the day before or after the target. For each of the operating parameters studied in the during characterization, a distribution was established based on the level of process control and in consultation with the process design scientists. Typically the distributions were centered on the set point with a range based on the NOR and shape based on subject matter expert consultation. Four of the factors (Reactor pH, temperature, DO and the seeding density) were set based on normal distributions, the harvest day was set based on a triangular distribution based on process experience. Triangular distributions were also useful for in-process holds where a defined distribution minimum, maximum and mode are easily elicited. Simulated operating parameters were generated over this joint distribution. This data was scaled, based on the same range as the range used to scale the characterization dataset and the scale parameter (from Eq. 13.1) was set to Commercial for the purpose of prediction to ensure small differences between scales do not bias the predictions at the commercial scale.

```
simulated_range=data.frame(pH=rnorm(20000,7,0.03),
                           Temperature=rnorm(20000,37,1),
                           DO=rnorm(20000,75,5),
                           Seed_Density=rnorm(20000,1,0.05),
                           Day=rtriangular(20000,9,10,11))
#Scaling the simulated data using
#the original bioreactor data ranges
scaled_sim=scale_data(simulated_range,use_ranges=range_brx)
#Setting the level to Commercial
scaled_sim$Scale="Commercial"
#Setting the scale as a factor using the original data levels
scaled_sim$Scale=factor(scaled_sim$Scale,
                levels=levels(d_brx$Scale))
```

The resulting distribution is then turned into a model matrix to account for the additional higher order terms included in the regression model. This can then be combined with the regression coefficients and random effects obtained from the MCMC output to obtain the posterior predictive distribution for PQA at this stage in the process, as shown in Equation 8 and code excerpt below.

$$Y_i = \beta_1 \mathbf{X}_1 + \beta_2[\mathbf{scale}] + \varepsilon_{\text{block},i} + \varepsilon_{\text{bioreactor},i} \tag{13.8}$$

where Y_i represents the value of the PQA for a future observation i, from a future block and bioreactor at commercial scale. Other terms are defined as above, except $\mathbf{X}_i$ is the simulated operating parameters and $[\mathbf{scale}]_i$ is set to commercial scale. Importantly, the residual variance is not included at this point as interest is in the true attribute level at this stage of the process rather than the measured attribute level.

```
X=model.matrix(as.formula(paste(fix_form_brx,"+ Scale")),
               scaled_sim)
#make predictions
pred_brx = apply(fit_brx$Sol*X,1,sum)
#add random effects
pred_brx=pred_brx+
          rnorm(20000,0,sqrt(fit_brx$VCV[,1]))+
          rnorm(20000,0,sqrt(fit_brx$VCV[,2]))
```

The simulation for each unit operation is generated by making predictions over the joint parameter estimate distribution using input variables sampled from the random distribution based on the NOR of the process. This results in a posterior predictive distribution which incorporates both the uncertainty in the parameter estimates and the variation in the process inputs. This process is repeated for the other unit operations until each unit operation is simulated, at which point the contribution of each unit operation is summed and the residual variance is added to simulate the drug substance PQA level. The residual variance can be estimated in several ways, often it can be the residual variance from the

DoE analysis or from stability studies. However, because the assay variation that is typically presented in regulatory applications is determined during assay validation, the intermediate precision of the assay may be used. In this case, additional simulations of an in-process hold step and a chromatography step are modeled in the same way as the bioreactor model. One difference is that where the output of the bioreactor model is the absolute level of PQA, the output of subsequent models is the change in PQA over the step so that the models can be combined. The residual assay variability is added at the end of the process and, in this specific example, is modeled using a normal distribution with standard deviation 0.2.

```
preds=data.frame(BRX=pred_brx,
                 Hold=pred_hold,
                 Chrom=pred_chrom)

preds$Process=apply(preds,1,sum)+rnorm(20000,0,0.2)
```

Figure 13.6 illustrates the comparison of the process model to the process data showing the model centered on the commercial scale data due to the fixed scale effect in the model but containing process variability attributable to variations of process parameters within their normal operating ranges. It should be noted that the combination of fixed effects may cause a shift in the posterior away from the observed mean of the data, especially if the design center point exists at an optimum. Specification ranges can be assessed using this method to determine what proportion of the simulated data is within the proposed specification. A consistent probability of an out of specification result for each product quality attribute ensures that specifications are consistently representative of process capability. It may be noted that the distribution of the observed data varies over a smaller range than the predicted distribution, which is consistent with the expectation that the full range of process variability may be as yet unobserved. Once additional at scale data is collected this assumption should be revisited.

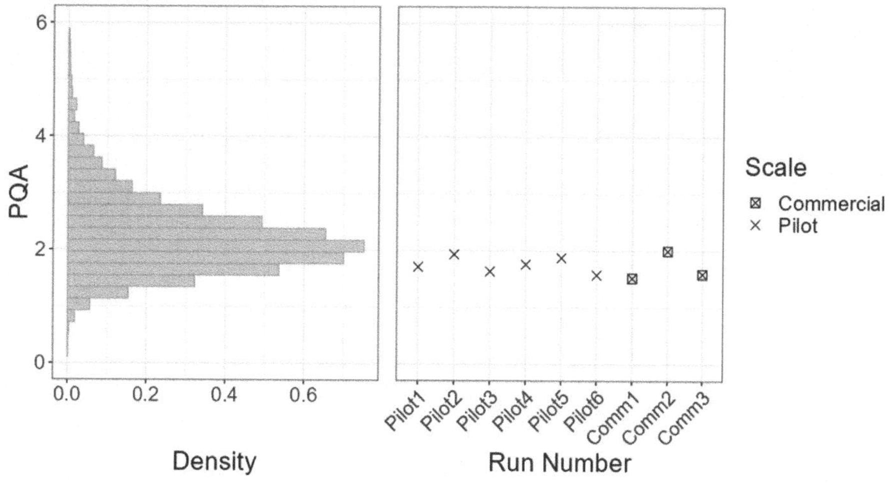

FIGURE 13.6
Comparison of process model to process data.

13.3 Case Study Part 2: Updating with Additional Data

The methodology described in Section 13.2 attempts to predict the long-term variability of the process earlier in the life cycle of the product, e.g., at time of first market application. As additional commercial scale batches are manufacture it becomes desirable to combine the initial prediction from the model in Section 13.2 with these additional batches to refine the estimate of long-term variability and, if appropriate, update the specifications. This can be done by treating the predictive distribution in Section 13.2 as a new prior distribution and combined with the additional batches to generate a new posterior predictive distribution. Methods exist to do this for a wide variety of parametric distributions. However, in the case of the process simulation, the output distribution need not follow any specific parametric distribution. Therefore, a method to update the distribution that does not require a distributional assumptions for the prior would give a more flexible methodology as this allows to account for features which would otherwise be challenging to model using a parametric distribution. One example of this would be the occurrence of shoulder integration issues in an assay method which can result in infrequent apparent outliers or shifts in the data when the threshold for peak detection is crossed. This would challenging to adequately model using a parametric distribution, but is not an issue using non-parametric methods. The method presented uses a smoothed local density function which allows the likelihood to be evaluated at each point along the range. Conjugate priors are placed on the likelihood of obtaining data at each point along the possible range of the attribute and updated with the new data. This method is relatively simple and computationally inexpensive. An example of this method is given below. Alternative methods exist for deriving likelihood-free posterior distributions which may also be of interest (Varin et al., 2011; Lintusaarii et al., 2017).

In this example, the process capability distribution for PQA is updated with commercial data from an additional 10 runs to assess how the initial distribution changes with the additional process data, illustrated in Figure 13.7.

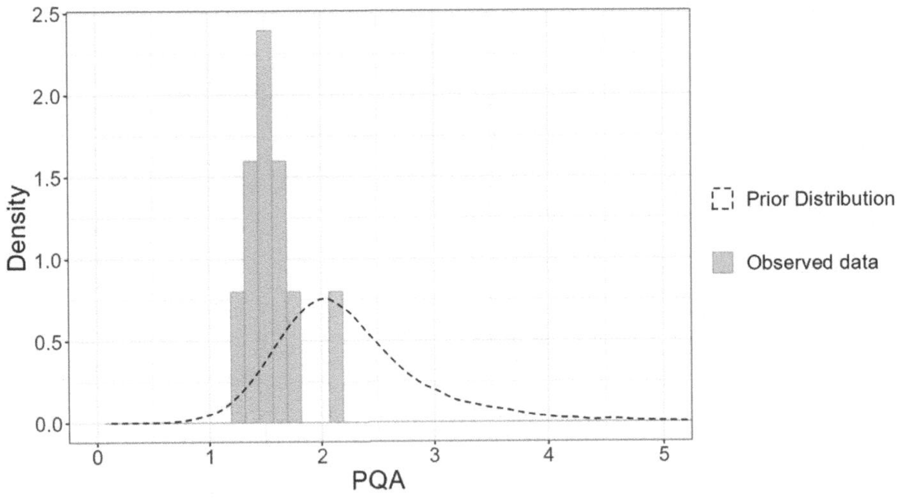

FIGURE 13.7
Comparison of process capability to new data. Existing process capability distribution (prior) shown as density plot outlined with a dashed line, overlaid with additional data shown as a histogram.

The approach detailed in this chapter is to assign a likelihood distribution to each possible outcome of the process output based on the distribution from the process capability model. As the results of product quality assays are often purities and reported to a rounded result, in this case one decimal place, there are 1001 possible results that could be returned by an assay of this type. The method discretizes the support of the distribution, so that a prior distribution can be put on each possible rounded result for the process output. As the desired output posterior is a distribution of the probability of a result occurring at each possible value, the observed probability can be seen as a binomial distribution with a conjugate beta prior obtained from the process simulation. As the beta distribution is defined by two hyperparameters (α, β), there is some flexibility in the choice of parameterization for the likelihood. While the mean is set to the probability of obtaining each value based on the process simulation, the choice of variance will determine the level of influence of the prior on the posterior distribution. In general, without additional knowledge, a high variance vague prior might be chosen so that the posterior is mostly driven by the new data. But this would reduce the information obtained from the process characterization studies. As additional information is available, it is more reasonable to weight the prior based on the relative number of lots used to construct the process model to the number of new lots to be added. In this example the prior distribution is weighted so that it is informative. If a vague prior is required, the beta distribution hyperparameters can be decreased proportionally so that the variance increases but the mean is still matches the prior estimate, or a uniform noninformative prior can be used by setting both hyperparameters to 1. The posterior can then be calculated analytically for each level over the support to obtain an updated distribution. Practically, it is desirable to apply a smoothing kernel to the observed probabilities so that weight is given for observations close to, as well as exactly at, the level of interest. A Gaussian function with variance equal to the level of assay variation is generally a good choice for this, although other functions may be used.

The beta-binomial is a simple example of the use of a conjugate prior distribution, which allows a closed-form algebraic solution to be obtained, rather than requiring a numerical solution. The reader is directed to Chapter 2 of Gelman et al. (2013) for more information. These solutions are convenient and illustrate the potential impact of the prior distribution on the computational cost of the method as well as on the result.

We are interested in the probability that a new datapoint will be observed with a given PQA measurement. Our prior distribution of the parameter p can be described by the beta distribution:

$$P(p) = \frac{p^{\alpha-1}(1-p)^{\beta-1}}{B(\alpha, \beta)} \tag{13.9}$$

where α and β are hyperparameters defining the distribution of p and $B(\cdot)$ is the beta function. The probability of observing a result (x) from a fixed number of trials, given the probability of success (p), is obtained from the binomial distribution:

$$P(x|p) = \binom{n}{s} p^s (1-p)^{n-s} \tag{13.10}$$

with n observations, s "successes" and p the probability of success.

To show that the beta distribution is a conjugate prior for the binomial distribution, we start with Bayes theorem:

$$P(p|x) = \frac{P(x|p)P(p)}{P(x)} \tag{13.11}$$

where:

- $P(p|x)$ is the posterior probability of the event, in this case the parameter, p given the data x
- $P(x|p)$ is the probability of the data given the parameter p
- $P(p)$ is the prior distribution of the parameter p
- $P(x)$ is the marginal probability of the data

Since the marginal probability $P(x)$ does not depend on the parameter p, it along with the binomial coefficient and the beta function can be combined into a single numeric normalizing constant and the posterior can be rewritten:

$$P(p|x) \propto p^s(1-p)^{1-s}p^{\alpha-1}(1-p)^{\beta-1} \quad (13.12)$$

$$\propto p^{s+\alpha-1}(1-p)^{\beta+n-s-1}. \quad (13.13)$$

When normalized, equation (13.13) becomes another another beta distribution with hyper-parameters:

$$\alpha' = \alpha + s \quad (13.14)$$

$$\beta' = \beta + n - s. \quad (13.15)$$

From this a posterior distribution on the probability of observing an event, for example that a lot will be produced with a PQA level of 2.5%, can be updated based on the observed data. The algorithm to perform this Bayesian updating method is given below:

1. Apply a smoothing function to the prior distribution to obtain an empirical density function. Add a small nominal probability to all values to eliminate areas of zero probability and renormalize the area of the distribution.

   Example: For this example, to create a smoothed prior distribution, we identify the range of potential values that the response can take, in this case values between 0 and 100, rounded to 0.1 intervals. For each of these values, we apply a smoothing function which calculates a likelihood at each point using the simulated distribution data from the process model, a smoothing kernel of 0.2 was used based on the assay variation, and the smoother was adjusted to compensate for edge effects at the floor and ceiling of the range.

   The method sets priors, obtains a likelihood and calculates posterior for every possible measured value of the PQA attribute. To illustrate the method more clearly, one can focus on one of these values and follow this though the method. For this example, the potential value of 1.5% is chosen. After rounding, 736 of the values from the process simulation were equal to 1.5% (about 3.7% of the total number of simulations). After smoothing and re-normalizing, the probability from the prior distribution is 3.8%.

```
d=sapply(prior.density$range, smooth,vec=prior,
         sd=sd.assay,floor=0,ceiling=100)
#Adding a minimal density to low probability events
d=d+prior.min.density/(length(d))
d=d/sum(d) #re-normalise the distribution
prior.density$density=d #Add data to data frame
```

2. For each possible result, set beta hyperpriors, with parameters α and β, such that the mean of the beta distribution is equal to the expected probability of the result. The variance can be set based on the number of commercial scale runs used to set the original distribution (in this case, $n = 3$).

   Example: Hyperparameters are set for every level, following from the previous step, the density at 1.5% is 0.038. There were 3 commercial scale lots used in the process model, compared to 10 lots that are being used to update the model, so the prior is given a weighting of 3 so that each lot is weighted equally. The α hyperparameter is calculated as 3 times the density (0.11) and the β hyperparameter is calculated as 3 minus alpha (2.89). The mean of this prior is 0.038 (3.8%) and the variance is such that 95% of the distribution is contained by the range of 0 to 0.35.

```
#Computing hyperpriors on each possible result
#From Beta distribution:
#a+b=n
#E(X)=a/(a+b)
#Var(X)=(ab)/((a+b)^2(a+b+1))

prior.density$alpha=prior.density$density*n.p
prior.density$beta=n.p-prior.density$alpha
```

3. From the additional observed data, gather the observed likelihoods of each possible result.

   Example: There were 3 results out of the 10 observations with a measured PQA level of 1.5%. However after the likelihood is smoothed this value decreases to 1.3. This is because the smoothing kernel used at this stage is the standard deviation of the observations. The reason for this is that with relatively small datasets the assay based kernel may not be wide enough to smooth between individual data points resulting in regions of lower density and a multimodal distribution. This effect may be the true distribution or a product of the small sample size. For this reason it is recommended that a larger kernel be used for more sparse data and that this be decreased as more data becomes available.

```
#### Observed likelihood
n.obs=length(observed.data)

#calculating smoothed observed likelihood
lik=sapply(prior.density$r, smooth,vec=observed.data,
           sd=sd.obs,floor=0,ceiling=100)

#normalizing the likelihood to the number of observations
lik=lik/(sum(lik)/n.obs)
```

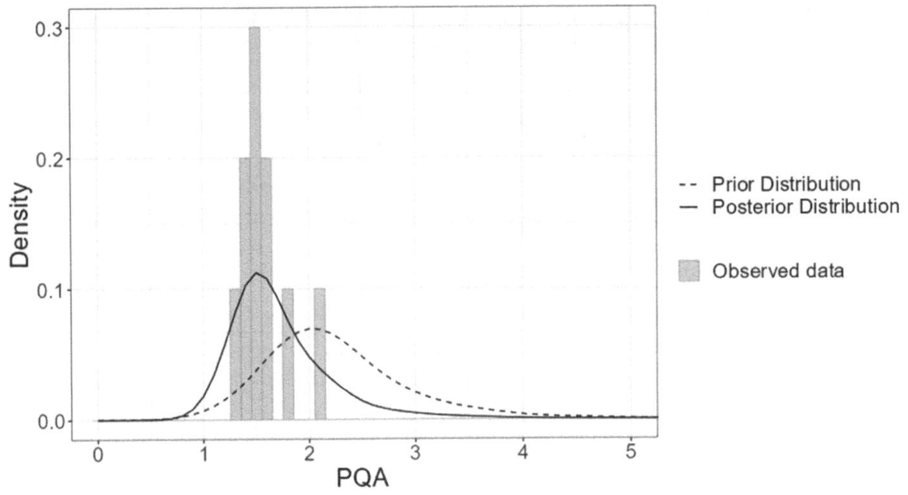

FIGURE 13.8
Comparison of prior, data, and posterior distributions.

4. Compute posterior hyperparameters and distribution for each result

Example: The posterior hyperparameters are calculated using Equations (13.14) and (13.15) which allows the calculation of the posterior distribution for each value over the range. Continuing from the previous step, the posterior hyperparameters were calculated as 1.46 and 11.5 for α and β respectively. This, in turn, increased our expectation of observing a result at 1.5% PQA from a frequency of 3.8% to 11.2% as well as decreasing the variance of the distribution.

```
#Calculating the posterior hyperparameters
post.density=data.frame(alpha=prior.density$alpha+lik)
post.density$beta=prior.density$beta+n.obs-lik

#And the posterior density
a=post.density$alpha
b=post.density$beta

#posterior probabilities
E.X.post=a/(a+b)
#variance of posterior probabilities
V.X.post=(a*b)/((a+b)^2*(a+b+1))
sum(E.X.post) #confirming distribution sums to 1
## [1] 1
```

Figure 13.8 illustrates the effect of the updating on the distribution. Intuitively, the distribution of the posterior is equal to a weighted average of the prior and the smoothed observed data, with weights equal to the number of batches in each group. As the number of batches increases the, distribution will more closely reflect to the distribution of the observed data. This method is very useful for updating empirical distributions and for updating process capability models with additional data without having to build a new model from scratch.

13.4 Conclusion

The use of Bayesian methods for studies involving simulations, such as the setting of process specifications, is attractive for a number of reasons. They can be easily modified to work with a wide range of model formulations, the results of a Bayesian analysis are typically in the form of a joint distribution of the statistics of interest, and they can incorporate prior knowledge explicitly into the analysis. This makes simulations much easier to set up and model than alternative methods, even for fairly simple models. The ability of Bayesian models to incorporate prior knowledge in the form of informative priors, and to give relative weights to the existing knowledge and new data, is not only a useful technique for updating models, but it aligns with how process developers are usually thinking as they update their expectations of the process as new data is collected. This eases the integration of these techniques and facilitates adoption and wider use.

It may be observed that a potential limitation to the process model method presented is that, as the commercial scale lots were all operated close to target and there are few commercial scale lots compared to the lab scale data, in effect the commercial data serves to center the posterior predictive distribution rather than contributing to the range of the distribution. This results in a distribution that is typically wider than the observed commercial scale data, which is consistent with the assumption that there is additional, as yet unobserved, variation in process inputs that should be accounted for. If instead the observed commercial data are considered to be representative of future process variation then the posterior predictive based primarily on the expected variation from the lab scale model may be too conservative. In this case the process model might be updated, as in Section 13.3 of this chapter, with the existing commercial data in order to better reflect the target distribution. The decision as to which model best represents the available data should be taken in conjunction with the process engineers and subject matter experts.

14

Calculating Statistical Tolerance Intervals Using SAS

Richard Lewis

Fellow, American Society for Quality

Buffy Hudson-Curtis

Research Statistics, GlaxoSmithKline

CONTENTS

14.1 Introduction

Tolerance intervals are frequently used in pharmaceutical development and manufacturing to assess and quantify past or future ranges of data produced by a process or system. One important application is using a relatively small sample from a population to assess the potential range of values in the population itself. This is expressed as an interval that captures a certain proportion of the data ($p, 0 < p < 1$) with a given level of confidence (usually written as $100(1-\alpha)\%, 0 < \alpha < 1$). While it is possible to use distribution free (i.e., nonparametric) methods to calculate tolerance intervals for any type of distribution (see Dixon and Massey (1969) or Meeker et al. (2017), for example), specifying the parametric form of the distribution allows for smaller sample sizes to be used. Consequently, we only consider parametric tolerance intervals in this chapter and further restrict our attention to normally distributed data.

Transformations, such as taking the square root or logarithm, can often be used to obtain data which is (approximately) normally distributed. Readers interested in non-normal distributions can refer to Young (2010), and the references therein. Note that one-sided tolerance limits are equivalent to confidence limits for population percentiles (see Patel (1986), for example). As a result, it is straightforward to use Bayesian methods to construct one-sided tolerance intervals; the endpoint of the interval is often referred to as a tolerance limit.

DOI: 10.1201/9781003255093-14

Typical applications of tolerance intervals include quantitating future ranges of data for the purpose of setting specifications, monitoring manufacturing processes and product quality, and assessing performance against an existing specification (e.g., content uniformity). For example, the application of tolerance intervals to content uniformity is discussed by Lewis and Novick (2012), Hudson-Curtis and Novick (2016) and Lewis and Fan (2016). Lewis and Fan (2016) use Bayesian tolerance intervals to obtain substantially better acceptance limits for content uniformity than those in ASTM Standard E2810 (2019), while Lewis (2020) uses tolerance intervals to obtain substantially better acceptance limits for dissolution than those in an ISPE Good Practice Guide on process validation (Guide, 2019). Parametric and nonparametric frequentist approaches for calculating one-sided and two-sided tolerance intervals are well documented in the literature (see Dixon and Massey (1969) or Meeker et al. (2017), for example). The calculations are relatively straightforward when the data are independent and identically distributed (*iid*), such as a random sample from a Normal distribution, but complexities arise when additional sources of variation are present, such as when observations are collected from several locations within a batch or from several different batches. In some situations, this necessitates the use of two (or more) variance components, such as between-location and within-location variation, or between-batch and within-batch variation. When sampling is balanced such that there is an equal number of observations per location or batch, a frequentist tolerance interval can be constructed using the appropriate variance components and an estimate for degrees of freedom. Also, Novick and Hudson-Curtis (2018) demonstrate how to calculate two one-sided tolerance intervals when two sources of variation are present, using a frequentist method called generalized pivotal quantities. In the case of unequal sample sizes, difficulties can arise with the frequentist approach (see Mee and Owen (1983), for example). A Bayesian approach for constructing tolerance intervals only requires specification of the prior and, as shown in Example 3, easily incorporates unequal sample sizes into the posterior distribution. The Bayesian approach can also provide additional benefit when prior information is available for the variance parameter(s).

This chapter will focus on three hands-on examples of constructing one-sided parametric tolerance intervals using Bayesian methods. The three examples illustrate a simple mean model, a one-way analysis of variance (ANOVA) model, and a one-way random-effects model. The approaches used for these three examples can be readily extended to additional scenarios. These examples assume normally distributed data and employ SAS statistical software. Other statistical packages provide similar capabilities (for example, see Young (2016) for implementations in R). Focusing on one-sided intervals is not a limitation, since two one-sided intervals may be used to construct a two-sided interval, with the added advantage that this approach controls the proportion of the population in each of the tails of the distribution. Although SAS `PROC MIXED` supports informative priors, all three examples use default noninformative Jeffreys priors. The Jeffreys priors for fixed effects are improper flat priors (that is, they are proportional to a constant), while the Jeffreys priors for variance components are proportional to the square root of the determinant of the expected information matrix (SAS Help Center). Jeffreys priors are invariant to the parameterization of the distribution parameters (see Box and Tiao (1973), for example). For example, using σ, σ^2 or $\ln(\sigma)$ to represent the spread of the normal distribution does not affect the probability of the corresponding subset of the parameter space. Although all three examples use noninformative priors, the second example illustrates a way to include prior information through additional data.

14.2 Population Quantiles and Tolerance Intervals

Population quantiles provide useful information about the range of data in a population. Consider a random variable Y, such as the drug content of individual tablets in a large batch of tablets, and let Q_p represent the p quantile of Y for $0 < p < 1$. Then by definition Q_p is the value such that $\Pr(Y \leq Q_p) = p$. Population quantiles can also be expressed as percentiles: the population quantile Q_p is the $100p^{th}$ percentile of the population. As an example, $\mu \pm 1.96\sigma$ are the 0.025 and 0.975 quantiles (or, equivalently the 2.5^{th} and 97.5^{th} percentiles) of a Normal distribution with mean μ and standard deviation σ. We often round 1.96 to 2 and say that 95% of the observations from a Normal distribution fall within $\mu \pm 2\sigma$. What can we say when we do not know the values of μ and σ, but have estimates $\bar{y}$ and s based on a sample of size n? Tolerance intervals provide an answer. For normally distributed data, tolerance intervals constructed using frequentist methods allow us to make a statement of the form "We are $100(1-\alpha)\%$ confident that a proportion p of the data fall within the interval $\bar{y} \pm ks$" where the factor k depends on α, p and n. The derivation of k is not simple; a more detailed discussion on how it is obtained can be found in Patel (1986).

Bayesian methods take a different approach than frequentist intervals, of course, and one-sided tolerance intervals are easier to construct than two-sided tolerance intervals (Wolfinger, 1998). One-sided Bayesian tolerance intervals are based on posterior probability statements about population quantiles and are straightforward to construct using a three-step method that will be illustrated in the examples below. For simple models (e.g., a random sample from a Normal distribution or balanced one-way layout) the frequentist and Bayesian intervals match very closely when a noninformative prior is used in constructing the Bayesian interval. In more complex situations, such as when there are random effects, unbalanced data, more than one source of variation or prior information about model parameters, frequentist intervals can be difficult to construct and the benefits of a Bayesian approach become clear. Example 2 addresses a situation with prior information about σ, and Example 3 addresses a situation with unbalanced data and two variance components.

14.2.1 Frequentist Approach

One-sided and/or two-sided tolerance intervals can be constructed for any probability distribution using nonparametric methods (see Meeker et al. (2017), for example), but parametric methods produce shorter intervals for a given sample size. Using frequentist methods, one-sided lower tolerance intervals for normally distributed data take the form $\bar{y} - ks$ and one-sided upper tolerance intervals take the form $\bar{y} + ks$, where there is an exact closed-form formula for the factor k (see Patel (1986), for example). There is no exact formula for two-sided tolerance intervals, but approaches for constructing them are discussed in Patel (1986) and Meeker et al. (2017). In addition, two one-sided $100(1-\alpha)\%$ confidence, $(1+p)/2$ coverage tolerance intervals can be used to construct an approximate two-sided $100(1-\alpha)\%$ confidence, p coverage tolerance interval. These intervals control the proportion of data in each of the tails, rather than the center of the distribution, which can make them particularly useful when the concern is in quantifying the number of units outside, rather than inside, of a range.

14.2.2 Bayesian Approach

Bayesian methods can also be used to construct tolerance intervals. The construction of one-sided Bayesian tolerance limits relies on the fact that one-sided confidence limits for population quantiles are equivalent to one-sided tolerance limits (see Patel (1986)). For example, a $100(1-\alpha)\%$ upper confidence limit for the population quantile Q_p is also a $100(1-\alpha)\%$ confidence, p coverage upper tolerance limit (UTL). Consequently, one-sided Bayesian tolerance limits can be obtained from percentiles of the posterior distribution of population quantiles. To illustrate this, suppose a random sample of n observations is obtained from a Normal distribution with mean μ and standard deviation σ. As mentioned above, a one-sided frequentist upper tolerance limit takes the form $\bar{y}+ks$ where the multiplier k has an exact closed-form solution. To calculate a one-sided Bayesian upper tolerance limit, one needs to 1) obtain a large sample from the joint posterior distribution for μ and σ^2, 2) calculate the population quantile $Q_p = \mu + z_p\sigma$ for each pair of μ and σ^2 in the sample (where z_p is the p quantile for the Standard Normal distribution), and 3) obtain the $100(1-\alpha)^{th}$ percentile of Q_p. Statistical software, such as SAS, provides a practical means for obtaining posterior samples to plug into Q_p which we illustrate in our examples. For one-sided Bayesian lower tolerance limits, the $100(\alpha)^{th}$ percentile of $Q_{1-p} = \mu - z_p\sigma$ can be used.

14.3 Examples

We demonstrate the construction of one-sided Bayesian tolerance intervals for normally distributed data through step-by-step examples that cover three useful models: a simple mean model, a one-way ANOVA model, and a one-way random-effects model. Although all three examples use SAS `PROC MIXED`'s default noninformative Jeffreys priors, as discussed in the Introduction, informative priors can also be used. Example 2 illustrates a data-based way to include prior information about σ despite using a noninformative prior. Introducing prior information into `PROC MIXED` via a specified distribution requires a dataset that describes the prior densities and the use of the `DATA=` option in the `PRIOR` statement; see the SAS Help Center for more information.

Example 1.
Construct an upper tolerance limit given a random sample from a Normal distribution with mean μ and standard deviation σ using frequentist and Bayesian methods. The model can be written as

$$Y_j = \mu + \varepsilon_j \tag{14.1}$$

where $\varepsilon_j \sim N(0, \sigma^2)$ for $j = 1, 2, ..., n$. The mean and variance of a future observation are μ and σ^2, respectively, and the p quantile is $\mu + z_p\sigma$.

This example will illustrate the three steps involved in constructing a one-sided Bayesian tolerance interval and also shows that frequentist and Bayesian methods typically yield similar tolerance limits for model (14.1) when using a noninformative prior distribution.

Example 2.
Construct upper tolerance limits given random samples from multiple groups, where group i is normally distributed with fixed mean μ_i and standard deviation σ. The model can be

written as

$$Y_{ij} = \mu_i + \varepsilon_{ij} \tag{14.2}$$

where $\varepsilon_{ij} \sim N(0, \sigma^2)$ for $i = 1, 2, ..., I$ and $j = 1, 2, ..., n_i$. The mean and variance of a future observation in the ith group are μ_i and σ^2, respectively, and the p quantile for the ith group is $\mu_i + z_p\sigma$.

This example will illustrate the ability to share information about a common parameter across multiple groups. In this example the common parameter is σ. This example will also illustrate a data-based way to include prior information about σ. For example, batches (i.e., groups) 1 to $I - 1$ could represent $I - 1$ historical batches while batch I could represent a more recent batch for which a tolerance interval is desired. Model (14.2) allows us to include the historical information about σ when constructing a tolerance interval for batch I.

Example 3.
Construct an upper tolerance limit given random samples from multiple groups, where group i is normally distributed with random mean $\mu_i = \mu + \delta_i$ and standard deviation σ. The model can be written as

$$Y_{ij} = \mu + \delta_i + \varepsilon_{ij} \tag{14.3}$$

where $\delta_i \sim N(0, \sigma_\delta^2)$ for $i = 1, 2, ..., I$, and where $\varepsilon_{ij} \sim N(0, \sigma_\varepsilon^2)$ for $i = 1, 2, ..., I$ and $j = 1, 2, ..., n_i$. The mean and variance of an observation in a future group are μ and $\sigma_\delta^2 + \sigma_\varepsilon^2$, respectively, and the p quantile for a future group is $\mu + z_p\sqrt{\sigma_\delta^2 + \sigma_\varepsilon^2}$.

This example will illustrate a situation with two variance components: within-group and between-group. The one-way random effects model is very useful when there are multiple batches that display both batch-to-batch and within-batch variability. It is also useful when there is a single observation per batch (which is common for homogenous batches of drug substance) and multiple production campaigns.

14.3.1 Example 1

One-sided frequentist and Bayesian tolerance limits for model (14.1) can easily be generated using several different software packages. We will illustrate the use of SAS to calculate a one-sided upper tolerance limit (UTL) with 95% confidence of 99% coverage ($\alpha = 0.05$ and $p = 0.99$). First, a frequentist UTL for normally distributed data can easily be obtained using the `INTERVALS` statement in SAS `PROC CAPABILITY`. Suppose the data are stored in a table named Data1 in a column labelled Response. Then, as shown below, specifying `TYPE=UPPER`, `P=0.99`, `ALPHA=0.05` and `METHOD=3` (which specifies a tolerance interval) requests SAS to calculate the desired UTL.

```
PROC CAPABILITY DATA=Data1 ;
INTERVALS Response / TYPE=UPPER P=0.99 ALPHA=0.05 METHOD=3 ;
RUN ;
```

It is also easy to construct a Bayesian UTL using the three steps discussed in the Population Quantiles and Tolerance Limits section.

First, obtain samples from the posterior distribution of μ and σ^2 using the `MIXED` procedure. SAS automatically includes an intercept term in the model and the error term is implicit, so the model statement is MODEL Response = / SOLUTION where the SOLUTION option is required for the Bayesian analysis.

```
PROC MIXED DATA=Data1 ;
MODEL Response = / SOLUTION ;
PRIOR / OUT=Posterior1 NSAMPLE=10000 SEED=6456443 ;
TITLE "Example 1" ;
RUN ;
PROC PRINT DATA=Posterior1 (OBS=20) ;
TITLE "First 20 Rows of Posterior1" ;
RUN ;
```

The PRIOR statement saves NSAMPLE=10,000 samples from the posterior distribution for μ and σ^2 to a dataset named Posterior1. The SEED= option allows one to reproduce the results with subsequent runs of the code. Note that SAS uses beta1 to represent μ and covp1 to represent σ^2. It is good practice to examine the posterior samples for the model parameters before proceeding to the second step. PROC MIXED uses an independence chain algorithm to generate the posterior samples, and the authors have never experienced poor convergence properties. Nonetheless, one should examine summary statistics, trend plots and histograms of the parameters as a check on convergence.

Second, use a DATA step to calculate the 99th percentile of a Normal distribution for each sample of μ and σ^2. This provides 10,000 samples from the posterior distribution for the 99th percentile, P99.

```
DATA Posterior ;
SET Posterior1 ;
SEED = 4896235 ;
z99 = PROBIT(0.99) ;
Mu = beta1 ;
Sigma = SQRT(covp1) ;
P99 = Mu + z99*Sigma ;
run ;
```

Third, use the UNIVARIATE procedure to obtain the 95th percentile of the samples for P99. The UNIVARIATE procedure also provides a histogram for P99 when a HISTOGRAM statement is included. The INSET option shown below places selected summary statistics in the northeast corner of the figure.

```
PROC UNIVARIATE DATA=Posterior ;
VAR P99 ;
HISTOGRAM ;
INSET N MEDIAN (6.2) MEAN (6.2) P95 (6.2) /
POS=NE HEADER="Summary Statistics" ;
TITLE ;
RUN ;
```

In order to illustrate the output generated using this code, $n = 20$ observations were generated from a $N(100, 5^2)$ distribution. The $p = 0.99$ quantile of this distribution is 111.6. The 20 observations are shown in Table 14.1; they have a mean of 99.883 and a standard deviation of 4.215. The `CAPABILITY` procedure was used to calculate a frequentist upper one-sided tolerance interval ($p = 0.99, \alpha = 0.05$); the UTL is 113.8. A Bayesian tolerance interval was calculated using the three steps outlined above, resulting in a UTL of 114.0. The two tolerance limits are shown in Table 14.2. Diagnostic plots are shown in Figures 14.1–14.4. The histograms show that the posterior samples for μ (`beta1`) and σ^2 (`covp1`) look reasonable: they have the shapes one would expect and there no extreme values. The trend plots showing the parameters vs the order simulated do not show any obvious trends or spikes. It is good practice to check these diagnostics, although the authors have not experienced any issues with convergence performing this analysis in SAS. Figure 14.5 provides a histogram of `P99` from the Bayesian analysis that shows that the 95th percentile of `P99` is 114.0. From a Bayesian perspective, the posterior probability that `P99` is less than 114.0 is 0.95. In this example, the frequentist and Bayesian tolerance intervals are similar due to the simplicity of model (14.1) and use of a noninformative prior. Indeed, the similarity of the intervals provides confidence in the Bayesian tolerance interval approach. In practice, it is convenient to simply use PROC CAPABILITY to generate tolerance intervals for data from model (14.1).

TABLE 14.1
Twenty observations from a $N(100, 5^2)$ distribution.

99.180	96.153	94.766	100.242
100.202	103.021	103.24	100.824
105.822	103.627	93.996	98.314
104.935	100.319	93.172	95.237
107.932	98.709	102.74	95.225

TABLE 14.2
Frequentist and Bayesian one-sided tolerance limits.

Approach	Upper Tolerance Limit
Frequentist	113.8
Bayesian	114.0

14.3.2 Example 2

One-sided Bayesian tolerance limits for Model (14.2) can easily be generated using several different software packages. These types of models may arise when there are multiple batches within one campaign that one is interested in, or when multiple analysts generate data from one batch. In this scenario, the batches (or analysts) are specifically of interest, and are considered fixed effects, rather than from some random population. Example 3 will discuss how tolerance intervals may be calculated when more than one random effect is believed to be present in the data. We will illustrate the use of SAS to calculate one-sided upper

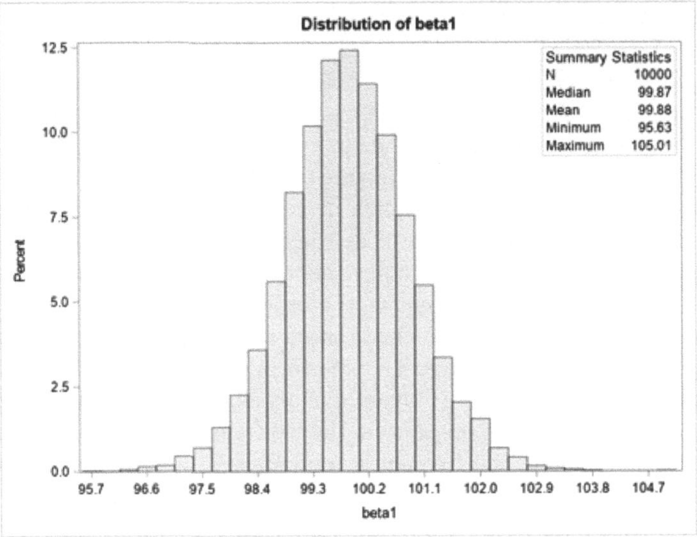

FIGURE 14.1
Distribution of μ (`beta1`) for Example 1.

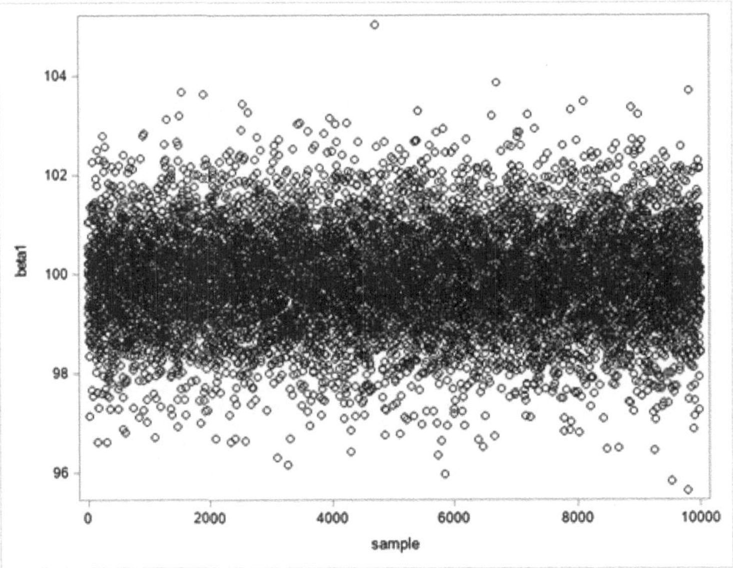

FIGURE 14.2
Trend plot of μ (`beta1`) for Example 1.

tolerance limits for each of three groups, with 95% confidence of 99% coverage ($\alpha = 0.05$ and $p = 0.99$).

First, obtain samples from the posterior distribution of the three means μ_i and σ^2 using the `MIXED` procedure. SAS automatically includes an intercept term in the model and the error term is implicit, so the model statement is `MODEL Response =Material / SOLUTION`

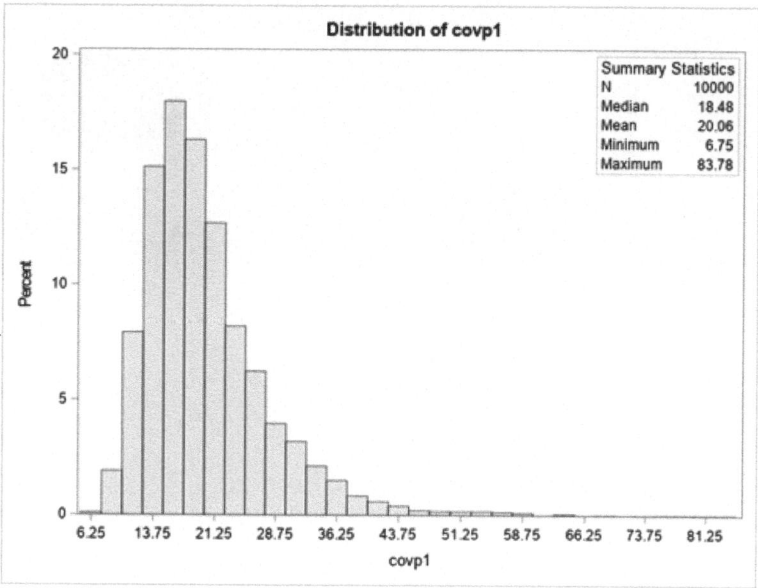

FIGURE 14.3
Distribution of σ^2 (`covp1`) for Example 1.

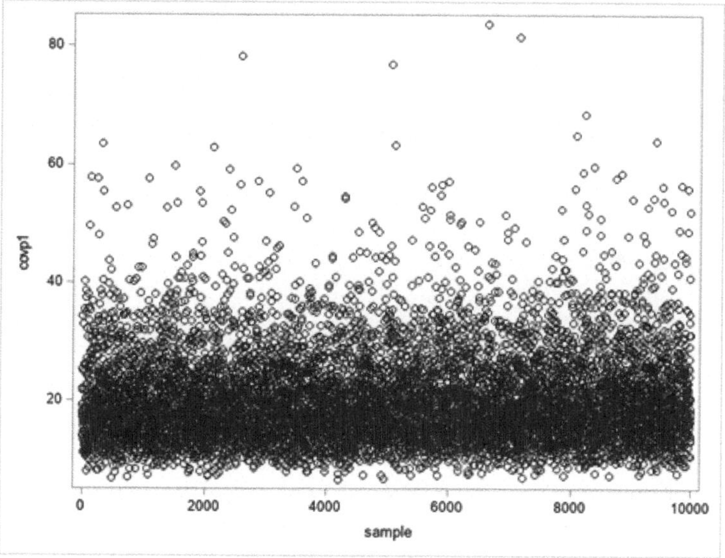

FIGURE 14.4
Trend plot of σ^2 (`covp1`) for Example 1.

where the `SOLUTION` option is required for the Bayesian analysis. The model as written in the SAS code is over-parameterized, because there is an intercept term in the model as well as a mean for each group. As a result, one must pay careful attention to how SAS parameterizes the fixed effects in the posterior dataset named `Posterior2`.

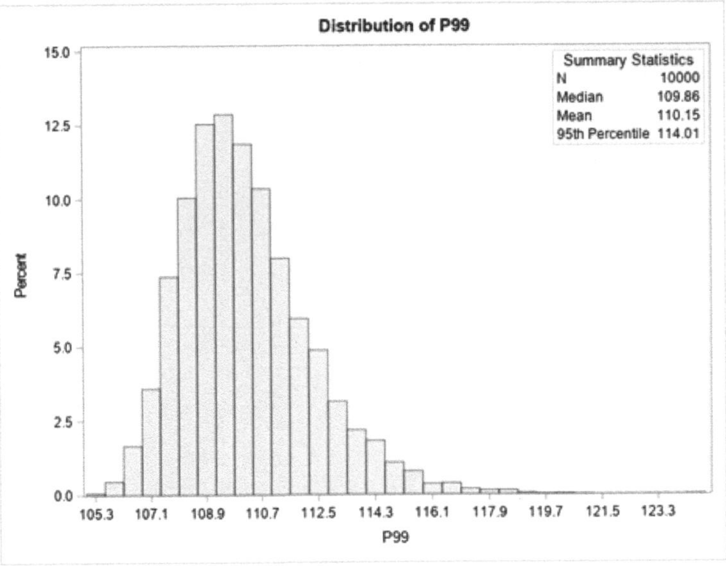

FIGURE 14.5
Posterior distribution of P99 for Example 1.

```
PROC MIXED DATA=Data2 ;
CLASS Material ;
MODEL Response = Material / SOLUTION ;
PRIOR / OUT=Posterior2 NSAMPLE=10000 SEED=6456443 ;
TITLE "Example 2" ;
RUN ;
PROC PRINT DATA=Posterior2 (OBS=20) ;
TITLE "First 20 Rows of Posterior2" ;
RUN ;
```

Second, use a DATA step to calculate the 99th percentile of a Normal distribution for each sample of the μ_i and σ^2. This provides samples from the posterior distribution for the 99th percentile, P99 for each group. When there are three groups, SAS uses beta1 to represent μ_3, beta1+beta2 to represent μ_1, beta1+beta3 to represent μ_2, and covp1 to represent σ^2. The example SAS code below shows how to construct Bayesian tolerance intervals assuming three groups labeled Material A, Material B and Material C.

```
DATA Posterior ;
SET Posterior2 ;
SEED = 4896235 ;
z99 = PROBIT(0.99) ;
Mu1 = beta1+beta2 ;
Mu2 = beta1+beta3;
Mu3 = beta1;
Sigma = SQRT(covp1) ;
```

```
P99_1 = Mu1 + z99*Sigma ;
P99_2 = Mu2 + z99*Sigma ;
P99_3 = Mu3 + z99*Sigma ;
RUN ;
```

Third, use the UNIVARIATE procedure to obtain the 95th percentile of the samples for P99. The UNIVARIATE procedure can also provide a histogram for P99.

```
PROC UNIVARIATE DATA=Posterior ;
VAR P99_1 P99_2 P99_3 ;
HISTOGRAM ;
INSET N MEDIAN (6.2) MEAN (6.2) P95 (6.2) /
POS=NE HEADER=\Summary Statistics" ;
TITLE ;
RUN ;
```

In order to illustrate the output generated using this code, $n = 30$ observations were generated. Ten observations were generated from each of a $N(95, 5^2)$, $N(100, 5^2)$, and $N(105, 5^2)$ distribution to represent data from batches with three different starting materials. The $p = 0.99$ quantiles of these three distributions are 106.6, 111.6, and 116.6, respectively. The observed data are shown in Table 14.3, summary statistics are shown in Table 14.4, and a boxplot of the data is provided in Figure 14.14. For discussion purposes, frequentist tolerance intervals were calculated individually for each group using the CAPABILITY procedure. The results are shown in Table 14.5.

TABLE 14.3
Data set from $N(95, 5^2)$, $N(100, 5^2)$, and $N(105, 5^2)$ distributions.

Material A	Material B	Material C
98.237	104.021	103.487
91.635	95.457	112.351
89.295	107.248	112.765
103.978	102.03	109.692
97.524	96.97	107.885
86.054	103.693	104.632
96.447	95.692	106.856
101.381	90.27	114.189
100.291	104.381	110.046
104.515	102.632	101.199

TABLE 14.4
Summary statistics.

Material	Mean	Standard Deviation
Material A	96.94	6.19
Material B	100.24	5.32
Material C	108.31	4.29

TABLE 14.5
Frequentist and Bayesian one-sided tolerance limits.

Approach	Material A	Material B	Material C
Frequentist Upper Tolerance Limit	121.6	121.4	125.4
Bayesian Upper Tolerance Limit	114.25	117.5	125.6

```
PROC CAPABILITY DATA=Data2 ;
BY Material ;
INTERVALS Response / TYPE=UPPER P=0.99 ALPHA=0.05 METHOD=3 ;
RUN ;
```

Each frequentist UTL is based on a single row of the summary statistics in Table 14.4. This has a noticeable impact on the frequentist tolerance intervals. For example, the observed mean and standard deviation for Material A are both greater than the true values, leading to a relatively high UTL. Similarly, the observed mean for Material C is greater than the true value, while the observed standard deviation is less that the true value; this leads to a relatively low UTL. Bayesian tolerance intervals were calculated using the results from the three-step procedure outlined above. Diagnostic plots are shown in Figures 14.6–14.13. The histograms show that the posterior samples for μ_1 (`beta1+beta2`), μ_2 (`beta1+beta3`), μ_3 (`beta1`) and σ^2 (`covp1`) look reasonable: they have the shapes one would expect and there no extreme values. The trend plots showing the parameters vs the order simulated do not show any obvious trends or spikes. The Bayesian tolerance limits are shown in Table 14.5, and the posterior distributions of the 99% quantiles for the three Materials are shown in Figures 14.15–14.17. The Bayesian UTLs are monotone increasing due to using a common posterior sample for σ^2. In addition, the Bayesian UTLs are closer to the true $p = 0.99$

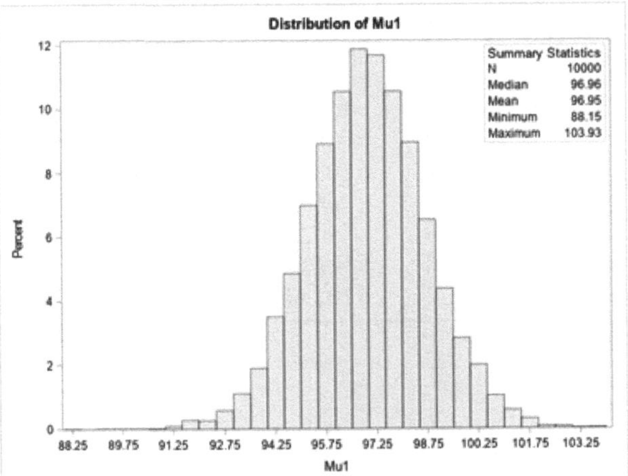

FIGURE 14.6
Distribution of μ_1 (`beta1 + beta2`) for Example 2.

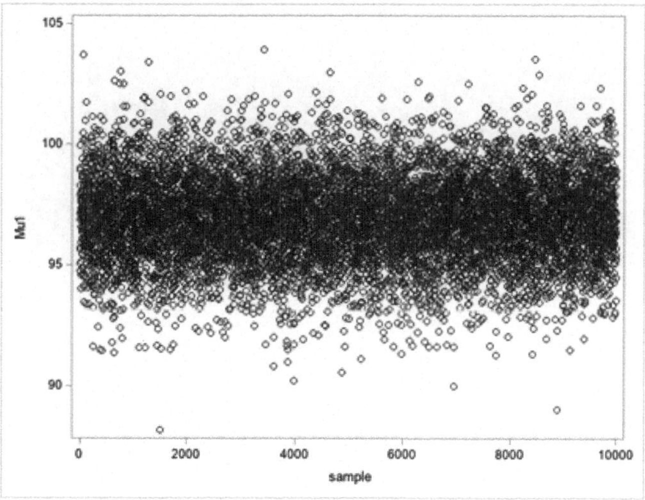

FIGURE 14.7
Trend plot of μ_1 (`beta1 + beta2`) for Example 2.

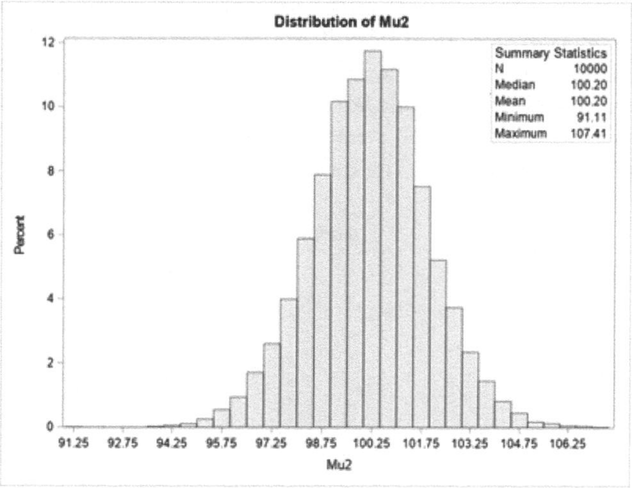

FIGURE 14.8
Distribution of μ_2 (`beta1 + beta3`) for Example 2.

quantiles except for Material C. This is due to sharing information about across the three groups, rather than using three separate estimates based on 10 observations each.

The differences between the frequentist and Bayesian intervals reflects the difference in approaches. In particular, the frequentist approach shown here analyzes each batch separately, while the Bayesian approach uses the entire dataset and shares information about σ^2 across the batches. One could of course use a frequentist approach more suited to the one-way ANOVA model, as discussed in Krishnamoorthy and Mathew (2009), but the authors prefer the simplicity of the Bayesian approach.

Note that Example 2 also illustrates a data-based way to include prior information about σ. For example, suppose Materials A and B represent two historical batches, while Material C represents a more recent batch for which a tolerance interval is desired. By including the

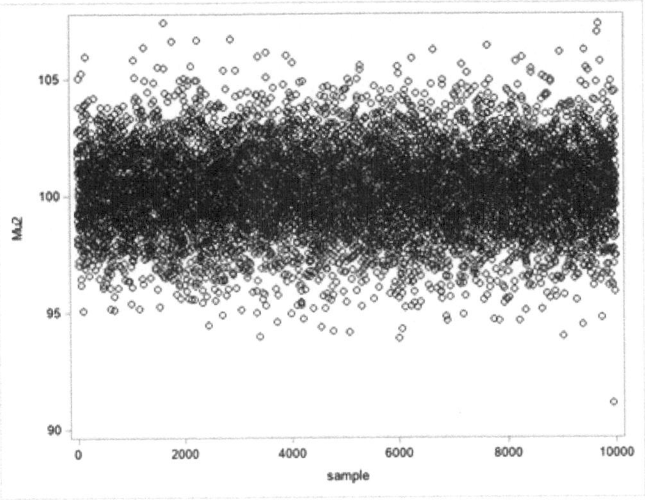

FIGURE 14.9
Trend plot of μ_2 (`beta1 + beta3`) for Example 2.

data for all three materials, model (14.2) allows one to incorporate historical information about σ when constructing a tolerance interval for Material C. An alternative is to use model (14.1) with a flat prior for μ and an informative prior for σ. The informative prior for σ would be based on the observed variability for Materials A and B, and remainder of the Bayesian analysis would only use the data for Material C.

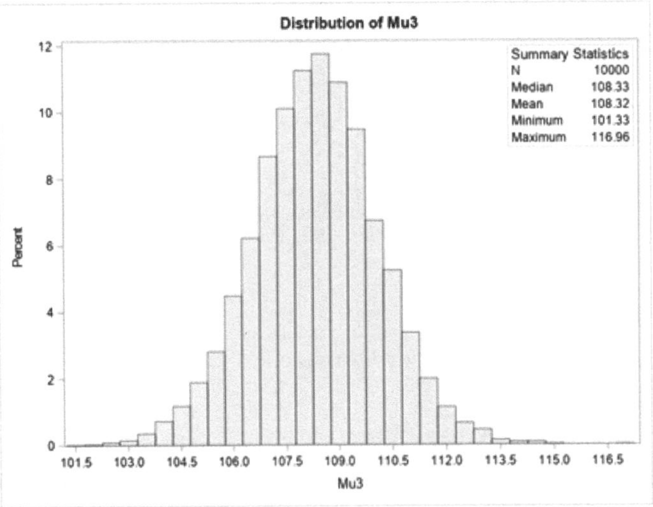

FIGURE 14.10
Distribution of μ_3 (`beta1`) for Example 2.

14.3.3 Example 3

Example 3 will demonstrate how to construct an upper tolerance limit given random samples from multiple groups, as in Example 2, but where the group means are considered to be

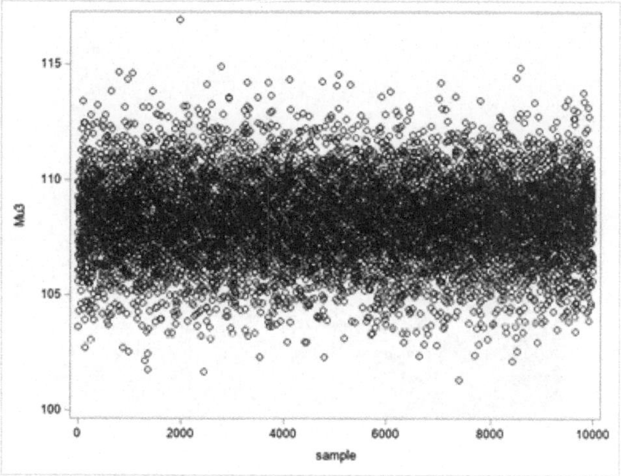

FIGURE 14.11
Trend plot of μ_3 (`beta1`) for Example 2.

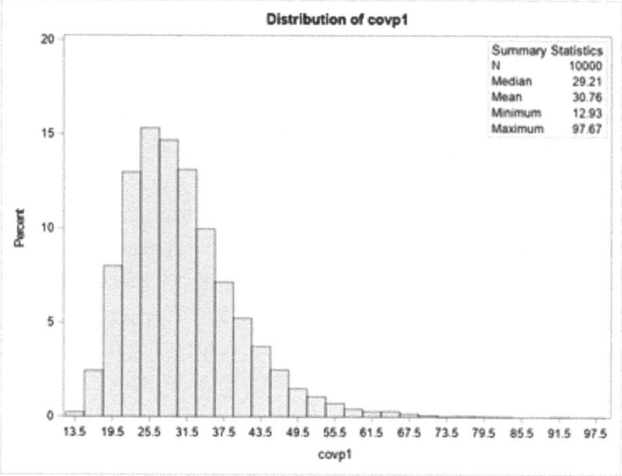

FIGURE 14.12
Distribution of σ^2 (`covp1`) for Example 2.

random rather than fixed. One-sided Bayesian tolerance limits for the one-way random effects model (model (14.3)) can easily be generated using several different software packages, while standard frequentist techniques require balanced data and knowledge of $\sigma_\delta^2/\sigma_\varepsilon^2$ (Mee and Owen, 1983). One could calculate separate tolerance intervals for each group using a frequentist approach, or improperly treat the data as iid and calculate a single tolerance interval. But, as neither of these approaches accurately reflects the model underlying the data, we will focus on a Bayesian approach. More specifically, we will illustrate the use of SAS to calculate one-sided 95% confidence, 99% coverage ($\alpha = 0.05$ and $p = 0.99$) upper tolerance limits for an observation from a future group. For this example, we shall let the groups represent production campaigns and let there be one observation per batch within each campaign. The mean and variance of an observation from a future campaign are μ and $\sigma_\delta^2 + \sigma_\varepsilon^2$, respectively, and the p quantile is $\mu + z_p\sqrt{\sigma_\delta^2 + \sigma_\varepsilon^2}$. The Bayesian approach requires the same three steps as Examples 1 and 2.

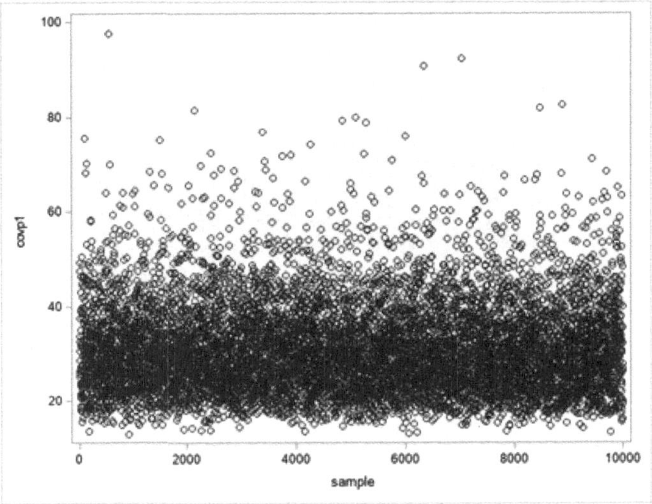

FIGURE 14.13
Trend plot of σ^2 (covp1) for Example 1.

First, obtain samples from the posterior distribution of μ, σ_δ^2, and σ_ε^2 using the MIXED procedure. SAS automatically includes an intercept term in the model and the error term is implicit, so the model statement is `MODEL Response = / SOLUTION` where the SOLUTION option is required for the Bayesian analysis. Campaign should be listed in a CLASS statement, and a random statement (see below) is needed for both sources of variation to be declared and estimated. Note that SAS uses beta1 to represent μ, covp1 to represent σ_δ^2, and covp2 to represent σ_ε^2. Note also that SAS uses transformed versions of variance parameters in its algorithm. The PTRANS option in the PRIOR statement shown below requests SAS to show how the transformed variance parameters relate to the non-transformed variance parameters.

```
PROC MIXED DATA=Data3 ;
CLASS Campaign ;
MODEL Response = / SOLUTION ;
RANDOM Campaign ;
PRIOR / OUT=Posterior3 NSAMPLE=10000 SEED=6456443 PTRANS ;
TITLE "Example 3" ;
RUN ;
PROC PRINT DATA=Posterior3 (OBS=20) ;
TITLE "First 20 Rows of Posterior3" ;
RUN ;
```

Second, use a DATA step to calculate the 99th percentile of a $N(\mu, \sigma_\delta^2 + \sigma_\varepsilon^2)$ distribution for each sample of μ, σ_δ^2, and σ_ε^2. This provides samples from the posterior distribution for the 99th percentile, P99.

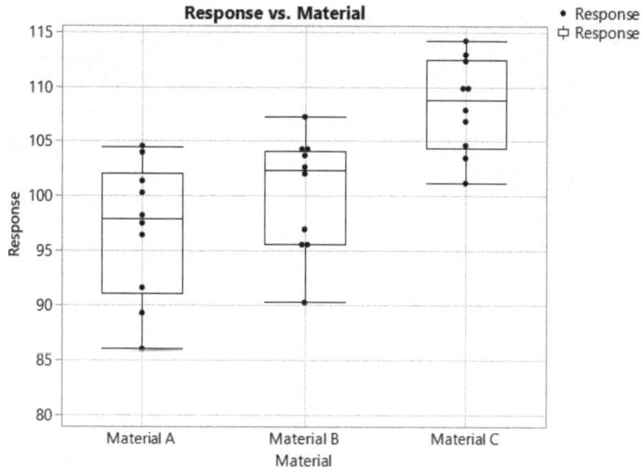

FIGURE 14.14
Boxplot of Example 2 data.

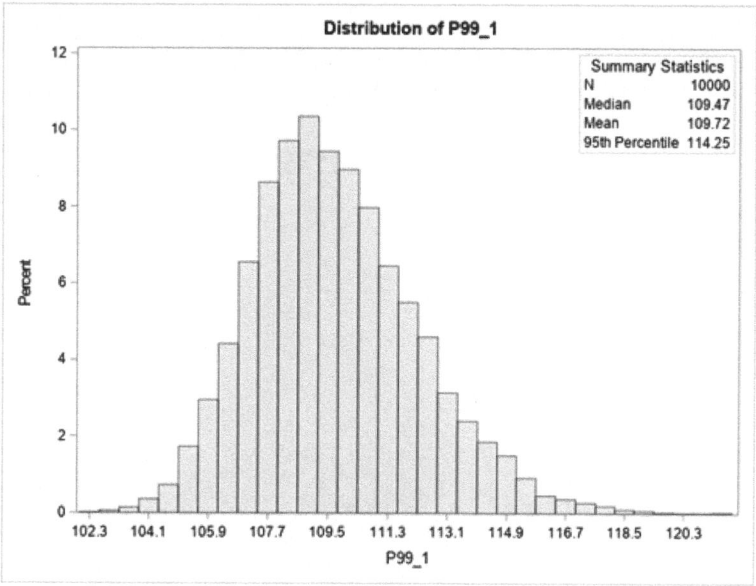

FIGURE 14.15
Posterior distribution of P99 for Material A, Example 2.

```
DATA Posterior ;
SET Posterior3 ;
SEED = 4896235 ;
z99 = PROBIT(0.99) ;
Mu = beta1 ;
SigmaTotal = SQRT(covp1 + covp2) ;
P99 = Mu + z99*SigmaTotal ;
RUN ;
```

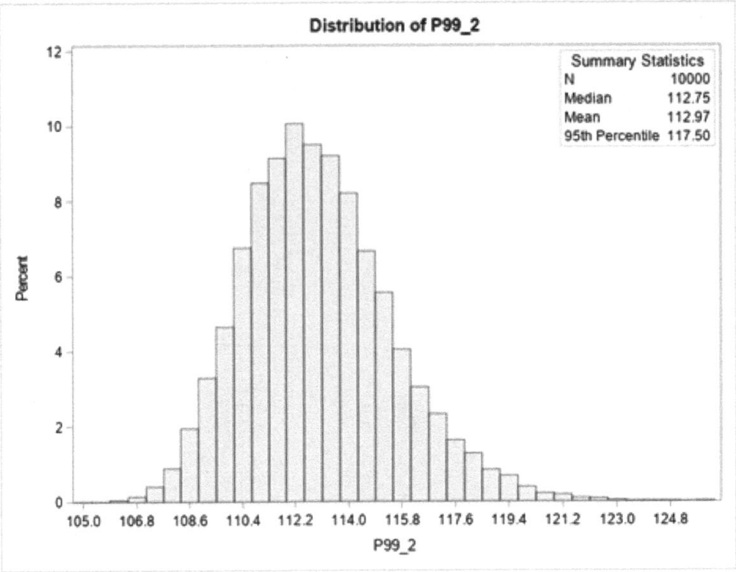

FIGURE 14.16
Posterior distribution of P99 for Material B, Example 2.

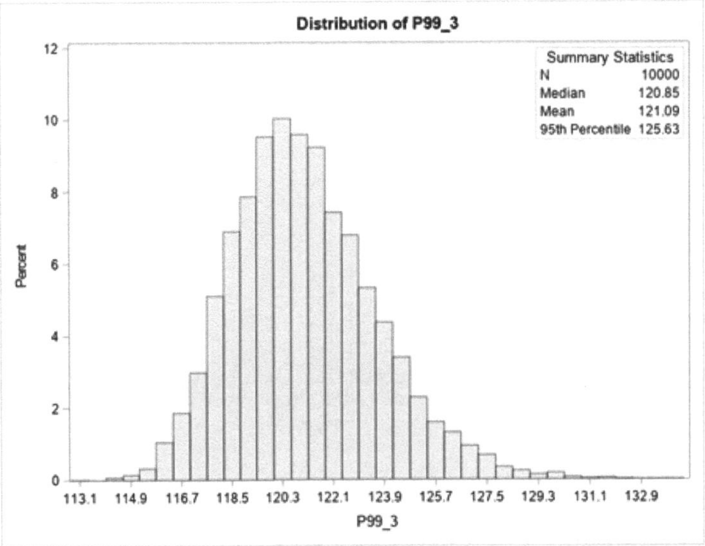

FIGURE 14.17
Posterior distribution of P99 for Material C, Example 2.

Third, use the `UNIVARIATE` procedure to obtain the 95th percentile of the samples for `P99`. The `UNIVARIATE` procedure also provides a histogram for `P99`.

```
PROC UNIVARIATE DATA=Posterior;
VAR P99 ;
HISTOGRAM ;
```

TABLE 14.6
Data set from five campaigns.

Campaign 1	Campaign 2	Campaign 3	Campaign 4	Campaign 5
95.661	98.830	96.665	98.198	95.922
102.529	94.887	106.234	98.186	102.956
103.135	103.362	103.735	107.872	101.596
99.827	94.117	104.317	99.987	96.806
		101.807	103.051	107.041
			106.445	92.589

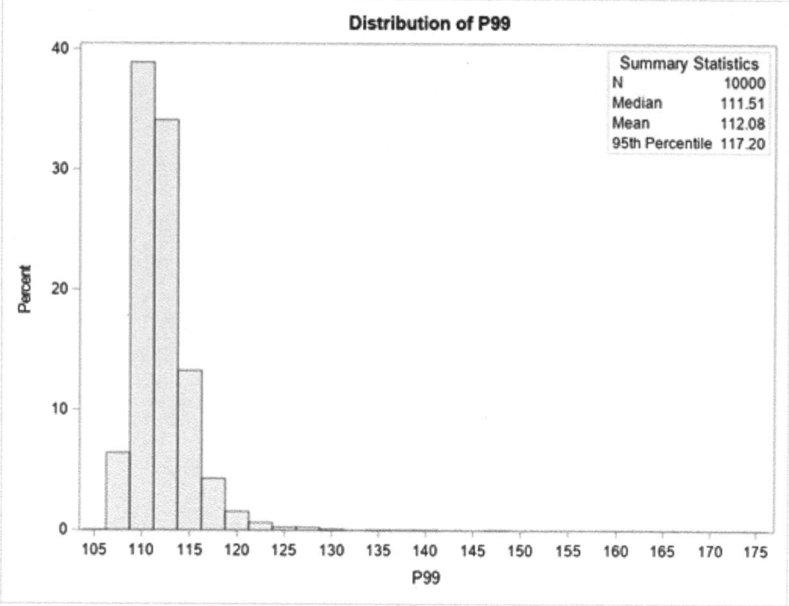

FIGURE 14.18
Posterior distribution of P99 for Example 3.

```
INSET N MEDIAN (6.2) MEAN (6.2) P95 (6.2) /
POS=NE HEADER="Summary Statistics" ;
TITLE ;
RUN ;
```

In order to illustrate the output generated using this code, $n = 25$ observations were generated from five campaigns, with $\mu = 100, \sigma_\delta = 5, \sigma_\varepsilon = 3, n_1 = 4, n_2 = 4, n_3 = 5, n_4 = 6$, and $n_5 = 6$. Here, σ_δ represents the between-campaign variability, and σ_ε the within-campaign (i.e., batch-to-batch) variability. There is one observation per batch, such as the relative potency of a batch of drug substance. The observations are shown in Table 14.6. The Bayesian tolerance interval was calculated using the results from the three-step procedure outlined above. Figure 14.18 provides a histogram of P99 from the Bayesian analysis that shows that the 95th percentile of P99 is 117.2. The Bayesian UTL is 117.2, while the true

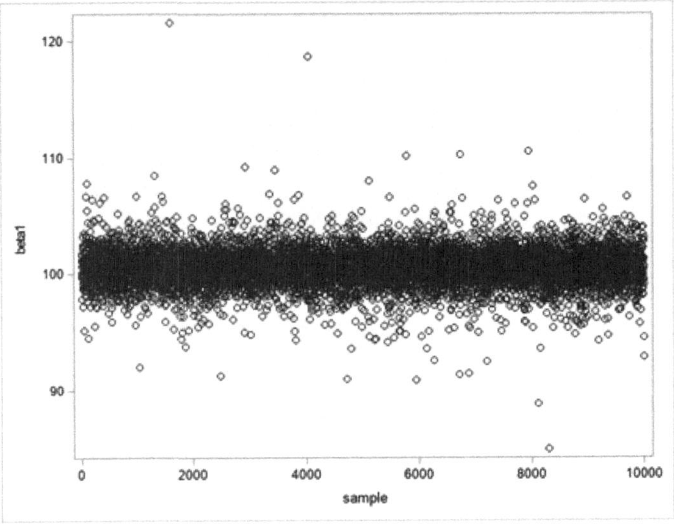

FIGURE 14.19
Trend plot of μ (`beta1`) for Example 3.

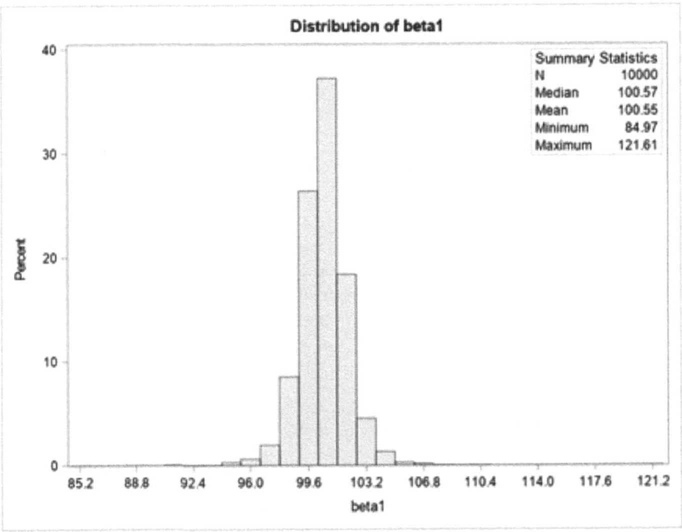

FIGURE 14.20
Distribution of μ (`beta1`) for Example 3.

$p = 0.99$ quantile is 113.6. In frequentist terms, this means one is 95% confident that 99% of future observations will be no greater than 113.6. The UTL may be useful for evaluating the performance of a process against specifications and provides a way to detect unusual observations in future batches and campaigns. If one is in interested in the performance of a particular batch and there is more than one observation per batch, the approach used in Example 2 may be more useful.

Diagnostic plots are shown in Figures 14.19–14.24. The histograms show that the posterior samples for μ (`beta1`), σ_δ^2 (`covp1`), and σ_ε^2 (`covp2`) look reasonable: they have the shapes one would expect and there are no unexpected extreme values. There are some large

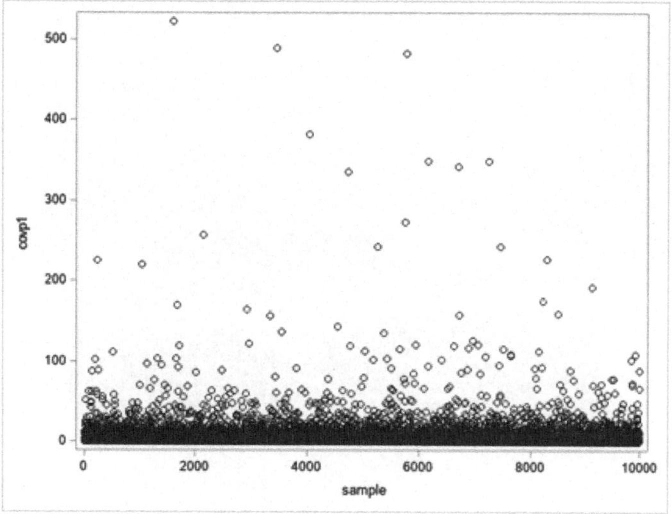

FIGURE 14.21
Trend plot of σ_δ^2 (covp1) for Example 3.

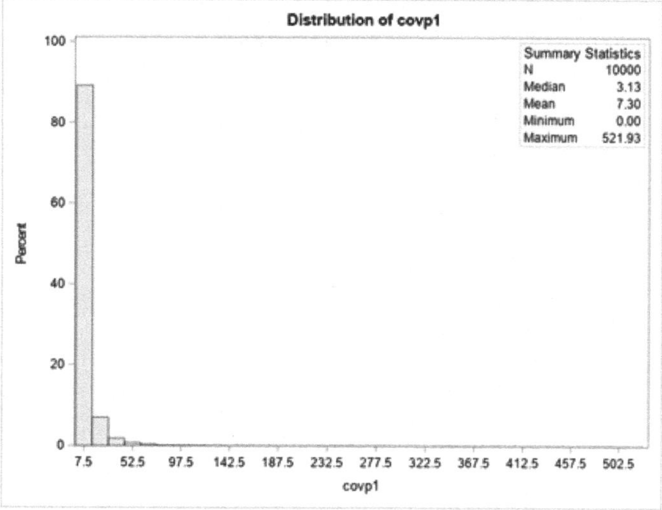

FIGURE 14.22
Distribution of σ_δ^2 (covp1) for Example 3.

values for σ_δ^2 (covp1), but this is not unexpected as there were only five campaigns available to estimate the magnitude of this source of variation. One would expect less variability in the samples for σ_δ^2 (covp1) as the number of campaigns increases. The trend plots showing the parameters vs the order simulated do not show any obvious trends or spikes. It is good practice to check these diagnostics, although the authors have not experienced any issues with convergence performing this analysis in SAS.

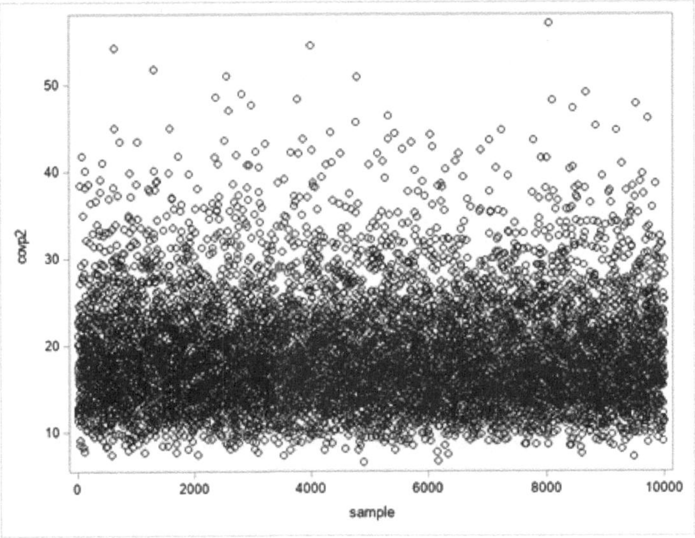

FIGURE 14.23
Trend plot of σ_ε^2 (covp2) for Example 3.

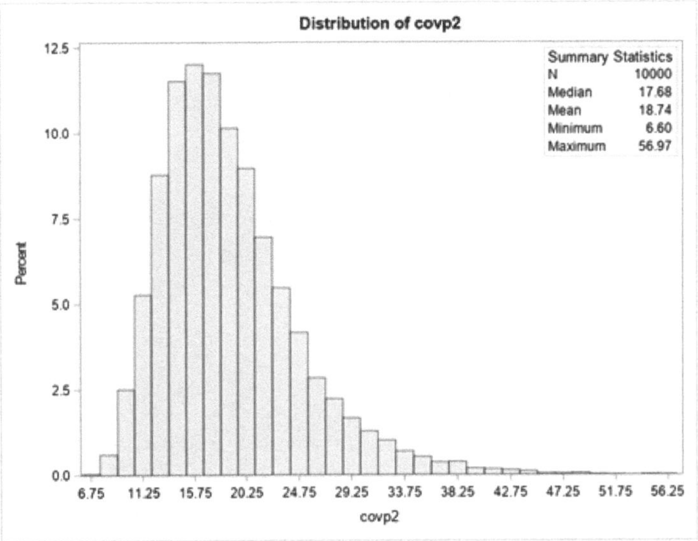

FIGURE 14.24
Distribution of σ_ε^2 (covp2) for Example 3.

14.4 Discussion

Tolerance intervals are a useful statistical tool. There are several important points to consider when constructing tolerance intervals. First, SAS PROC CAPABILITY provides frequentist tolerance intervals for model (14.1) and it is convenient to use these tolerance intervals when there is no prior information about μ or σ. Second, while frequentist methods also work well in many other situations, appropriate assumptions and formulas need to be derived for each type of model, a process which may be time consuming or unwieldly. A Bayesian approach uses the same three steps for each type of model, easily handles unbalanced data and, as shown in Example 2, can also incorporate prior information through a data-based approach (rather than specifying an informative prior). The Bayesian approach shown in this chapter can easily be extended to any linear mixed model that SAS `PROC MIXED` can handle. More complicated models can be handled using SAS `PROC MCMC` (for Markov Chain Monte Carlo). Third, Bayesian tolerance intervals for additional types of observations, such as the mean of several observations, can also be constructed. One simply needs to be able to calculate the p quantile of the item of interest from the model parameters. Fourth, when constructing Bayesian tolerance intervals, it is good practice to check the model assumptions and the convergence of the posterior distribution. As shown in Example 1, SAS can be used to generate summary statistics, histograms and trend plots for the parameters in the posterior distribution. The observed data should be examined, as well. Finally, Bayesian methodology described in this chapter can also be used to generate other types of statistical intervals, such as prediction intervals (Hamada et al., 2004). Prediction intervals are useful for predicting the behavior of a specific number of future observations, rather than focusing on population quantiles. For instance, a frequentist prediction interval may be used to predict what range a future observation may fall within with a given level of confidence. Again, with more complex data structures, such as multiple batches generated for multiple campaigns, the technical aspects of constructing such an interval can create some difficulties. However, as shown in this chapter with tolerance intervals, the Bayesian methodology allows the practitioner to generate prediction intervals for the many complex situations that may arise.

15

A Bayesian Application in Process Monitoring – Establishing Limits for Dosage Units in Early Phase Process Control

Yanbing Zheng, James Reynolds, Man Tang, Mark Johnson and Hesham Fahmy
Data and Statistical Sciences, AbbVie Inc.

CONTENTS

15.1 Introduction

Statistical process control (SPC), typically used for quality control, has a long history of use within manufacturing. Shewhart developed statistical measures to identify non-random trends reflective of results from a source outside the normal process that significantly impacts process performance ("special cause" variation) vs results from noise associated with non-assignable sources that occur naturally within the process ("common cause" variation) (Shewhart, 1931; Deming, 1986). Douglas Montgomery and Donald Wheeler, current quality scientists, also endorsed use of statistical process measures to characterize process performance of attribute results governed by normal and non-normal distributional observations (Wheeler and Chambers, 1992; Wheeler, 1993; Montgomery, 2020). Today, statistical process control methods are considered key elements within multiple manufacturing contexts. In the pharmaceutical industry, process control is essential to developing new processes, improving existing processes, and ensuring consistent processes that yield products with satisfactory quality.

Control charts play a major role in process monitoring. Constructing a control chart generally occurs in two phases. The Phase I control chart is typically based on a limited amount of current data often consisting of process validation and process performance batches. This can be supplemented with historical data from similar manufacturing and analytical

DOI: 10.1201/9781003255093-15

processes when appropriate. Phase II establishes control limits once additional batches are available and are based on the common cause variation of the current process. This common cause variation can include batch-to-batch variation and within-batch variation and additional relevant variance components.

Traditional methods for statistical process monitoring usually rely on long-run stability to establish a pattern by which further sample data would be compared. Obviously, short production runs would impact the performance of such methods because it is impossible to obtain sufficient insight to control limits due to limited measurements. The lack of information within a production run may be partly offset by previous experience, such as historical data and experts' knowledge. Over the past decades, Bayesian statistics, an approach to modeling and analysis which integrates a prior distribution and current sample data, has rapidly become a popular methodology in statistical process monitoring (Colosimo and Del Castillo, 2006; Marcellus, 2007). Under a Bayesian approach, process parameters are considered as random variables. An obvious advantage of the Bayesian approach in statistical process monitoring is the ability to incorporate prior information. An additional benefit of the Bayesian approach is it uses the predictive sample to compute probability when the sampling distribution is unknown or intractable. Bayesian posterior inference can be derived by combining the potential prior information from these sources and the likelihood function, compensating for the limited measurements. The process stability can be assessed through monitoring the posterior probability distributions of these parameters over time or computing the fraction outside of the specification limit based on the posterior predictive distribution (Peterson and Yahyah, 2009; Apley, 2012; Tan and Shi, 2012). Much work has been done applying the Bayesian approach to statistical process control and monitoring, considering various types of control charts for attributes and continuous variables and proposing approaches to determine the optimal decision parameters in chart design, such as sampling interval, sample sizes and control limits (e.g., Girshick and Rubin (1952); Menzefricke (2002); Tagaras and Nikolaidis (2002); Bayarri and García-Donato (2005); Kooli and Limam (2009)). Numerical examples have shown that the Bayesian techniques can be economically optimal compared to the traditional charts in dealing with the control chart design issue (Calabrese, 1995; Makis, 2008).

This chapter presents a Bayesian application in which in-process control limits are established for uniformity of dosage units (UDU) based on weight variation in the early phase (phase I) of drug development. Blend and content uniformity are important measures of in-process batch assessment. These in-process controls provide assurance that the current process is stable and that product will perform to quality expectations. Since USP, General Chapter $< 905 >$ (2014) permits the assessment of uniformity of dosage units by weight variation, it is important to control weight during tablet manufacturing. In this chapter, the control limits determined using the Bayesian method will be compared to typical practices (including $\pm 5\%$ of target based on prior experiences of the scientists, $\pm 3\sigma$ and Monte Carlo simulation). The Bayesian control limits presented will be based on the posterior predictive distribution of the charted variable (i.e., individual weight unit).

The remainder of this chapter is as follows. In Section 15.2, we present statistical models for UDU by weight. Bayesian applications are described in Section 15.3 with a new method proposed to determine control limits. In Section 15.4, we compare the performance of statistical methods on control limits setup and offer some concluding remarks. A final discussion is provided in Section 15.5.

15.2 Statistical Models

15.2.1 Mixed Effects Model for UDU by Weight

Here we consider a real application of Bayesian inference for process monitoring in the early phase of drug development. Tablet weight data are fitted using a mixed effects model, where time is considered as a categorical variable with fixed effect and batch as a categorical variable with random effect. The mixed effects model is presented as

$$Y_{ijk} = \alpha + \beta_i + t_j + \gamma_{ij} + \varepsilon_{ijk}, \tag{15.1}$$

where $i = 1, 2, ..., I$, $j = 1, ..., T$, and $k = 1..., K$. I is the number of batches, T is the number of time points, and K is the number of replicates for each time point. Here Y_{ijk} denotes the tablet weight for the kth tablet from the ith batch at the jth time point, α is the overall population mean for the first time point, $t_1 = 0$, t_j is the difference between the mean for the jth time point and the mean the first time point, $j = 2, ..., T$, β_i *i.i.d.* $\sim N(0, \sigma_\beta^2)$ is the random effect added by the ith batch, γ_{ij} *i.i.d.* $\sim N(0, \sigma_\gamma^2)$ is the random effect added by the ith batch at the jth time point, ε_{ijk} *i.i.d.* $\sim N(0, \sigma_\varepsilon^2)$ is the random error. The time points are fixed at the same intervals for all batches. And it is assumed that the sampling time points are sufficiently spaced to be independent of each other.

To assist programming, model (15.1) is rewritten in the matrix format. Let $\mathbf{Y}_{ij.} = (Y_{ij1}, ..., Y_{ijK})'$ and $\mathbf{Y} = (\mathbf{Y}'_{11.}, \mathbf{Y}'_{12.}, ..., \mathbf{Y}'_{1T.}, \mathbf{Y}'_{21.}, ..., \mathbf{Y}'_{IT.})'$. Let $\boldsymbol{\eta} = (\alpha, t_2, ..., t_T)'$, $\boldsymbol{\beta} = (\beta_1, ..., \beta_I)'$, $\boldsymbol{\gamma} = (\gamma_{11}, ..., \gamma_{1T}, \gamma_{21}, ..., \gamma_{IT})'$ and $\mathbf{u} = (\boldsymbol{\beta}', \boldsymbol{\gamma}')'$. Then the conditional expectation of $\mathbf{Y}$ given random effects would be

$$\boldsymbol{\mu} = \mathbb{E}(\mathbf{Y}|\boldsymbol{\beta}, \boldsymbol{\gamma}) = \mathbf{X}\boldsymbol{\eta} + \mathbf{Z}\mathbf{u}, \tag{15.2}$$

where $\mathbf{X}$ is the design matrix for the fixed effects, $\boldsymbol{\eta}$, and $\mathbf{Z}$ is the design matrix for the random effects, $\mathbf{u}$.

15.2.2 Bayesian Model

In Bayesian framework, non-informative priors and power priors (Ibrahim and Chen, 2000) were considered for posterior analysis. The power prior has been widely used in many applications (e.g., Duan et al. (2006), Viele et al. (2014), Ibrahim et al. (2015), Faya et al. (2020)), and is intended to be an informative prior that controls the amount of informativeness from historical data. Let the data for the current batches be denoted by $\mathbf{D}$ with likelihood $L(\boldsymbol{\theta}|\mathbf{D})$, where $\boldsymbol{\theta} = (\boldsymbol{\eta}, \sigma_\beta^2, \sigma_\gamma^2, \sigma_\varepsilon^2)'$ is a vector of model parameters. Let the data for historical batches be denoted by $\mathbf{D}_0$ with likelihood $L(\boldsymbol{\theta}|\mathbf{D}_0)$. The power prior is defined as

$$\pi(\boldsymbol{\theta}|\mathbf{D}_0, a) \propto L(\boldsymbol{\theta}|\mathbf{D}_0)^a \pi_0(\boldsymbol{\theta}), \tag{15.3}$$

where $\pi_0(\boldsymbol{\theta})$ is an initial prior for $\boldsymbol{\theta}$ before incorporating information from historical data $\mathbf{D}_0$ and a is the power parameter, $0 \leq a \leq 1$. Under this prior, the posterior distribution of $\boldsymbol{\theta}$ is

$$\pi(\boldsymbol{\theta}|\mathbf{D}, \mathbf{D}_0, a) \propto L(\boldsymbol{\theta}|\mathbf{D}) L(\boldsymbol{\theta}|\mathbf{D}_0)^a \pi_0(\boldsymbol{\theta}). \tag{15.4}$$

Values of a weight the information from historical batches relative to current batches. An a near zero limits the information from historical batches, while an a value near 1 allows complete borrowing of information from historical batches. If the "historical" data were from the same process for the same product using $a = 1$ would be wholly appropriate. However, "historical" data from a different product with the same platform and same weight (e.g., different API) could necessitate more caution with $a = 0.5$. In this example, non-informative priors were implemented with $a = 0$ in (15.3) and power priors with $a = 0.5$ in (15.3) to partially include historical information. As an informative prior, the power prior offers a simple calculation in that it is just the likelihood function raised to a power and thus shares all the properties that likelihood functions have, which makes it more attractive in results interpretation and model/variable selection. In addition, the power prior is very flexible in controlling the role of historical data via adjusting the power parameter.

Two different initial non-informative priors (π_0) were used:

1. a non-informative constant prior $\pi_0(\tilde{\boldsymbol{\theta}}) \propto 1$ where $\tilde{\boldsymbol{\theta}} = (\boldsymbol{\eta}, \sigma_\beta, \sigma_\gamma, \sigma_\varepsilon)'$, subsequently referred to as the constant prior and
2. a non-informative constant prior for fixed effects $\pi_0(\boldsymbol{\eta}) \propto 1$ multiplied by a non-informative Jeffreys' prior for the variance components

$$\pi_0(\boldsymbol{\theta}) = \pi_0(\boldsymbol{\eta}) \times \pi_0(\sigma_\beta^2, \sigma_\gamma^2, \sigma_\varepsilon^2) \propto \frac{1}{\sigma_\varepsilon^2(K\sigma_\gamma^2 + \sigma_\varepsilon^2)(TK\sigma_\beta^2 + K\sigma_\gamma^2 + \sigma_\varepsilon^2)}, \qquad (15.5)$$

hereafter referred to as the Jeffreys' prior.

The Jeffreys' prior, which was determined with the aid of symbolic matrix computation in MATLAB Release 2020b (2020), is recognized as the inverse product of the expected mean squares of the random batch, β_i, and batch-by-time interaction, γ_{ij}, and error ε_{ijk}. Overall, there are four priors considered in this chapter: 1) power prior with $a = 0.5$ and constant initial prior π_0; 2) power prior with $a = 0.5$ and Jeffreys' initial prior π_0; 3) constant prior π_0 (Note: $a = 0$); 4) Jeffreys' prior π_0 (Note: $a = 0$). The use of multiple priors enables the assessment of the Bayesian inference to the choice of prior.

Markov chain Monte Carlo (MCMC) would be implemented to obtain posteriors of model parameters. Although all the priors are improper, it can be shown that each prior results in a proper posterior distribution. With $a = 0$ in (15.3), the constant prior determines the scaling constant for the likelihood thus effectively demonstrating its propriety. Concerning the use of Jeffreys' prior, the prior beliefs can be updated with the likelihood either before or after integrating out the fixed effects (since the prior only involves the variance components). Heuristically, extending the results for the balanced one-way random effects model (see Searle et al. (1992)), based on the partitioning of the sums of squares, the restricted likelihood can be written as

$$L(\sigma_\beta^2, \sigma_\gamma^2, \sigma_\varepsilon^2|\mathbf{D}) \propto \frac{\exp\left(-\frac{SS_\varepsilon}{2\sigma_\varepsilon^2}\right)\exp\left(-\frac{SS_\gamma}{2(K\sigma_\gamma^2+\sigma_\varepsilon^2)}\right)\exp\left(-\frac{SS_\beta}{2(TK\sigma_\beta^2+K\sigma_\gamma^2+\sigma_\varepsilon^2)}\right)}{\sigma_\varepsilon^{2\times\frac{1}{2}(IT(K-1))}(K\sigma_\gamma^2+\sigma_\varepsilon^2)^{\frac{1}{2}((T-1)(I-1))}(TK\sigma_\beta^2+K\sigma_\gamma^2+\sigma_\varepsilon^2)^{\frac{1}{2}(I-1)}}, \qquad (15.6)$$

where the subscripts on the sum of squares (SS) indicate error (ε), batch by time interaction (γ), and batch (β). The posterior distribution for variance components can be written as

$$p(\sigma_\beta^2, \sigma_\gamma^2, \sigma_\varepsilon^2|\mathbf{D}) \propto \pi_0(\sigma_\beta^2, \sigma_\gamma^2, \sigma_\varepsilon^2)L(\sigma_\beta^2, \sigma_\gamma^2, \sigma_\varepsilon^2|\mathbf{D}). \qquad (15.7)$$

The posterior can be shown to be proportional to a triple integral of three inverted-gamma-type distributions with constrained limits of integration resulting from the hierarchy of the expected mean squares. This triple integral (representing the posterior) is less than or equal to the product of three independent integrals of inverted-gamma distributions. Since the product of the three independent known distributions is finite, the posterior is proper (see the chapter's Appendix). Whereas the above details are provided for $a = 0$, results from Carvalho and Ibrahim (2021) are relied upon for $0 < a \leq 1$. Note that the restricted likelihood provided in this paragraph is only for theoretical proof purpose and not directly programmed.

15.3 Application of Bayesian Inference

15.3.1 The Data

In this example, the data consist of 10 tablets sampled from each of 7 times points from 5 current batches. The batch sizes were the same with the sampling times also being the same for each batch. In addition, 5 historical batches from which to elicit prior distributions were also available. The current data and historical data are displayed in Section 15.4 where the control limits are included. In the frequentist framework, `lmer` function from R package `lme4` can be used to fit the mixed effect model with restricted maximum likelihood (REML) as the default parameter estimation method. The results of the mixed model analysis are shown below in the R output. The particular data analyzed did not exhibit a detectable time effect (notwithstanding neglecting possible multiplicity) at the 0.05 significance level in `lmer`. The process generating the data can be described as stable. Also, for these particular data, the residual variance is the largest variance component, and the batch-to-batch component is the smallest.

R output for REML estimates of parameters for model (15.1):

```
# Example Data
# Group=1 corresponds to current batches and
# Group=2 historical batches

> dat[1:10,]
   Time Batch value Group
1     1     1 449.8     1
2     1     1 446.2     1
3     1     1 450.7     1
4     1     1 448.4     1
5     1     1 452.1     1
6     1     1 447.6     1
> dim(dat)
[1] 700   4

> library(lme4)
> datCurrent=dat[dat$Group==1,] #data for current batches
> datCurrent$Time = as.factor(datCurrent$Time)
> datCurrent$Batch = as.factor(datCurrent$Batch)
> fitReml = lmer(value ~ Time + (1|Batch) + (1|Batch:Time),
                 data=datCurrent) # Time is considered as fixed
```

```
    # class effect and batch and batch-by-time interaction
    # are considered as random effects. The form of lmer
    # function is slightly different from model (12.1) format,
    # but the output is consistent with model (12.1) format.

> summary(fitReml)
Linear mixed model fit by REML ['lmerMod']
Formula: value1 ~ Time + (1 | Batch) + (1 | Batch:Time)
   Data: datCurrent

REML criterion at convergence: 1810.2

Scaled residuals:
    Min      1Q  Median      3Q     Max
-2.8486 -0.6383  0.0532  0.5704  3.1749

Random effects:
 Groups     Name        Variance Std.Dev.
 Batch:Time (Intercept) 2.3988   1.5488
 Batch      (Intercept) 0.8436   0.9185
 Residual               9.4385   3.0722
Number of obs: 350, groups:  Batch:Time, 35; Batch, 5

Fixed effects:
            Estimate Std. Error t value
(Intercept)  447.866      0.915 489.462
Time2          1.256      1.156   1.086
Time3          0.588      1.156   0.509
Time4          0.078      1.156   0.067
Time5         -0.100      1.156  -0.086
Time6         -0.248      1.156  -0.214
Time7         -0.076      1.156  -0.066

Correlation of Fixed Effects:
      (Intr) Time2  Time3  Time4  Time5  Time6
Time2 -0.632
Time3 -0.632  0.500
Time4 -0.632  0.500  0.500
Time5 -0.632  0.500  0.500  0.500
Time6 -0.632  0.500  0.500  0.500  0.500
Time7 -0.632  0.500  0.500  0.500  0.500  0.500

> library(lmerTest)
> anova(fitReml)
Type III Analysis of Variance Table with Satterthwaite's
                                                  method
     Sum Sq Mean Sq NumDF DenDF F value Pr(>F)
Time 23.804  3.9674     6    24  0.4203 0.8581
```

15.3.2 Posterior Samples via MCMC in R

The `rstan` package (Stan Development Team, 2021a) in R was used for Bayesian modeling and inference. The `rstan` package provides an R interface to Stan. The following is Rstan code for Bayesian inference with a power prior with $a = 0.5$ and the Jeffreys' initial prior π_0 as an example. Overall, our `rstan` program includes four blocks: a data block to specify data used in the program, a parameter block to specify parameters of the model, a transformed parameters block to specify parameter transformation, and a model block to specify the model. The `stan` function implements Bayesian inference via Stan with the default and preferred "NUTS" algorithm. NUTS refers to the No-U-Turn sampler variant of Hamiltonian Monte Carlo (Betancourt, 2017; Hoffman and Gelman, 2014). The constant prior is assumed by the `stan` function if there is no specific prior is specified.

```
library(rstan)

## design matrix for fixed effects
X <- model.matrix(~ as.factor(Time), data = dat)

## design matrix for random effects gamma
Z1 <- cbind(X[,1]-apply(X[,2:7], 1, sum), X[,2:7])

stanDat <- list(Batch=as.integer(dat$Batch),
                Group=as.integer(dat$Group),
                y=dat$value, N=nrow(dat), I=10, T=7, K=10,
                X=X, Z1=Z1, a=0.5)
                ## 10 batches (5 current, 5 historical),
                ## 7 time points, and 10 replicates for
                ## each time point and each batch

# rstan program

scode <- "

data {

int<lower=1> N;
int<lower=1> I;
int<lower=1> T;
int<lower=1> K;
vector[N] y;
matrix[N,T] X;
matrix[N,T] Z1;
int<lower=1,upper=2> Group[N];
int<lower=1,upper=I> Batch[N];
real<lower=0,upper=1> a;

}

parameters {

vector[T] eta;/* fixed effects */
vector[I] beta; /* random effect added by batch */
vector[I] gamma1; /* random effect added by batch*(time point 1) */
```

```
vector[I] gamma2; /* random effect added by batch*(time point 2) */
vector[I] gamma3; /* random effect added by batch*(time point 3) */
vector[I] gamma4; /* random effect added by batch*(time point 4) */
vector[I] gamma5; /* random effect added by batch*(time point 5) */
vector[I] gamma6; /* random effect added by batch*(time point 6) */
vector[I] gamma7; /* random effect added by batch*(time point 7) */

/* residual variance */
real<lower=0> sigma_e2;
/* variance for random effect added by batch */
real<lower=0> sigma_beta2;
/* variance for random effect added by batch*time */
real<lower=0> sigma_gamma2;

}

transformed parameters {

real<lower=0> sigma_e;
real<lower=0> sigma_beta;
real<lower=0> sigma_gamma;

sigma_e = sqrt(sigma_e2);
sigma_beta = sqrt(sigma_beta2);
sigma_gamma = sqrt(sigma_gamma2);

}

model {

real mu;    /* Conditional Expectation of Y given beta and gamma */

beta ~ normal(0, sigma_beta);
gamma1 ~ normal(0, sigma_gamma);
gamma2 ~ normal(0, sigma_gamma);
gamma3 ~ normal(0, sigma_gamma);
gamma4 ~ normal(0, sigma_gamma);
gamma5 ~ normal(0, sigma_gamma);
gamma6 ~ normal(0, sigma_gamma);
gamma7 ~ normal(0, sigma_gamma);

for (i in 1:N){

mu = X[i,]*eta + beta[Batch[i]] + gamma1[Batch[i]]*Z1[i,1]+
          gamma2[Batch[i]]*Z1[i,2]+gamma3[Batch[i]]*Z1[i,3] +
          gamma4[Batch[i]]*Z1[i,4]+gamma5[Batch[i]]*Z1[i,5] +
          gamma6[Batch[i]]*Z1[i,6]+ gamma7[Batch[i]]*Z1[i,7];

if (Group[i] == 2)
target += a*normal_lpdf(y[i]|mu, sigma_e);

if (Group[i] == 1)
target += normal_lpdf(y[i]|mu, sigma_e);
```

```
}

target += -log(sigma_e2)-log(K*sigma_gamma2+sigma_e2)-
         log(T*K*sigma_beta2+K*sigma_gamma2+sigma_e2);
         /* add Jeffreys' initial prior for variance components;
         assume constant initial prior for fixed effects */

}
"

fitppj <- stan(model_code=scode, data=stanDat, iter=10000)
```

We used the default setting of warmup and number of Markov chains for the `stan` function in MCMC: run four Markov chains and for each Markov chain and take half of iterations as warm up. For thinning, we used the default recommended unthinned option as thinning throws away information (Stan Development Team, 2021a). We set number of iterations to be 10000 for each chain to ensure good effective sample size (ESS), which measures the effectiveness of MCMC sample chains (Geyer, 2011). The following is R output from the `print` function for the posterior summary:

```
# Output for power prior with Jeffreys' initial prior
> print(fitppj, pars = c("eta", "beta", "gamma1", "gamma2",
"gamma3", "gamma4", "gamma5", "gamma6", "gamma7", "sigma_e",
"sigma_beta", "sigma_gamma"), probs = c(0.025, 0.5, 0.975),
digits = 3)
Inference for Stan model:
4 chains, each with iter=10000; warmup=5000; thin=1;
post-warmup draws per chain=5000, total post-warmup draws=20000  .

                mean se_mean    sd    2.5%     50%   97.5% n_eff Rhat
eta[1]       447.088   0.008 0.677 445.752 447.099 448.404  7439    1
eta[2]         2.663   0.009 0.882   0.947   2.654   4.417  9367    1
eta[3]         1.896   0.009 0.875   0.208   1.885   3.630  9184    1
eta[4]         0.904   0.009 0.873  -0.806   0.902   2.635  9388    1
eta[5]         0.984   0.009 0.873  -0.727   0.971   2.722  9583    1
eta[6]         0.531   0.009 0.878  -1.168   0.529   2.266  9785    1
eta[7]         0.903   0.009 0.882  -0.785   0.900   2.640 10154    1
......
sigma_e          3.227   0.001 0.106   3.029   3.225   3.441 23251    1
sigma_beta       0.750   0.006 0.379   0.167   0.702   1.615  4421    1
sigma_gamma      1.526   0.003 0.243   1.079   1.517   2.028  6463    1
```

For comparison, we also print the posterior summary for noninformative Jeffreys' prior ($a = 0$). We can see that after accounting for information from historical batches, power prior with Jeffreys' initial prior gives slightly lower posterior mean of variances for random batch and batch-time interaction.

```
> print(fitnpj, pars = c("eta", "beta", "gamma1", "gamma2", "gamma3",
"gamma4", "gamma5", "gamma6", "gamma7", "sigma_e", "sigma_beta",
"sigma_gamma"), probs = c(0.025, 0.5, 0.975), digits = 3)
Inference for Stan model:
4 chains, each with iter=10000; warmup=5000; thin=1;
post-warmup draws per chain=5000, total post-warmup draws=20000.

               mean   se_mean    sd     2.5%      50%    97.5%   n_eff  Rhat
eta[1]      447.858    0.016 1.039 445.847 447.860 449.862   4143 1.000
eta[2]        1.266    0.015 1.220  -1.103   1.260   3.694   6522 1.000
eta[3]        0.603    0.015 1.215  -1.774   0.600   3.006   6428 1.001
eta[4]        0.100    0.015 1.217  -2.267   0.095   2.520   6333 1.001
eta[5]       -0.079    0.015 1.226  -2.489  -0.084   2.336   6474 1.000
eta[6]       -0.239    0.015 1.217  -2.670  -0.236   2.128   6390 1.000
eta[7]       -0.058    0.015 1.229  -2.472  -0.057   2.349   6289 1.000
......
sigma_e       3.077    0.001 0.123   2.846   3.074   3.328  25179 1.000
sigma_beta    1.083    0.017 0.729   0.210   0.930   2.950   1938 1.001
sigma_gamma   1.637    0.006 0.336   1.061   1.607   2.370   2756 1.001
```

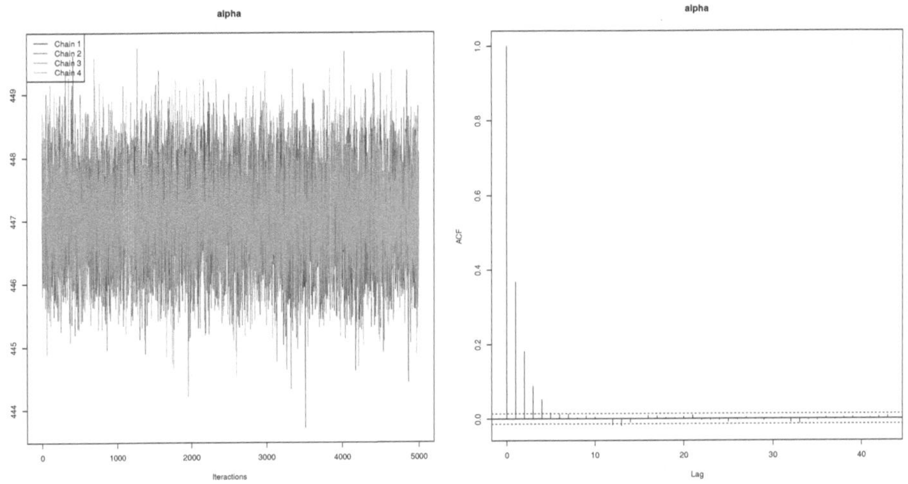

FIGURE 15.1
Trace plot and ACF plot for the intercept α using power prior with Jeffreys' initial prior (with $a = 0.5$)

From the trace plot and autocorrelation function (acf) plot (Figure 15.1 with the intercept α, i.e. `eta[1]` in stan output, as an example) and density plots (Figure 15.2), we can see the chains mixed well for our example. Rhat statistic was calculated for convergence diagnostics (Vehtari et al., 2021). The Rhat function produces a R-hat convergence diagnostic, which compares the between- and within-chain estimates for model parameters and other univariate quantities of interest. If chains have not mixed well (i.e., the between- and within-chain estimates do not agree), then R-hat is larger than 1. `n_eff` in the posterior summary is the ESS measure. Small effective sample size would indicate poor mixing of MCMC chains. Stan recommends ESS of at least 400 when running 4 chains.

R code to generate the trace plot and the acf plot:

```
# Trace plot
out = as.array(fitppj)
plot.ts(out[,,"eta[1]"], main="alpha", xlab="Iteractions",
        ylab="", plot.type="single", col=grey.colors(8))
legend("topleft", legend=c("Chain 1", "Chain 2", "Chain 3",
       "Chain 4"), col=grey.colors(8), lty=1)

# acf plot
acf(c(extract(fitppj, pars="eta[1]", permuted=FALSE)),
    main="alpha")
```

R code to generate density plots:

```
library(ggpubr)

out = as.matrix(fitppj) # power prior with Jeffreys' initial prior
chain = rep(1:4, each=5000)
outplot = data.frame(cbind(out[,c(1,91,92,93)], chain))
outplot$alpha=outplot$eta.1.
outplot$chain=as.factor(outplot$chain)

out1 = as.matrix(fitnpj) # Noninformative prior - Jeffreys' prior
outplot1 = data.frame(cbind(out1[,c(1,91,92,93)], chain))
outplot1$alpha=outplot1$eta.1.
outplot1$chain=as.factor(outplot1$chain)

a=ggplot(outplot, aes(x=alpha, lty=chain))+geom_density()+
  xlim(c(445,455))+theme(axis.title=element_text(size=16))
b=ggplot(outplot, aes(x=sigma_beta, lty=chain))+geom_density()+
  xlim(c(0,10))+theme(axis.title=element_text(size=16))
c=ggplot(outplot, aes(x=sigma_gamma, lty=chain))+geom_density()+
  xlim(c(0,5))+theme(axis.title=element_text(size=16))
d=ggplot(outplot, aes(x=sigma_e, lty=chain))+geom_density()+
  xlim(c(0,5))+theme(axis.title=element_text(size=16))

e=ggplot(outplot1, aes(x=alpha, lty=chain))+geom_density()+
  xlim(c(445,455))+theme(axis.title=element_text(size=16))
f=ggplot(outplot1, aes(x=sigma_beta, lty=chain))+geom_density()+
  xlim(c(0,10))+theme(axis.title=element_text(size=16))
g=ggplot(outplot1, aes(x=sigma_gamma, lty=chain))+geom_density()+
  xlim(c(0,5))+theme(axis.title=element_text(size=16))
h=ggplot(outplot1, aes(x=sigma_e, lty=chain))+geom_density()+
  xlim(c(0,5))+theme(axis.title=element_text(size=16))

ggarrange(a,b,c,d,e,f,g,h, labels=c("(a)","(b)","(c)","(d)",
          "(e)","(f)","(g)","(h)"),ncol=4,nrow=2)
```

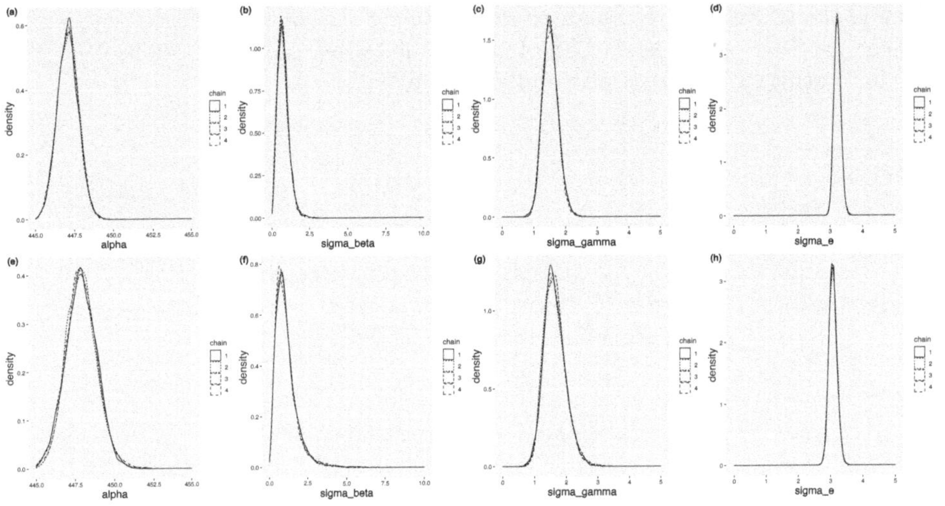

FIGURE 15.2
Density plots of posterior samples for Jeffreys' initial prior with (top (a)-(d), with $a = 0.5$) and without (bottom (e)-(h), with $a = 0$) power prior.

Sensitivity analysis was conducted to evaluate the impact of the choice of the initial prior $\pi_0(\boldsymbol{\theta})$ on the Bayesian inference. Density plots of the posterior samples from two initial priors were compared in Figures 15.3 and 15.4. The two initial priors result in similar density curves. In general, a sensitivity analysis is recommended in Bayesian inference to make sure results are consistent when changing initial noninformative priors.

15.3.3 Bayesian Inference from Posterior Predictive Samples

Under a Bayesian framework, Wolfinger (1998) proposed a simulation-based approach for determining Bayesian tolerance intervals for a variance component model. Hamada et al. (2004) considered Bayesian prediction intervals that contain a proportion of a finite number of observations with a specified probability. For our study, with limited data, we constructed control limits using the idea of the Bayesian prediction intervals from Hamada et al. (2004). With probability (confidence) 0.9973, control limits proposed would cover 100% of finite sample observations Y_{ijk} with $i = 1, 2, ..., I$, $j = 1, ..., T$, and $k = 1, ..., K$.

Specifically, posterior predictive samples were generated from model (15.1) based on posterior samples of model parameter. For each posterior predictive sample that contains data for five current batches, seven time points and ten replicates per each time point, a minimum and maximum were calculated (`q.min`, `q.max`).

R code for calculating `q.min` and `q.max`:

```
library(ggplot2)

out = as.matrix(fitppj)

y<-list()

for (i in 1:20000){
```

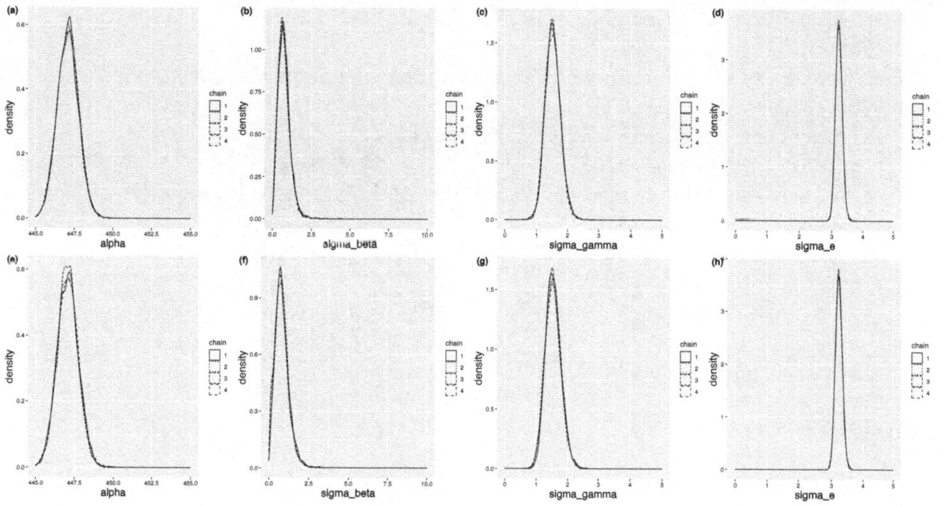

FIGURE 15.3
Density plots of posterior samples for power prior ($a = 0.5$) with Jeffreys' initial prior (top (a)-(d)) and with constant initial prior (bottom (e)-(h)).

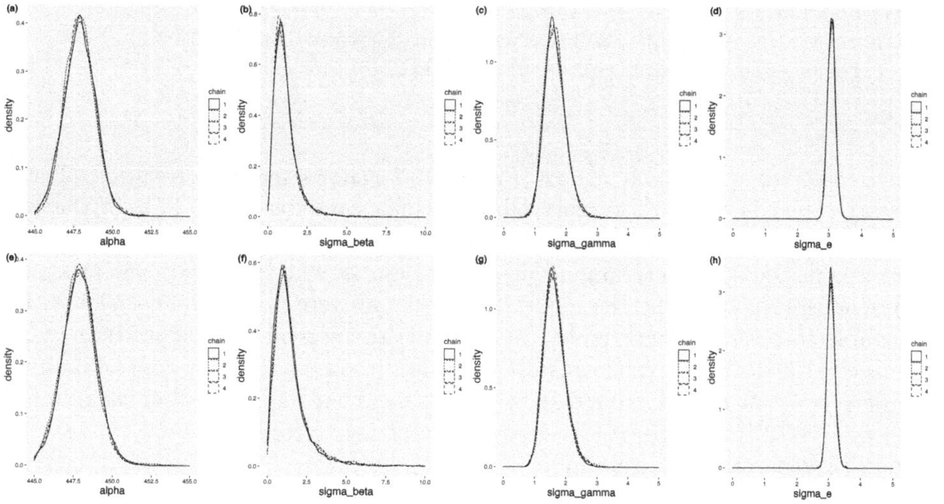

FIGURE 15.4
Density plots of posterior samples for two noninformative priors ($a = 0$): Jeffreys' prior (top (a)-(d)) and constant prior (bottom (e)-(h)).

```
  y_int <- rep(rnorm(5*7,sd= out[i,93]),each=10)
  y_batch <- rnorm(5,sd=out[i,92])
  y1<-as.vector(rnorm(70,mean=X[1:70,]%*%out[i,1:7],sd=out[i,91])) +
      y_batch[1]+y_int[1:70]
  y2<-as.vector(rnorm(70,mean=X[1:70,]%*%out[i,1:7],sd=out[i,91])) +
      y_batch[2]+y_int[71:140]
  y3<-as.vector(rnorm(70,mean=X[1:70,]%*%out[i,1:7],sd=out[i,91])) +
      y_batch[3]+y_int[141:210]
  y4<-as.vector(rnorm(70,mean=X[1:70,]%*%out[i,1:7],sd=out[i,91])) +
      y_batch[4]+y_int[211:280]
  y5<-as.vector(rnorm(70,mean=X[1:70,]%*%out[i,1:7],sd=out[i,91])) +
      y_batch[5]+y_int[281:350]
  y[[i]]<-as.data.frame(c(y1, y2, y3, y4, y5))

  y[[i]]$Batch<-rep(1:5, each=70)
  time<-rep(1:7, each=10)
  y[[i]]$Time<-rep(time, 5)

  colnames(y[[i]])<-c("value", "Batch", "Time")

}

q.min<-unlist(lapply(y, function(x) min(x[, "value"])))
q.max<-unlist(lapply(y, function(x) max(x[, "value"])))

# R code for generating the scatter plot of q.min and q.max
qvec <- data.frame(cbind(q.min, q.max))
ggplot(qvec, aes(x=q.max, y=q.min)) +
  geom_point(color="grey") +
  stat_ellipse(level=0.95, color=1, linetype=1, lwd=1.2) +
  theme(panel.grid.major=element_blank(),
  panel.grid.minor=element_blank(), panel.background=element_blank(),
  panel.border=element_rect(color="black", fill=NA, size=1))
```

A scatterplot of `q.min` and `q.max` (Figure 15.5) shows minor correlation. The circle in the scatter plot is the 95% density ellipse, which contains about 95% of the (`q.min`, `q.max`) points. Narrower ellipse represents higher correlation. The minor correlation in the quantiles was neglected in determining the control limits. The stability of the process mentioned previously may be why the quantiles calculated were not highly correlated. It may be reasonable to postulate that under a detectable time trend, the quantiles may exhibit significant correlation which would require attention when determining control limits. Control limits were set at the $((1-0.9973)/2)^{th}$ quantile of the distribution of the minima and the $((1+0.9973)/2)^{th}$ quantile of the distribution of the maxima.

R code for generating control limits:

```
lwr<-quantile(q.min, prob=1-pnorm(3))
uppr<-quantile(q.max, prob=pnorm(3))
```

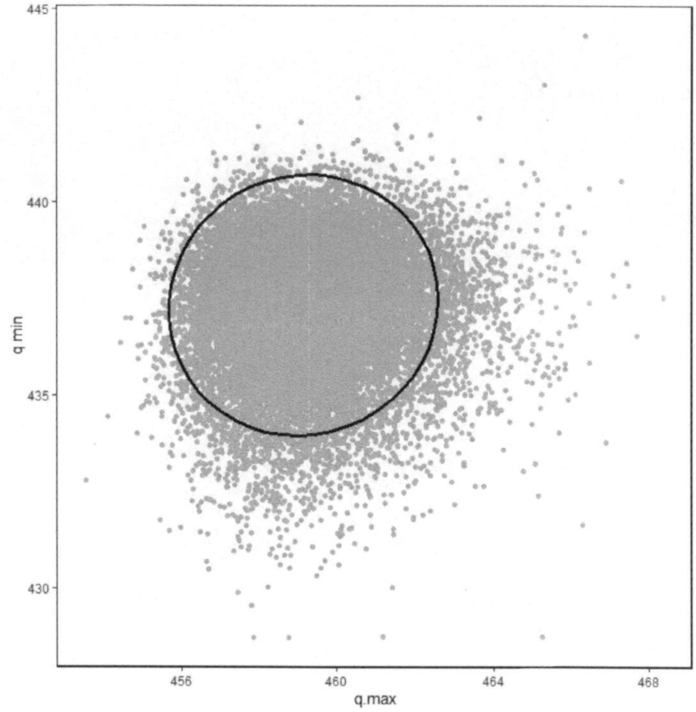

FIGURE 15.5
Scatterplot of q.min and q.max with density ellipse.

15.4 Results

Control limits were developed under the Bayesian framework together with limits from two typical approaches and a frequentist approach: (1) Mean $\pm 3\sigma$, where Mean and σ are the overall mean and standard deviation of data from current batches respectively; (2) Mean $\pm 5\%$ of the Mean; and (3) Monte Carlo simulation based on REML estimates of model parameters. That is, after obtaining REML estimates of parameters for model (15.1), we generated random samples from model (15.1) with parameters set at REML estimates. Control limits are then established using the same "quantile of quantiles" method as in the Bayesian setting. Figures 15.6 and 15.7 report the control limits determined using these different methods, where Figure 15.6 compares the control limits directly and Figure 15.7 incorporates data from current and historical batches.

R code for generating control limits for methods (1)–(3):

```
## Method (1)

mean(datCurrent$value) - 3*sd(datCurrent$value)
mean(datCurrent$value) + 3*sd(datCurrent$value)

## Method (2)
```

```
mean(datCurrent$value)*0.95
mean(datCurrent$value)*1.05

## Method (3)

varvector = as.data.frame(VarCorr(fitReml))
sigma_beta = varvector$sdcor[2]
sigma_gamma = varvector$sdcor[1]
sigma_e = varvector$sdcor[3]
eta = fitReml@beta

y<-list()

for (i in 1:20000){

  y_int <- rep(rnorm(5*7,sd=sigma_gamma),each=10)
  y_batch <- rnorm(5,sd=sigma_beta)
  y1<-as.vector(rnorm(70,mean=X[1:70,]%*%eta, sd=sigma_e))+
      y_batch[1] +y_int[1:70]
  y2<-as.vector(rnorm(70,mean=X[1:70,]%*%eta, sd=sigma_e))+
      y_batch[2] +y_int[71:140]
  y3<-as.vector(rnorm(70,mean=X[1:70,]%*%eta, sd=sigma_e))+
      y_batch[3] +y_int[141:210]
  y4<-as.vector(rnorm(70,mean=X[1:70,]%*%eta, sd=sigma_e))+
      y_batch[4] +y_int[211:280]
  y5<-as.vector(rnorm(70,mean=X[1:70,]%*%eta, sd=sigma_e))+
      y_batch[5] +y_int[281:350]
  y[[i]]<-as.data.frame(c(y1, y2, y3, y4, y5))

  y[[i]]$Batch<-rep(1:5, each=70)
  time<-rep(1:7, each=10)
  y[[i]]$Time<-rep(time, 5)

  colnames(y[[i]])<-c("value", "Batch", "Time")

}

q.min<-unlist(lapply(y, function(x) min(x[, "value"])))
q.max<-unlist(lapply(y, function(x) max(x[, "value"])))

lwr<-quantile(q.min, prob=1-pnorm(3))
uppr<-quantile(q.max, prob=pnorm(3))
```

The traditional approach, Mean $\pm 3\sigma$, yields the narrowest control limits among the approaches studied and is not recommended when limited data are available, owing to the large sample nature of such limits. Further, the frequentist approach using Monte Carlo simulation based on REML estimates does not consider parameter estimation uncertainty and thus yields narrower limits than those based on either of the Bayesian approaches investigated. The ad hoc method Mean ±5% of the Mean provides the widest control limits. For power prior, complete borrowing with $a = 1$ gives very close limits to $a = 0.5$ in this example (not shown here). In general, historical data could be from different process or different products with similar characteristics. In these cases, rather than using complete borrowing, it may be appropriate to discount the borrowing information using an intermediate value for the power parameter a.

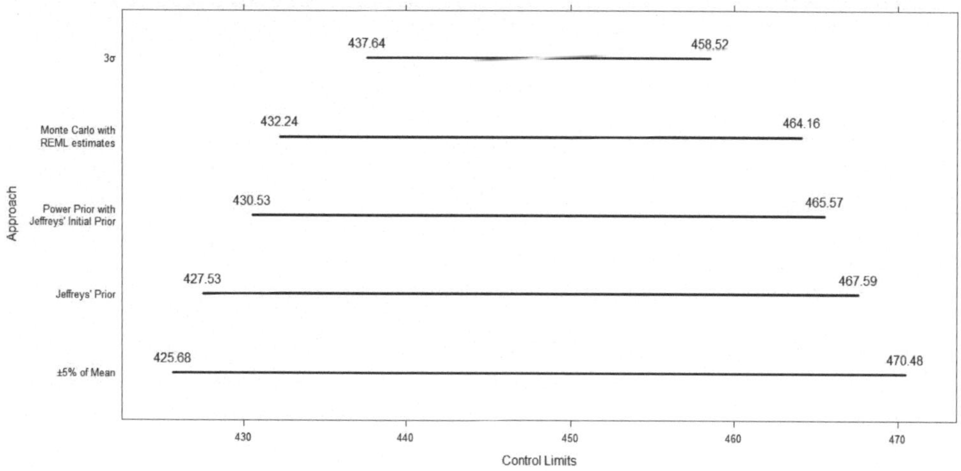

FIGURE 15.6
Control limits based on different methods.

R code for Figure 15.6 generation:

```
library(reshape); library(lattice);
library(gridExtra); library(grid);

# Limits developed were saved in the file "Control Limits.csv".
# There are 3 columns in the file: Approach (5 approaches),
#  LCL (lower control limits), and UCL (upper control limits).
CL<-read.csv(file="Control Limits.csv", header=TRUE)
ORDER<-c("3*Sigma", "REML", "Power prior","Jeffrey prior","5%*Mean")
LABEL<-rev(c(paste("3", "\u03C3", sep=""),
      "Monte Carlo with\n REML estimates",
      "Power Prior with\n Jeffreys' Inital Prior",
      "Jeffreys' Prior", paste("\u00B1", "5% of Mean", sep="")))
CL.Ordered <- CL[match(ORDER, CL$Approach), ]
CL.Ordered_m<-melt(CL.Ordered, id.vars=c("Approach"),
                measure.vars=c("LCL", "UCL"))
trellis.par.set(box.umbrella = list(lty = 1, lwd=3, col="black"),
box.rectangle=list(lwd=3, col="black"))

mypanel<-function(x,y,...){
     panel.bwplot(x,y,coef=0,box.ratio=0, col="black", pch="")
     panel.text(CL.Ordered$LCL[1], x=CL.Ordered$LCL[1],
     y=5.2, cex=1)
```

```
    panel.text(CL.Ordered$UCL[1], x=CL.Ordered$UCL[1],
    y=5.2, cex=1)
    panel.text(CL.Ordered$LCL[2], x=CL.Ordered$LCL[2],
    y=4.2, cex=1)
    panel.text(CL.Ordered$UCL[2], x=CL.Ordered$UCL[2],
    y=4.2, cex=1)
    panel.text(CL.Ordered$LCL[3], x=CL.Ordered$LCL[3],
    y=3.2, cex=1)
    panel.text(CL.Ordered$UCL[3], x=CL.Ordered$UCL[3],
    y=3.2, cex=1)
    panel.text(CL.Ordered$LCL[4], x=CL.Ordered$LCL[4],
    y=2.2, cex=1)
    panel.text(CL.Ordered$UCL[4], x=CL.Ordered$UCL[4],
    y=2.2, cex=1)
    panel.text(CL.Ordered$LCL[5], x=CL.Ordered$LCL[5],
    y=1.2, cex=1)
    panel.text(CL.Ordered$UCL[5], x=CL.Ordered$UCL[5],
    y=1.2, cex=1)
}
bwplot(factor(Approach, levels=rev(ORDER), labels=c(LABEL)) ~ value,
CL.Ordered_m, ylab="Approach", xlab="Control Limits", col="black",
pch="", panel=mypanel)
```

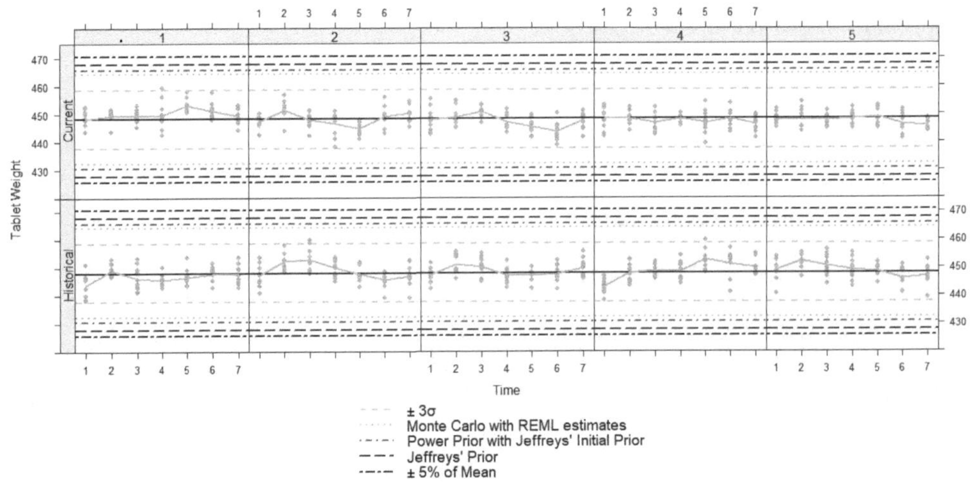

FIGURE 15.7
Tablet weight data with control limits based on different methods.

R code for Figure 15.7 generation:

```
library(lattice); library(latticeExtra)
Data=dat
Data$BatchDesc<-ifelse(Data$Batch %in% 1:5, "Current", "Historical")
```

```
Data$BatchNo<-ifelse(Data$Batch %in% 6:10, Data$Batch-5, Data$Batch)
LABEL1<-c(paste("\u00B1", " 3", "\u03C3", sep=""),
      "Monte Carlo with REML estimates",
      "Power Prior with Jeffreys' Initial Prior",
      "Jeffreys' Prior", paste("\u00B1", " 5% of Mean", sep=""))

mypanel<-function(x, y, ...){
     panel.xyplot(x, y, ...)
     panel.abline(h=c(CL.Ordered$LCL[1], mean(datCurrent$value),
        CL.Ordered$UCL[1]), col=c("grey80", "black", "grey80"),
        lty=c(2, 1, 2), lwd=2)
     panel.abline(h=c(CL.Ordered$LCL[2], CL.Ordered$UCL[2]),
        col=c("grey75", "grey75"), lty=c(3, 3), lwd=2)
     panel.abline(h=c(CL.Ordered$LCL[3], CL.Ordered$UCL[3]),
        col=c("grey45", "grey45"), lty=c(4, 4), lwd=2)
     panel.abline(h=c(CL.Ordered$LCL[4], CL.Ordered$UCL[4]),
        col=c("grey20", "grey20"), lty=c(5, 5), lwd=2)
     panel.abline(h=c(CL.Ordered$LCL[5], CL.Ordered$UCL[5]),
        col=c("black", "black"), lty=c(6, 6), lwd=2)
     panel.linejoin(x, y, horizontal = FALSE, lwd=2, col=c("grey"))
}
useOuterStrips(xyplot(value~Time | factor(BatchNo)*factor(BatchDesc),
as.table=TRUE, par.strip.text=list(cex=1), layout=c(5,2,1),
data=Data, pch=16, type=c("p"), col="grey", panel=mypanel,
ylim=c(420, 475), ylab="Tablet Weight", key=list(space="bottom",
lines=list(col=c("grey80", "grey75", "grey45", "grey20", "black"),
lty=c(2,3,4,5,6), lwd=2), text=list(c(LABEL1), cex=1.2))))
```

15.5 Discussion

In this chapter, we presented an example of establishing control limits for weight variation in early phase production, with limited data available, within a Bayesian framework. A linear mixed effects model was fit to the data. The mixed effects model was augmented using a noninformative prior and an informative power prior incorporating historical information for Bayesian inference of model parameters. The frequentist approach using REML estimates and the Bayesian approach using noninformative prior only include the information from five current batches, while the power prior approach also considers information from five historical batches. Incorporating informative historical data by updating the power prior with current data, provides tighter control limits compared to the Bayesian approach with noninformative prior. Control limits were constructed based on the idea of a Bayesian prediction interval using posterior predictive samples. Comparisons were made to other methods. The Bayesian approaches provided reasonable control limits compared to two typical approaches (Mean $\pm 3\sigma$ and Mean $\pm 5\%$ of the Mean) and the frequentist use of Monte Carlo simulations based on REML estimates. The typical approach Mean $\pm 3\sigma$ and the frequentist approach provided limits which were too narrow because they do not account for the uncertainty in the parameter estimates. In general, wider control limits would be more desirable to avoid too many false alarms but may not be acceptable to regulatory agencies unless good justification is provided. Bayesian methods provide good justification while incorporating relevant uncertainties. When sample size is small, the ability to borrow historical data using the power prior is very advantageous. In our example, the ad hoc method Mean ±5% of the Mean provides the widest control limits. However, there is no underlying statistical justification for this method.

We observed that with a limited number of batches (e.g., 2-3 batches), treating batch as a random effect with non-informative constant prior in the Bayesian setting could result in large batch-to-batch variation estimate, which is consistent with the findings in Gelman (2006). In addition, as Gelman (2006) points out, constant prior on variance would result in the miscalibration toward higher values.

Other ways to incorporate prior knowledge include the empirical Bayesian methods using historical data to infer prior distribution and hierarchical models by establishing the hyperpriors. Further research could explore these methods in `rstan` and compare the estimated control limits with the ones obtained in this chapter.

The `stan_lmer` function in `rstanarm` R package provides a convenient way for Bayesian inference of linear mixed effects models. The package allows the user to select priors from provided families and the default priors are intended to be weekly informative by adjusting the scales of the priors. This program is not implemented in our project due to the limited prior selection.

15.6 Appendix

The posterior can be expressed as

$$p(\sigma_\beta^2, \sigma_\gamma^2, \sigma_\varepsilon^2 | \mathbf{D}) \propto \pi_0(\sigma_\beta^2, \sigma_\gamma^2, \sigma_\varepsilon^2) L(\sigma_\beta^2, \sigma_\gamma^2, \sigma_\varepsilon^2 | \mathbf{D}) \tag{15.8}$$

with the following prior

$$\pi_0(\sigma_\beta^2, \sigma_\gamma^2, \sigma_\varepsilon^2) \propto \frac{1}{\sigma_\varepsilon^2 (K\sigma_\gamma^2 + \sigma_\varepsilon^2)(TK\sigma_\beta^2 + K\sigma_\gamma^2 + \sigma_\varepsilon^2)} \tag{15.9}$$

and the following likelihood

$$L(\sigma_\beta^2, \sigma_\gamma^2, \sigma_\varepsilon^2 | \mathbf{D}) \propto \frac{\exp\left(-\frac{SS_\varepsilon}{2\sigma_\varepsilon^2}\right) \exp\left(-\frac{SS_\gamma}{2(K\sigma_\gamma^2 + \sigma_\varepsilon^2)}\right) \exp\left(-\frac{SS_\beta}{2(TK\sigma_\beta^2 + K\sigma_\gamma^2 + \sigma_\varepsilon^2)}\right)}{\sigma_\varepsilon^{2\times\frac{1}{2}(IT(K-1))} (K\sigma_\gamma^2 + \sigma_\varepsilon^2)^{\frac{1}{2}((T-1)(I-1))} (TK\sigma_\beta^2 + K\sigma_\gamma^2 + \sigma_\varepsilon^2)^{\frac{1}{2}(I-1)}}. \tag{15.10}$$

The posterior is proper if

$$\int_0^\infty \int_0^\infty \int_0^\infty p(\sigma_\beta^2, \sigma_\gamma^2, \sigma_\varepsilon^2 | \mathbf{D}) d\sigma_\beta^2, d\sigma_\gamma^2, d\sigma_\varepsilon^2 < \infty. \tag{15.11}$$

Using the transformation $F : \mathbb{R}^3 \longrightarrow \mathbb{R}^3$

$$l_1 = \sigma_\varepsilon^2 \qquad 0 \leq l_1 < \infty \tag{15.12}$$

$$l_2 = K\sigma_\gamma^2 + \sigma_\varepsilon^2 \qquad l_1 \leq l_2 < \infty \tag{15.13}$$

$$l_3 = TK\sigma_\beta^2 + K\sigma_\gamma^2 + \sigma_\varepsilon^2 \qquad l_2 \leq l_3 < \infty, \tag{15.14}$$

the Jacobian of the transformation is

$$J_F\left(\frac{l_1, l_2, l_3}{\sigma_\varepsilon^2, \sigma_\gamma^2, \sigma_\beta^2}\right) = \begin{pmatrix} \frac{\partial l_1}{\partial \sigma_\varepsilon^2} & \frac{\partial l_1}{\partial \sigma_\gamma^2} & \frac{\partial l_1}{\partial \sigma_\beta^2} \\ \frac{\partial l_2}{\partial \sigma_\varepsilon^2} & \frac{\partial l_2}{\partial \sigma_\gamma^2} & \frac{\partial l_2}{\partial \sigma_\beta^2} \\ \frac{\partial l_3}{\partial \sigma_\varepsilon^2} & \frac{\partial l_3}{\partial \sigma_\gamma^2} & \frac{\partial l_3}{\partial \sigma_\beta^2} \end{pmatrix} = \begin{pmatrix} 1 & 0 & 0 \\ 1 & K & 0 \\ 1 & K & KT \end{pmatrix} \tag{15.15}$$

the determinant of which is a constant (since it is a linear transformation). The integral of the posterior, I_1, can then be written as

$$I_1 \propto |J_F| \int_0^\infty \int_{l_1}^\infty \int_{l_2}^\infty \frac{1}{l_1 l_2 l_3} \frac{\exp\left(-\frac{SS_\varepsilon}{2l_1}\right)\exp\left(-\frac{SS_\gamma}{2l_2}\right)\exp\left(-\frac{SS_\beta}{2l_3}\right)}{l_1^{\frac{1}{2}(IT(K-1))} l_2^{\frac{1}{2}((T-1)(I-1))} l_3^{\frac{1}{2}(I-1)}} dl_3 dl_2 dl_1 \tag{15.16}$$

or as

$$I_1 \propto \int_0^\infty \frac{\exp\left(-\frac{SS_\varepsilon}{2l_1}\right)}{l_1 l_1^{\frac{1}{2}(n_1)}} \int_{l_1}^\infty \frac{\exp\left(-\frac{SS_\gamma}{2l_2}\right)}{l_2 l_2^{\frac{1}{2}(n_2)}} \int_{l_2}^\infty \frac{\exp\left(-\frac{SS_\beta}{2l_3}\right)}{l_3 l_3^{\frac{1}{2}(n_3)}} dl_3 dl_2 dl_1 \tag{15.17}$$

where n_i is the degrees of freedom associated with the particular sum-of-squares.

The inverted gamma has distribution

$$f(x; a, b) = \frac{\exp\left(-\frac{b}{x}\right) \frac{1}{x}^{a+1}}{G(a) b^a}, \qquad 0 \leq x \leq \infty. \tag{15.18}$$

The integral of a product of three independent inverted gamma distributions is

$$I_2 \propto \prod_{i=1}^{3} \int_0^\infty \frac{\exp\left(-\frac{SS_i}{2l_i}\right)}{l_i l_i^{\frac{1}{2}(n_i)}} dl_i < \infty, \tag{15.19}$$

with $b = SS_i/2$ and $a = n_i/2$.

Since $I_1 \leq I_2$ due to the order $l_1 \leq l_2 \leq l_3$, and I_2 is finite, I_1 is a proper integral.

Bibliography

A-Mab (2009). A-Mab: A case study in bioprocess development. Technical report, CMC Biotech Working Group.

Abadi, M., Agarwal, A., Barham, P., Brevdo, E., Chen, Z., Citro, C., Corrado, G. S., Davis, A., Dean, J., Devin, M., Ghemawat, S., Goodfellow, I., Harp, A., Irving, G., Isard, M., Jia, Y., Jozefowicz, R., Kaiser, L., Kudlur, M., Levenberg, J., Mané, D., Monga, R., Moore, S., Murray, D., Olah, C., Schuster, M., Shlens, J., Steiner, B., Sutskever, I., Talwar, K., Tucker, P., Vanhoucke, V., Vasudevan, V., Viégas, F., Vinyals, O., Warden, P., Wattenberg, M., Wicke, M., Yu, Y., and Zheng, X. (2015). TensorFlow: Large-scale machine learning on heterogeneous systems. Software available from tensorflow.org.

Allaire, J. and Tang, Y. (2022). *tensorflow: R Interface to 'TensorFlow'*. R package version 2.8.0.

Allen, P. V., Dukes, G. R., and Gerger, M. E. (1991). Determination of release limits: A general methodology. *Pharmaceutical Research*, 8(9):1210–1213.

Almeida, A., Loy, A., and Hofmann, H. (2018). ggplot2 compatible quantile-quantile plots in R. *The R Journal*, 10(2):248–261.

Altan, S., Dong, Y., Gorko, M. A., Hartvig, N. V., Johnson, M., Larner, G., and Sherling, S. (2018). Understanding internal release limits. *Pharmaceutical Technology*, 42(20):30–39.

Amadeo, I., Mauro, L., Ortií, E., and Forno, G. (2014). Establishment of a design space for biopharmaceutical purification processes using DoE. *Protein Downstream Processing*, 1129:11–27.

Apley, D. W. (2012). Posterior distribution charts: a Bayesian approach for graphically exploring a process mean. *Technometrics*, 54(3):279–293.

ASTM Standard E2810 (2019). Standard practice for demonstrating capability to comply with the test for uniformity of dosage units. Technical report, ASTM International.

Auguie, B. (2017). *gridExtra: Miscellaneous Functions for "Grid" Graphics*. R package version 2.3.

Bancroft, T. A. (1964). Analysis and inference for incompletely specified models involving the use of preliminary test(s) of significance. *Biometrics*, 20(3):427–442.

Bates, D., Maechler, M., Bolker, B., and Walker, S. (2015). Fitting linear mixed-effects models using lme4. *Journal of Statistical Software*, 67(1):1–48.

Bäth, R. (2018). *bayesboot: An Implementation of Rubin's (1981) Bayesian Bootstrap*. R package version 0.2.2.

Bayarri, M. J. and García-Donato, G. (2005). A Bayesian sequential look at u-control charts. *Technometrics*, 47(2):142–151.

Benaroya, H., Han, S. M., and Nagurka, M. (2015). *Probability Models in Engineering and Science (vol. 192)*. CRC Press, Boca Raton.

Bernardo, J. M. and Irony, T. Z. (1996). A general multivariate Bayesian process capability index. *The Statistician*, 45(3):487–502.

Bernardo, J. M. and Smith, A. F. (2009). *Bayesian Theory (Vol. 405): Wiley Series in Probability and Statistics*. John Wiley & Sons, New York, NY.

Betancourt, M. (2017). A conceptual introduction to Hamiltonian Monte Carlo. *arXiv preprint arXiv:1701.02434*.

Betancourt, M., Byrne, S., Livingstone, S., and Girolami, M. (2017). The geometric foundations of Hamiltonian Monte Carlo. *Bernoulli*, 23(4A):2257–2298.

Bezanson, J., Edelman, A., Karpinski, S., and Shah, V. B. (2017). Julia: A fresh approach to numerical computing. *SIAM Review*, 59(1):65–98.

Borman, P. J., Chatfield, M. J., Damjanov, I., and Jackson, P. (2009). Design and analysis of method equivalence studies. *Analytical Chemistry*, 81(24):9849–9857.

Box, G. E. P. and Tiao, G. C. (1973). *Bayesian Inference in Statistical Analysis*. Addison-Wesley, Reading, MA.

Brunelle, J. (2016). FDA recommendations for comparability studies to support manufacturing changes. Technical report, CASSS Midwest Discussion Group.

Brutti, P., De Santis, F., and Gubbiotti, S. (2008). Robust Bayesian sample size determination in clinical trials. *Statistics in Medicine*, 27:2290–2306.

Burdick, R., LeBlond, D., Pfahler, L., Quiroz, J., Sidor, L., Vukovinsky, K., and Zhang, L. (2017). *Statistical Applications for Chemistry, Manufacturing and Controls (CMC) in the Pharmaceutical Industry*. Springer, Cham, Switzerland.

Burdick, R. K. (2015). Comments on analytical similarity session. Technical report, FDA-Industry Statistics Workshop, Washington D.C.

Burdick, R. K. and Ramírez, J. G. (2015). Statistical issues in biosimilar analytical assessment: Perspective on FDA ODAC analysis. Technical report, DIA/FDA Statistics 2015 Forum, Washington D.C.

Bürkner, P., Gabry, J., Weber, S., Johnson, A., Modrak, M., Badr, H. S., Weber, F., Ben-Schachar, M. S., and Rabel, H. (2021). *brms: Bayesian regression models using STAN*. R package version 2.16.3.

Bürkner, P.-C. (2017). brms: An R package for Bayesian multilevel models using Stan. *Journal of Statistical Software*, 80:1–28.

Bürkner, P.-C., Gabry, J., Kay, M., and Vehtari, A. (2021). posterior: Tools for working with posterior distributions. R package version 1.1.0.

Calabrese, J. M. (1995). Bayesian process control for attributes. *Management Science*, 41(4):637–645.

Capen, R., Christopher, D., Forenzo, P., Huynh-Ba, K., LeBlond, D., Liu, O., O'Neil, J., Patterson, N., Quinlan, M., Rajagopalan, R., Schwenke, J., and Stroup, W. (2018). Evaluating current practices in shelf life estimation. *The American Association of Pharmaceutical Scientists: PharmSciTech*, 19(2):668–680.

Carlin, B. and Louis, T. (2008). *Bayesian Methods for Data Analysis, Third Edition.* CRC Press, Boca Raton.

Carpenter, B., Gelman, A., Hoffman, M., Lee, D., Goodrich, M. B., Brubaker, M., Guo, J., Li, P., and Riddell, A. (2017). Stan: A probabilistic programming language. *Journal of Statistical Software*, 76(1):1–32.

Carvalho, L. M. and Ibrahim, J. G. (2021). On the normalized power prior. *Statistics in Medicine*, 40(24):5251–5275.

Casella, G. and George, E. I. (1992). Explaining the Gibbs sampler. *The American Statistician*, 46(3):167–174.

Chatfield, M., Borman, P., and Damjanov, I. (2011). Evaluating change during pharmaceutical product development and manufacture – comparability and equivalence. *Quality Reliability Engineering*, 27:629–640.

Chen, F. (2011). The RANDOM statement and more: Moving on with PROC MCMC. In *Proceedings of the SAS Global Forum 2011 Conference. Cary, NC: SAS Institute Inc.* SAS Institute Inc.

Chen, F. (2014). Bayesian modeling using the MCMC procedure. In *Proceedings of the SAS Global Forum 2008 Conference, SAS Institute Inc.* Citeseer.

Chen, J. J., Hwang, J. S., and Tsong, Y. (1995). Estimation of the shelf-life of drugs with mixed effects models. *Journal of Biopharmaceutical Statistics*, 5(1):131–140.

Chen, Y. and Ye, K. (2011). A Bayesian hierarchical approach to dual response surface modeling. *Journal of Applied Statistics*, 38(9):1963–1975.

Chow, S. C. (2014). On assessment of analytical similarity in biosimilar studies. *Drug Designing*, 3(3):1–4.

Chow, S. C. (2015). Challenging issues in assessing analytical similarity in biosimilar studies. *Biosimilars*, pages 33–39.

Chow, S. C. and Liu, J. P. (2008). *Design and Analysis of Bioavailability and Bioequivalence Studies, Third Edition.* Chapman & Hall/CRC, London, United Kingdom.

Christensen, R., Johnson, W., Branscum, A., and Hanson, T. (2011). *Bayesian Ideas and Data Analysis.* CRC Press, Boca Raton.

Civoli, F., Kasinath, A., Cai, X., Wadhwa, M., Exley, A., Oldfield, P., and Alvandkouhi, S. (2019). Recommendations for the development and validation of immunogenicity assays in support of biosimilar programs. *The American Association of Pharmaceutical Scientists*, 22:1–9.

Clark, S. J. and Perry, J. N. (1994). Small sample estimation for Taylor's power law. *Environmental and Ecological Statistics*, 1(4):287–302.

Colosimo, B. M. and Del Castillo, E. (2006). *Bayesian Process Monitoring, Control and Optimization.* CRC Press, Boca Raton.

Conrad, B. (2005). Impossibility theorems for elementary integration. In *Academy Colloquium Series.* Clay Mathematics Institute, Cambridge, MA.

Costa, P. and Sousa Lobo, J. M. (2001). Modeling and comparison of dissolution profiles. *European Journal of Pharmaceutical Sciences*, 13(2):123–133.

Cowles, M. (2013). *Applied Bayesian Statistics.* Springer, New York.

Crisp, A., Miller, S., Thompson, D., and Best, N. (2018). Practical experiences of adopting assurance as a quantitative framework to support decision making in drug development. *Pharmaceutical Statistics*, 17(4):317–328.

Dawson, R. (2011). How significant is a boxplot outlier. *Journal of Statistics Education*, 19(2):1–12.

de Valpine, P., Turek, D., Paciorek, C. J., Anderson-Bergman, C., Lang, D. T., and Bodik, R. (2017). Programming with models: writing statistical algorithms for general model structures with NIMBLE. *Journal of Computational and Graphical Statistics*, 26(2):403–413.

Deming, W. E. (1986). *Out of the Crisis.* Massachusetts Institute of Technology Center for Advanced Engineering, Cambridge, MA.

Denwood, M. J. (2016). runjags: An R package providing interface utilities, model templates, parallel computing methods and additional distributions for MCMC models in JAGS. *Journal of Statistical Software*, 71(9):1–25.

Depaoli, S., Clifton, J. P., and Cobb, P. R. (2016). Just another Gibbs sampler (JAGS) flexible software for mcmc implementation. *Journal of Educational and Behavioral Statistics*, 41(6):628–649.

Depaoli, S. and van de Schoot, R. (2017). Improving transparency and replication in Bayesian statistics: The WAMBAS-checklist. *Psychological Methods*, 22(2):240–261.

Devanarayan, V. (2017). Practical advice & insights on immunogenicity cut points and some assay validation parameters. Technical report, Training Course European Immunogenicity Platform (EIP) Symposium Lisbon, Portugal.

Devanarayan, V., Smith, W. C., Brunelle, R. L., Seger, M. E., Krug, K., and Bowsher, R. R. (2017). Recommendations for systematic statistical computation of immunogenicity cut points. *American Association of Pharmaceutical Scientists*, 19:1487–1498.

Dillon, J. V., Langmore, I., Tran, D., Brevdo, E., Vasudevan, S., Moore, D., Patton, B., Alemi, A., Hoffman, M., and Saurous, R. A. (2017). Tensorflow distributions. *arXiv preprint arXiv:1711.10604.*

Dixon, W. J. and Massey, F. J. (1969). *Introduction to Statistical Analysis, Third Edition.* McGraw-Hill, New York, NY.

Dokoumetzidis, A., Papadopoulou, V., and Macheras, P. (2006). Analysis of dissolution data using modified versions of Noyes-Whitney equation and the Weibull function. *Pharmaceutical Research*, 23(2):256–261.

Dong, X., Tsong, Y., and Shen, M. (2015). Statistical considerations in setting product specifications. *Journal of Biopharmaceutical Statistics*, 25(2):280–294.

Draper, N. R. and Smith, H. (1998). *Applied Regression Analysis (vol. 326).* John Wiley & Sons, Hoboken, NJ.

Duan, Y., Ye, K., and Smith, E. P. (2006). Evaluating water quality using power priors to incorporate historical information. *Environmetrics*, 17(1):95–106.

Duane, S., Kennedy, A. D., Pendleton, B. J., and Roweth, D. (1987). Hybrid Monte Carlo. *Physics Letters B*, 195(2):216–222.

Egan, W. and Schofield, T. (2009). Basic principles of stability. *Biologicals*, 37(6):379–386.

EMA (2010a). Guideline on immunogenicity assessment of therapeutic proteins. Technical report, European Medicines Agency, London, England.

EMA (2010b). Guideline on the investigation of bioequivalence (CMP/EWP/QWP/1401/98 Rev.1/Corr **). Technical report, European Medicines Agency, London, England.

EMA (2021). Reflection paper on statistical methodology for comparative assessment of quality attributes in drug development. Technical report, European Medicines Agency Paper Draft, London, England.

Faya, P. and Berry, D. (2022). Bayesian methods in CMC - Has the time come for a regulatory guidance? *ASA Biopharmaceutical Report*, 28(3):6–9.

Faya, P., Novick, S., Seaman, Jr. J. W., Peterson, J. J., Pourmohamad, T., Banton, D., and Zheng, Y. (2022). Continuous method validation: beyond one-time studies to characterize analytical methods. *Statistics in Biopharmaceutical Research*, pages 1–9.

Faya, P., Seaman, Jr. J., and Stamey, J. D. (2016). Bayesian assurance and sample size determination in the process validation life-cycle. *Journal of Biopharmaceutical Statistics*, 27(1):159–174.

Faya, P., Seaman Jr. J. W., and Stamey, J. D. (2020). Power priors for sample size determination in the process validation life cycle. In Lakshminarayanan, M. and Natanegara, F., editors, *Bayesian Applications in Pharmaceutical Development*. Chapman and Hall/CRC, New York.

Faya, P., Sondag, P., Novick, S., Banton, D., Seaman, Jr. J. W., Stamey, J. D., and Boulanger, B. (2021). The current state of Bayesian methods in nonclinical pharmaceutical statistics: Survey results and recommendations from the DIA/ASA-BIOP Nonclinical Bayesian Working Group. *Pharmaceutical Statistics*, 20(2):245–255.

FDA (1995). Guidance for industry: Extended release oral dosage forms: Development, evaluation, and application of in vitro/in vivo correlations. Technical report, U.S. Department of Health and Human Services, FDA. Center of Drug Evaluation and Research (CDER), Rockville, MD.

FDA (1997a). Guidance for industry: Dissolution testing of immediate release solid oral dosage forms. Technical report, U.S. Department of Health and Human Services, FDA. Center of Drug Evaluation and Research (CDER), Rockville, MD.

FDA (1997b). Guidance for industry: Immediate release solid oral dosage forms. Scale-up and postapproval changes: Chemistry, manufacturing and controls, in vitro dissolution testing and in vivo bioequivalence documentation. Technical report, U.S. Department of Health and Human Services, FDA. Center of Drug Evaluation and Research (CDER), Rockville, MD.

FDA (1997c). Guidance for industry: SUPAC-MR: Modified release solid oral dosage forms. scale-up and postapproval changes: Chemistry, manufacturing and controls; in vitro dissolution testing and in vivo bioequivalence documentation. Technical report, U.S. Department of Health and Human Services, FDA. Center of Drug Evaluation and Research (CDER), Rockville, MD.

FDA (2000). Guidance for industry: Waiver of in vivo bioavailability and bioequivalence studies for immediate- release solid oral dosage forms based on biopharmaceutics classification system. Technical report, U.S. Department of Health and Human Services, FDA. Center of Drug Evaluation and Research (CDER), Rockville, MD.

FDA (2003). Guidance for industry: Bioavailability and bioequivalence studies for orally administered drug products – general considerations. Technical report, U.S. Department of Health and Human Services, FDA. Center of Drug Evaluation and Research (CDER), Rockville, MD.

FDA (2004). Pharmaceutical CGMPs for the 21st century – A risk based approach. Technical report, U.S. Department of Health and Human Services, FDA. Center of Drug Evaluation and Research (CDER), Rockville, MD.

FDA (2010). Guidance for industry: Guidance for the use of Bayesian statistics in medical device clinical trials. Technical report, U.S. Department of Health and Human Services, FDA. Center of Drug Evaluation and Research (CDER), Rockville, MD.

FDA (2011). Guidance for industry: Pprocess validation: General principles and practices. Technical report, U.S. Department of Health and Human Services, FDA. Center of Drug Evaluation and Research (CDER), Rockville, MD.

FDA (2015a). Code of federal regulations - title 21 - food and drugs. Technical report, U.S. Department of Health and Human Services, FDA. Center of Drug Evaluation and Research (CDER), Rockville, MD.

FDA (2015b). FDA briefing document for the Oncologic Drugs Advisory Committee ODAC meeting held on january 7, 2015. Technical report, U.S. Department of Health and Human Services, FDA. Center of Drug Evaluation and Research (CDER), Rockville, MD.

FDA (2015c). Guidance for industry: Biosimilars: Questions and answers regarding implementation of the Biologics Price Competition and Innovation Act of 2009. Technical report, U.S. Department of Health and Human Services, FDA. Center of Drug Evaluation and Research (CDER), Rockville, MD.

FDA (2015d). Guidance for industry: Quality considerations in demonstrating biosimilarity to a reference protein. Technical report, U.S. Department of Health and Human Services, FDA. Center of Drug Evaluation and Research (CDER), Rockville, MD.

FDA (2015e). Guidance for industry: Scientific considerations in demonstrating biosimilarity to a reference product. Technical report, U.S. Department of Health and Human Services, FDA. Center of Drug Evaluation and Research (CDER), Rockville, MD.

FDA (2016). Guidance for industry: Comparability protocols for human drugs and biologics: chemistry, manufacturing, and controls information. Technical report, U.S. Department of Health and Human Services, FDA. Center of Drug Evaluation and Research (CDER), Rockville, MD.

FDA (2018). Guidance for industry: Statistical approaches to evaluate analytical similarity. Technical report, U.S. Department of Health and Human Services, FDA. Center of Drug Evaluation and Research (CDER), Rockville, MD.

FDA (2019a). Guidance for industry: Development of therapeutic protein biosimilars: comparative analytical assessment and other quality-related considerations. Technical report, U.S. Department of Health and Human Services, FDA. Center of Drug Evaluation and Research (CDER), Rockville, MD.

FDA (2019b). Guidance for industry: Immunogenicity testing of therapeutic protein products – developing and validating assays for anti-drug antibody detection. Technical report, U.S. Department of Health and Human Services, FDA. Center of Drug Evaluation and Research (CDER), Rockville, MD.

FDA (2021). Guidance for industry: Chemistry, manufacturing, and controls changes to an approved application: certain biological products. Technical report, U.S. Department of Health and Human Services, FDA. Center of Drug Evaluation and Research (CDER), Rockville, MD.

Feinberg, M., Boulanger, B., Dewe, W., and Hubert, P. (2004). New advances in method validation and measurement uncertainty aimed at improving the quality of chemical data. *Communications in Statistics – Simulation and Computation*, 380(3):502–514.

Finkler, C. and Krummen, L. (2016). Introduction to the application of QbD principles for the development of monoclonal antibodies. *Biologicals*, 44(5):282–290.

Flegal, J., Haran, M., and Jones, G. (2008). Markov chain Monte Carlo: can we trust the third significant figure? *Statistical Science*, 23(2):250–260.

Fong, Y., Rue, H., and Wakefield, J. (2010). Bayesian inference for generalized linear mixed models. *Biostatistics*, 11(3):397–412.

Gabry, J. and Mahr, T. (2021). bayesplot: Plotting for Bayesian models. R package version 1.8.1.

Ge, H., Xu, K., and Ghahramani, Z. (2018). Turing: a language for flexible probabilistic inference. In *International Conference on Artificial Intelligence and Statistics*, pages 1682–1690. PMLR.

Gelfand, A. E. (2000). Gibbs sampling. *Journal of the American Statistical Association*, 95(452):1300–1304.

Gelfand, A. E. and Smith, A. F. (1990). Sampling-based approaches to calculating marginal densities. *Journal of the American Statistical Association*, 85(410):398–409.

Gelman, A. (2006). Prior distributions for variance parameters in hierarchical models (comment on article by browne and draper). *Bayesian Analysis*, 1(3):515–534.

Gelman, A., Carlin, J., Stern, H., Dunson, D., Vehtari, A., and Rubin, D. (2013). *Bayesian Data Analysis, Third Edition*. Chapman & Hall/CRC Texts in Statistical Science. Taylor & Francis.

Gelman, A. and Rubin, D. B. (1992). Inference from iterative simulation using multiple sequences. *Statistical Science*, 7(4):457–472.

Gelman, A. and Shirley, K. (2011). Inference from simulations and monitoring convergence. In Brooks, S., Gelman, A., Jones, G., and Meng, X., editors, *Handbook of Markov Chain Monte Carlo*, pages 163–174. CRC Press, Boca Raton.

Geman, S. and Geman, D. (1984). Stochastic relaxation, gibbs distributions, and the Bayesian restoration of images. *IEEE Transactions on Pattern Analysis and Machine Intelligence*, (6):721–741.

Geyer, C. (2011). Introduction to Markov chain Monte Carlo. In Brooks, S., Gelman, A., Jones, G., and Meng, X., editors, *Handbook of Markov Chain Monte Carlo*, pages 3–48. CRC Press, Boca Raton.

Gilks, W. R. and Wild, P. (1992). Adaptive rejection sampling for Gibbs sampling. *Journal of the Royal Statistical Society: Series C (Applied Statistics)*, 41(2):337–348.

Girshick, M. A. and Rubin, H. (1952). A Bayes approach to a quality control model. *The Annals of Mathematical Statistics*, 23(1):114–125.

Golding, N. (2019). greta: simple and scalable statistical modelling in R. *Journal of Open Source Software*, 4(40):1601.

Goodrich, B., Gabry, J., Ali, I., and Brilleman, S. (2020). rstanarm: Bayesian applied regression modeling via Stan. R package version 2.21.1.

Goudie, R. J., Turner, R. M., De Angelis, D., and Thomas, A. (2020). MultiBUGS: a parallel implementation of the BUGS modelling framework for faster Bayesian inference. *Journal of Statistical Software*, 95.

Grangeia, H. B., Silva, C., Simões, S. P., and Reis, M. S. (2020). Quality by design in pharmaceutical manufacturing: A systematic review of current status, challenges and future perspectives. *European Journal of Pharmaceutics and Biopharmaceutics*, 147:19–37.

Graybill, F. A. (1976). *Theory and Application of the Linear Model.* Wadsworth Publishing Company, Belmont, CA.

Grubbs, F. E. (1950). Sample criteria for testing outlying observations. *The Annals of Mathematical Statistics*, 21(1):27–58.

Gufstafson, P. (2004). *Measurement Error and Misclassification in Statistics and Epidemiology.* Chapman and Hall.

Guide, I. G. P. (2019). Practical implementation of the lifecycle approach to process validation. Technical report, International Society for Pharmaceutical Engineering.

Hadfield, J. D. (2010). MCMC methods for multi-response generalized linear mixed models: The MCMCglmm R package. *Journal of Statistical Software*, 33(2):1–22.

Hamada, M., Johnson, V., Moore, L. M., and Wendelberger, J. (2004). Bayesian prediction intervals and their relationship to tolerance intervals. *Technometrics*, 46(4):452–459.

Hanning, J. (2009). On generalized fiducial inference. *Statistica Sinica*, 19(2):491–544.

Harris, C. R., Millman, K. J., van der Walt, S. J., Gommers, R., Virtanen, P., Cournapeau, D., Wieser, E., Taylor, J., Berg, S., Smith, N. J., Kern, R., Picus, M., Hoyer, S., van Kerkwijk, M. H., Brett, M., Haldane, A., del Río, J. F., Wiebe, M., Peterson, P., Gérard-Marchant, P., Sheppard, K., Reddy, T., Weckesser, W., Abbasi, H., Gohlke, C., and Oliphant, T. E. (2020). Array programming with NumPy. *Nature*, 585(7825):357–362.

Hastings, W. K. (1970). Monte carlo sampling methods using Markov chains and their applications. *Biometrika*, 57(1):97–109.

Hawkins, D. M. (1980). *Identification of Outliers*. Chapman & Hall, London, United Kingdom.

Hoffelder, T. (2016). A false sense of security? Can tiered approach be trusted to accurately classify immunogenicity samples? *Journal of Pharmaceutical and Biomedical Analysis*, 128(5):166–173.

Hoffelder, T. (2018). Comparison of dissolution profiles: a statistician's perspective. *Therapeutic Innovation & Regulatory Science*, 52(4):423–429.

Hoffman, M. D. and Gelman, A. (2014). The No-U-Turn sampler: Adaptively setting path lengths in Hamiltonian Monte Carlo. *Journal of Machine Learning Research*, 15:1593–1623.

Hudson-Curtis, B. and Novick, S. (2016). Content uniformity. In Zhang, L., editor, *Nonclinical Statistics for Pharmaceutical/Biotechnology Industries*, pages 631–651. Springer, Berlin.

Hyndman, R. J. and Fan, Y. (1996). Sample quantiles in statistical packages. *The American Statistician*, 50(4):361–365.

Ibrahim, G. and Chen, M. (2000). Power prior distributions for regression models. *Statistical Science*, 15(1):46–60.

Ibrahim, G., Chen, M., Gwon, Y., and Chen, F. (2015). The power prior: theory and applications. *Statistics in Medicine*, 34(28):3274–3749.

ICH E9 (1998). Guidance for industry: E9 statistical principles for clinical trials. Technical report, U.S. Department of Health and Human Services, FDA. Center of Drug Evaluation and Research (CDER), Rockville, MD.

ICH Q10 (2009). Guidance for industry: Q10 pharmaceutical quality systems. Technical report, U.S. Department of Health and Human Services, FDA. Center of Drug Evaluation and Research (CDER), Rockville, MD.

ICH Q11 (2012). Guidance for industry: Q11 development and manufacture of drug substances (chemical entities and biotechnological/biological entities). Technical report, U.S. Department of Health and Human Services, FDA. Center of Drug Evaluation and Research (CDER), Rockville, MD.

ICH Q14 (2022). Guidance for industry: Q14 analytical procedure development (draft). Technical report, U.S. Department of Health and Human Services, FDA. Center of Drug Evaluation and Research (CDER), Rockville, MD.

ICH Q1A(R2) (2003). Guidance for industry: Q1A(R2) stability testing of new drug substances and products. Technical report, U.S. Department of Health and Human Services, FDA. Center of Drug Evaluation and Research (CDER), Rockville, MD.

ICH Q1E (2003). Guidance for industry: Q1E evaluation of stability data. Technical report, U.S. Department of Health and Human Services, FDA. Center of Drug Evaluation and Research (CDER), Rockville, MD.

ICH Q2(R2) (2022). Guidance for industry: Q2(R2) validation of analytical procedures (draft). Technical report, U.S. Department of Health and Human Services, FDA. Center of Drug Evaluation and Research (CDER), Rockville, MD.

ICH Q5E (2005). Guidance for industry: Q5E comparability of biotechnological/biological products subject to changes in their manufacturing process. Technical report, U.S. Department of Health and Human Services, FDA. Center of Drug Evaluation and Research (CDER), Rockville, MD.

ICH Q8 (2005). Guidance for industry: Q8 pharmaceutical development. Technical report, U.S. Department of Health and Human Services, FDA. Center of Drug Evaluation and Research (CDER), Rockville, MD.

ICH Q8(R2) (2009). Guidance for industry: Q8 (R2) pharmaceutical development. Technical report, U.S. Department of Health and Human Services, FDA. Center of Drug Evaluation and Research (CDER), Rockville, MD.

ICH Q9 (2005). Guidance for industry: Q9 quality risk management. Technical report, U.S. Department of Health and Human Services, FDA. Center of Drug Evaluation and Research (CDER), Rockville, MD.

Jennrich, R. I. (1969). Asymptotic properties of non-linear least squares estimators. *The Annals of Mathematical Statistics*, 40(2):633–643.

JMP (2022). *JMP, Version 16*. SAS Institute Inc., Cary, NC.

Juárez, M. A. and Steel, M. F. J. (2010). Model-based clustering of non-Gaussian panel data based on skew-t distributions. *Journal of Business & Economic Statistics*, 28(1):52–66.

Kampstra, P. (2008). Beanplot: A boxplot alternative for visual comparisons of distribution. *Journal of Statistical Software*, 28(1):1–9.

Kass, R. E. and Raftery, A. E. (1995). Bayes factors. *Journal of the American Statistical Association*, 90(430):773–795.

Katz, D., Azen, S. P., and Schumitzky, A. (1981). Bayesian approach to the analysis of nonlinear models: Implementation and evaluation. *Biometrics*, 37(1):137–142.

Kiermeier, A., Jarrett, R. G., and Verbyla, A. P. (2004). A new approach to estimating shelf-life. *Pharmaceutical Statistics: The Journal of Applied Statistics in the Pharmaceutical Industry*, 3(1):3–11.

Komsta, L. (2022). *outliers: Tests for outliers*. R package version 0.15.

Kooli, I. and Limam, M. (2009). Bayesian np control charts with adaptive sample size for finite production runs. *Quality and Reliability Engineering International*, 25(4):439–448.

Krishnamoorthy, K. and Mathew, T. (2009). *Statistical Tolerance Regions: Theory, Applications, and Computation*. John Wiley & Sons, Hoboken, NJ.

Kruschke, J. K. (2015). *Doing Bayesian Data Analysis, Second Edition: A Tutorial with R, JAGS, and Stan*. Academic Press/Elsevier, Burlington, MA.

Kruschke, J. K. (2021). Bayesian analysis reporting guidelines. *Nature Human Behaviour*, 5:1282–1291.

Kryzwinski, M. and Altman, N. (2014). Visualizing samples with box plots. *Nature Methods*, 11(2):119–120.

Kubiak, R. J., Zhang, J., Ren, P., Yang, H., and Roskos, L. K. (2018). Excessive outlier removal may result in cut points that are not suitable for immunogenicity assessments. *Journal of Immunological Methods*, 463:105–111.

Kumar, R., Carroll, C., Hartikainen, A., and Martín, O. A. (2019). ArviZ a unified library for exploratory analysis of Bayesian models in Python, 1–5.

Kuznetsova, A., Brockhoff, P. B., and Christensen, R. H. (2017). lmerTest package: tests in linear mixed effects models. *Journal of Statistical Software*, 82:1–26.

Labes, D., Schütz, H., and Lang, B. (2022). *PowerTOST: Power and Sample Size for (Bio)Equivalence Studies.* R package version 1.5-4.

LeBlond, D., Altan, S., Novick, S., Peterson, J., Shen, Y., and Yang, H. (2015). In vitro dissolution curves comparisons: A critique of current practices. *Dissolution Technologies*, 23:14–23.

Lebrun, P., Giacoletti, K., Scherder, T., Rozet, E., and Boulanger, B. (2015). A quality by design approach for longitudinal quality attributes. *Journal of Biopharmaceutical Statistics*, 25(2):247–259.

Lee, H. Y., Wu, P. C., and Lee, Y. J. (2010). stab: An R package for drug stability data analysis. *Computer Methods and Programs in Biomedicine*, 100(2):140–148.

Lee, J. F., Litten, J. B., and Grampp, G. (2012). Comparability and biosimilarity: considerations for healthcare providers. *Current Medical Research and Opinion*, 28(6):1053–1058.

Lesaffre, E. and Lawson, A. (2012). *Bayesian Biostatistics.* Wiley, New York.

Lewandowski, D., Kurowicka, D., and Joe, H. (2009). Generating random correlation matrices based on vines and extended onion method. *Journal of Multivariate Analysis*, 100(9):1989–2001.

Lewis, R. A. (2020). Dissolution acceptance limits based on parametric tolerance intervals. In *JSM Proceedings, Statistics in Genomics and Genetics Section.* Joint Statistical Meetings.

Lewis, R. A. and Fan, A. (2016). Improved acceptance limits for ASTM Standard E2810. *Statistics in Biopharmaceutical Research*, 8(1):40–48.

Lewis, R. A. and Novick, S. J. (2012). A generalized pivot quantity approach to the parametric tolerance interval test for dose-content uniformity batch testing. *Statistics in Biopharmaceutical Research*, 4(1):28–36.

Liao, J. J. Z. and Darken, P. F. (2013). Comparability of critical quality attributes for establishing biosimilarity. *Statistics in Medicine*, 32(3):52–66.

Limentani, G. B., Ringo, M. C., Ye, F., and Berquist, M. L. (2005). Beyond the t-test: statistical equivalence and testing. *Analytical Chemistry*, 77(11):221A–226A.

Lintusaarii, J., Gutman, M. U., Dutta, R., Kaski, S., and Coriandor, J. (2017). Fundamentals and recent developments in approximate Bayesian computation. *Systematic Biology*, 66(1):66–82.

Lopez-Ruiz, R., Lopez, J., and Calbet, X. (2012). Exponential wealth distribution: A new approach from functional iteration theory. In *ESIAM Proceedings 36*, pages 189–196. ESIAM.

Lunn, D., Jackson, C., Best, N., Thomas, A., and Spiegelhalter, D. (2013). *The BUGS Book: A Practical Intrduction to Bayesian Analysis.* CRC Press, Boca Raton.

Lunn, D., Spiegelhalter, D., Thomas, A., and Best, N. (2009). The BUGS project: Evolution, critique and future directions. *Statistics in Medicine*, 28(25):3049–3067.

Lunn, D., Thomas, A., Best, N., and Spiegelhalter, D. (2000). WinBUGS–a Bayesian modelling framework: Concepts, structure, and extensibility. *Statistics and Computing*, 10:325–337.

Makis, V. (2008). Multivariate Bayesian control chart. *Operations Research*, 25(4):487–496.

Marcellus, R. L. (2007). Bayesian statistical process control. *Quality Engineering*, 20(1):113–127.

Marjou, R. K., Barash, S., and Brisbane, C. E. (2018). Evaluation of a biologic formulation using customized design of experiment and novel multidimensional robustness diagrams. *Journal of Pharmacuetical Sciences*, 107(3):797–806.

Martin, A. D., Quinn, K. M., and Park, J. H. (2011). MCMCpack: Markov chain Monte Carlo in R. *Journal of Statistical Software*, 42(9):22.

Martins, T. G., Simpson, D., Lindgren, F., and Rue, H. (2013). Bayesian computing with INLA: new features. *Computational Statistics & Data Analysis*, 67:68–83.

MATLAB Release 2020b (2020). The Mathworks, Inc., Natick Massachusetts, United States.

McCormac, P., Warren, J., Beumer-Sassi, A., Sanders, I., Sun, J., Maranga, L., Cheng, A., Richardson, J., Sharma, S., Henke, D., Hung, J., and Singh, N. (2021). Project a-gene: A case study-based aproach to integrating QbD principles in gene therapy CMC programs. Technical report, Alliance for Regenerative Medicine and the National Institute for Innovation in Manufacturing Biopharmaceuticals.

McElreath, R. (2020). *Statistical Rethinking: A Bayesian Course with Examples in R and Stan, Second Edition.* CRC Press, Boca Raton.

Mee, R. W. and Owen, D. B. (1983). Improved factors for one-sided tolerance limits for balanced one-way ANOVA random model. *Journal of the American Statistical Association*, 78(384):901–905.

Meeker, W. Q., Hahn, G. J., and Escobar, L. A. (2017). *Statistical Intervals: A Guide for Practitioners, and Researchers, Second Edition.* Wiley, Hoboken, NJ.

Menzefricke, U. (2002). On the evaluation of control chart limits based on predictive distributions. *Communications in Statistics-Theory and Methods*, 31(8):1423–1440.

Millard, S. P. (2013). *EnvStats: An R Package for Environmental Statistics.* Springer.

Minitab, LLC (2022). *Minitab.* State College, PA.

Miro-Quesada, G., Del Castillo, E., and Peterson, J. J. (2011). A Bayesian approach for multiple response surface optimization in the presence of noise variables. *Journal of Applied Statistics*, 31(3):251–270.

Mockus, L. and LeBlond, D. (2020). Bayesian methods for in vitro dissolution drug testing and similarity comparisons. In Lessaffre, E., Baio, G., and Boulanger, B., editors, *Bayesian Methods in Pharmaceutical Research*, pages 421–447. CRC Press, Boca Raton.

Mollenhoff, K., Dette, H., Kotzagiorgis, E., and Volgushev, S. (2018). Regulatory assessment of drug dissolution profiles comparability via maximum deviation. *Statistics in Medicine*, 37:2968–2981.

Montes, R. O., Burdick, R. K., and Leblond, D. J. (2019). Simple approach to calculate random effects model tolerance intervals to set release and shelf-life specification limits of pharmaceutical products. *PDA Journal of Pharmaceutical Science and Technology*, 73(1):39–59.

Montgomery, D. C. (2017). *Design and Analysis of Experiments.* John Wiley & Sons, Hoboken, NJ.

Montgomery, D. C. (2020). *Introduction to Statistical Quality Control.* John Wiley & Sons, Hoboken, NJ.

Moore, J. W. and Flanner, H. H. (1996). Mathematical comparison of distribution profiles. *Pharmaceutical Technology*, 20(6):64–74.

Morita, S., Thall, P., and Müller, P. (2008). Determining the effective sample size of a parametric prior. *Biometrics*, 6(3):595–602.

Morita, S., Thall, P., and Müller, P. (2010). Evaluating the impact of prior assumptions in Bayesian biostatistics. *Statistics in Biosciences*, 2:1–17.

Morita, S., Thall, P., and Müller, P. (2012). Prior effective sample size in conditionally independent hierarchical models. *Bayesian Analysis*, 6(3):591–614.

Murphy, J. and Hofer, J. (2002). Establishing shelf life, expiry limits, and release limits. *Drug Information Journal*, 36(4):769–781.

Narayanan, H., Dingfelder, F., Morales, I. C., Patel, B., Heding, K. E., Bjelke, J. R., Egebjerg, T., Butté, A., Sokolov, M., Lorenzen, N., and Arosio, P. (2021). Design of biopharmaceutical formulations accelerated by machine learning. *Molecular Pharmaceutics*, 18:3843–3853.

Neal, R. (1995). *Bayesian Learning for Neural Networks.* PhD thesis, University of Toronto.

Neal, R. M. (2003). Slice sampling. *The Annals of Statistics*, 31(3):705–767.

Neal, R. M. (2011). MCMC using Hamiltonian dynamics. In Brooks, S., Gelman, A., Jones, G. L., and Meng, X.-L., editors, *Handbook of Markov Chain Monte Carlo*, pages 113–162. Chapman and Hall/CRC.

Neuenschwander, B., Branson, M., and Spiegelhalter, D. (2009). A note on the power prior. *Statistics in Medicine*, 28:3562–3566.

Ng, H. K. T., Ling, M. H., and Chan, P. S. (2018). A gamma process modeling approach for the comparison of dissolution profiles. *Drug Development and Industrial Pharmacy*, 44(4):553–562.

Novick, S. and Hudson-Curtis, B. (2018). Content uniformity testing for stratified samples via parametric tolerance interval testing. *Journal of Biopharmaceutical Statistics*, 28(3):463–474.

Novick, S., Shen, Y., Yang, H., Peterson, J., LeBlond, D., and Altan, S. (2015). Dissolution curve comparisons through the f_2 parameter, a Bayesian extension of the f_2 statistic. *Journal of Biopharmaceutical Statistics*, 25(2):351–371.

Novick, S. J., Christian, E., Farmer, E., and Tejada, M. (2021). A Bayesian statistical approach to continuous qualification of a bioassay. *PDA Journal of Pharmaceutical Science and Technology*, 75(1):8–23.

Ocaña, J., Frutos, G., and Sánchez, P. (2009). Using the similarity factor f_2 in practice: A critical revision and suggestions for its standard error estimation. *Chemometrics and Intelligent Laboratory Systems*, 99:49–56.

O'Hagan, A., Stevens, J. W., and Campbell, M. J. (2005). Assurance in clinical trial design. *Pharmaceutical Statistics*, 4(3):187–201.

Owen, D. B. (1965). A special case of a bivariate non-central t-distribution. *Biometrika*, 52(3–4):437–446.

Patel, J. K. (1986). Tolerance limits – a review. *Communication in Statistics – Theory and Methods*, 15(9):2719–2762.

Peng, H. and Lu, Y. (2012). Model selection in linear mixed effect models. *Journal of Multivariate Analysis*, 109:109–129.

Peterson, J. J. (2008). A Bayesian approach to the ICH Q8 definition of design space. *Journal of Biopharmaceutical Statistics*, 18(5):959–975.

Peterson, J. J. and Lief, K. (2010). The ICH Q8 definition of design space: A comparison of the overlapping means and the Bayesian predictive approaches. *Statistics in Biopharmaceutical Research*, 2(2):249–259.

Peterson, J. J. and Yahyah, M. (2009). A Bayesian design space approach to robustness and system suitability for pharmaceutical assays and other processes. *Statistics in Biopharmaceutical Research*, 1(4):441–449.

Plummer, M. (2003). JAGS: A program for analysis of Bayesian graphical models using gibbs sampling. In *Proceedings of the 3rd International Workshop on Distributed Statistical Computing*, volume 124, pages 1–10. Vienna, Austria.

Plummer, M. (2021). *rjags: Bayesian Graphical Models using MCMC.* R package version 4-12.

Plummer, M., Best, N., Cowles, K., and Vines, K. (2006). CODA: Convergence diagnosis and output analysis for MCMC. *R News*, 6(1):7–11.

Podcseck, F. (1993). Comparison of in vitro dissolution profiles by calculating the mean dissolution time (MDT) or mean residence time (MRT). *International Journal of Pharmaceutics*, 97(1–3):93–100.

Pourmohamad, T., Oliva Avilés, C. M., and Richardson, R. (2022). Gaussian process modeling for dissolution curve comparisons. *Journal of the Royal Statistics Society: Series C*, 71(2):331–351.

Quinlan, M., Stroup, W., Schwenke, J., and Christopher, D. (2013). Evaluating the performance of the ICH guidelines for shelf life estimation. *Journal of Biopharmaceutical Statistics*, 23(4):3–11.

R Core Team (2021). *R: A Language and Environment for Statistical Computing.* R Foundation for Statistical Computing, Vienna, Austria.

Rasmussen, C. E. and Williams, C. K. I. (2006). *Gaussian Processes for Machine Learning.* The MIT Press, Cambridge, MA.

Rigby, R. A. and Stasinopoulos, M. D. (2005). Generalized additive models for location, scale, and shape. *Applied Statistics*, 54(3):507–554.

Rigby, R. A., Stasinopoulos, M. D., Heller, G. Z., and De Bastiani, F. (2020). *Distributions for Modelling Location, Scale, and Shape: Using Gamlss in R.* CRC Press, Boca Raton.

Robert, C. (2007). *The Bayesian Choice, Second Edition.* Springer-Verlag, New York.

Robert, C. P. and Casella, G. (2004). *Monte Carlo Statistical Methods, Second Edition.* Springer.

Roos, M., Martins, T., Held, L., and Rue, H. (2015). Sensitivity analysis for Bayesian hierarchical models. *Bayesian Analysis*, 10(2):321–349.

Rosner, B. (1975). On the detection of many outliers. *Technometrics*, 17(2):221–227.

Rosner, G., Laud, P., and Johnson, W. (2021). *Bayesian Thinking in Biostatistics.* CRC Press, Boca Raton.

Rozet, E., Lepbrun, P., Hubert, P., Debrus, B., and Boulanger, B. (2013). Design spaces for analytical methods. *TrAC Trends in Analytical Chemistry*, 42:157–167.

Rue, H., Martino, S., and Chopin, N. (2009). Approximate Bayesian inference for latent Gaussian models by using integrated nested Laplace approximations. *Journal of the Royal Statistical Society: Series B (Statistical Methodology)*, 71(2):319–392.

Salvatier, J., Wiecki, T. V., and Fonnesbeck, C. (2016). Probabilistic programming in Python using PyMC3. *PeerJ Computer Science*, 2:e55.

Saranadasa, H. and Krishnamoorthy, K. (2005). A multivariate test for similarity of two dissolution profiles. *Journal of Biopharmaceutical Statistics*, 15:265–278.

Sathe, P. M., Tsong, Y., and Shah, V. P. (1996). In-vitro dissolution profile comparison: Statistics and analysis, model dependent approach. *Pharmaceutical Research*, 13:1799–1803.

Satterthwaite, F. E. (1946). An approximate distribution of estimates of variance components. *Biometrics Bulletin*, 2(6):110–114.

Schlain, B., Amaravadi, L., Donley, J., Wickramasekera, A., Bennett, D., and Subramanyam, M. (2010). A novel gamma-fitting statistical method for anti-drug antibody assays to establish assay cut points for data with non-normal distribution. *Journal of Immunological Methods*, 352(1):161–168.

Schrieber, S. J., Putnam, W. S., Chow, E. C. Y., Cieslak, J., Zhuang, Y., Martin, S. W., Hanson, P., Maggio, F., and Rosado, L. A. R. (1998). Comparability considerations and challenges for expedited development programs for biological products. *Drugs in R&D*, 20:889–896.

Schuetzenmeister, A. and Dufey, F. (2020). *VCA: Variance Component Analysis.* R package version 1.4.3.

Schuirmann, D. J. (1987). A comparison of the two one-sided tests procedure and the power approach for assessing th equivalence of average bioavailability. *Journal of Pharmacokinetics and Biopharmaceutics*, 15:657–680.

Seaman, J. III, Seaman, J. Jr., and Stamey, J. (2012). Hidden dangers of specifying noninformative priors. *The American Statistician*, 66(2):77–84.

Seaman Jr., J. W., Stamey, J. D., Kahle, D. J., and Blair, S. (2020). A brief guide to Bayesian model checking. In Lakshminarayanan, M. and Natanegara, F., editors, *Bayesian Applications in Pharmaceutical Development.* Chapman and Hall/CRC, New York.

Searle, S. R., Casella, G., and McCulloch, C. E. (1992). *Variance Components.* John Wiley & Sons, Hoboken, NJ.

Shah, V. P., Tsong, Y., Sathe, P., and Liu, J. (1998). In vitro dissolution profile comparison – statistics and analysis of the similarity factor, f_2. *Pharmaceutical Research*, 15(6):889–896.

Shankar, G., Devanarayan, V., Amaravadi, L., Barrett, Y. C., Bowsher, R., Finco-Kent, D., Fiscella, M., Gorovits, B., Kirschner, S., Moxness, N., Parish, T., Quarmby, V., Smith, H., Smith, W., Zuckerman, L. A., and Koren, E. (2008). Recommendations for the validation of immunoassays used for detection of host antibodies against biotechnology products. *Journal of Pharmaceutical and Biomedical Analysis*, 48(5):1267–1281.

Shen, M., Dong, X., and Tsong, Y. (2015). Equivalence margin determintaion for analytical biosimilar assessment. Technical report, 2015 FDA Industry Statstics Workshop.

Shen, Y., Psioda, M. A., and Ibrahim, J. G. (2021). Bayesppd: An R package for Bayesian sample size determination using the power and normalized power prior for generalized linear models. *arXiv preprint arXiv:2112.14616.*

Shen, Y., Psioda, M. A., and Ibrahim, J. G. (2022). *BayesPPD: Bayesian Power Prior Design.* R package version 1.0.4.

Shewhart, W. A. (1931). *Economic Control of Quality Manufactured Product.* Macmillan and Co Ltd, London.

Smith, A. F. and Gelfand, A. E. (1992). Bayesian statistics without tears: a sampling-resampling perspective. *The American Statistician*, 23(2):84–88.

Spiegelhalter, D., Abrams, K., and Myles, J. (2004). *Bayesian Approaches to Clinical Trials and Health-Care Education.* Wiley, Chichester, England.

Spiegelhalter, D., Thomas, A., Best, N., and Lunn, D. (2014). *OpenBUGS user manual, version 3.2.3.*

Stab-e-Lity (2022). *Stab-e-Lity by PharmaLex.* PharmaLex GmbH, Mont-Saint-Guibert, Belgium.

Stan Development Team (2021a). *RStan: the R interface to Stan.* R package version 2.21.3.

Stan Development Team (2021b). Stan modeling language users guide and reference manual. Version 2.28.

Stokes, M., Chen, F., and Gunes, F. (2014). An introduction to Bayesian analysis with SAS/STAT® software. In *Proceedings of the SAS Global Forum 2014 Conference, SAS Institute Inc.* Citeseer.

Sturtz, S., Ligges, U., and Gelman, A. (2005). R2WinBUGS: A package for running WinBUGS from R. *Journal of Statistical Software*, 12(3):1–16.

Tabora, J. E., Lora Gonzales, F., and Tom, J. W. (2019). Bayesian probabilistic modeling in pharmaceutical process development. *AIChE Journal*, 65(11):1–11.

Tagaras, G. and Nikolaidis, Y. (2002). Comparing the effectiveness of various Bayesian X control charts. *Operations Research*, 50(5):878–888.

Tan, C. (2019). New paradigm to derive and assess ADA cut points. Technical report, 2019 Regulatory-Industry Statistics Workshop, Rockville, Md.

Tan, M. H. and Shi, J. (2012). A Bayesian approach for interpreting mean shifts in multivariate quality control. *Technometrics*, 54(3):294–307.

Temple, J. R. and Robertson, J. R. (2021). Conditional assurance: the answer to the questions that should be asked within drug development. *Pharmaceutical Statistics*, 20(6):1102–1111.

Thomas, A., O'Hara, B., Ligges, U., and Sturtz, S. (2006). Making BUGS open. *R News*, 6(1):12–17.

Thompson, L., Chu, J., Xu, J., Li, X., Nair, R., and Tiwari, R. (2021). Dynamic borrowing from a single prior data source using the conditional power prior. *Journal of Biopharmaceutical Research*, 31(4):403–424.

Tsong, Y., Shen, M., and Dong, X. (2015). Development of statistical approaches for analytical biosimilarity evaluation. Technical report, DIA/FDA Statistics 2015 Forum, Washington D.C.

Tukey, J. (1977). *Exploratory Data Analysis*. Addison-Wesley, Reading, MA.

Ushey, K., Allaire, J., and Tang, Y. (2021). *reticulate: Interface to 'Python'*. R package version 1.22.

USP, General Chapter $< 1711 >$ (2016). Ophthalmic products-performance tests. Technical report, USP-NF US Pharmacopeial Covention, Rockville, MD.

USP, General Chapter $< 711 >$ (2011). Dissolution. Technical report, USP-NF US Pharmacopeial Covention, Rockville, MD.

USP, General Chapter $< 724 >$ (2018). Drug release. Technical report, USP-NF US Pharmacopeial Covention, Rockville, MD.

USP, General Chapter $< 905 >$ (2014). Uniformity of dosage units. Technical report, USP-NF US Pharmacopeial Covention, Rockville, MD.

van den Brand, T. (2021). *ggh4x: Hacks for 'ggplot2'*. R package version 0.2.1.

Van Den Heuvel, E. R. (2010). A comparison of estimation methods on the coverage probability of Satterthwaite confidence intervals for assay precision with unbalanced data. Communications in Statistics—Simulation and Computation®, 39(4), 777–794.

Varin, C., Reid, N., and Firth, D. (2011). An overview of composite likelihood methods. *Statistica Sinica*, 21:5–42.

Vehtari, A., Gelman, A., Simpson, D., Carpenter, B., and Bürkner, P. (2021). Rank-normalization, folding, and localization: An improved $\hat{R}$ for assessing convergence of MCMC (with discussion). *Bayesian Analysis*, 16(2):667–718.

Viele, K., Berry, S., Neuenschwander, B., Amzal, B., Chen, F., Enas, N., Hobbs, B., Ibrahim, J. G., Kinnersley, N., Lindborg, S., Micallef, S., Roychoudhury, S., and Thompson, L. (2014). Use of historical control data for assessing treatment effects in clinical trials. *Pharmaceutical Statistics*, 13(1):41–54.

Wagner, J. G. (1975). *Fundamentals of Clinical Pharmacokinetics.* Drug Intelligence Pub. Inc., Hamilton, Illinois.

Wang, W. and Ohtake, S. (2019). Science and art of protein formulation development. *International Journal of Pharmaceutics*, 568:118505.

Weerahandi, S. (2004). *Generalized Inference in Repeated Measures: Exact Methods in MANOVA and Mixed Models.* John Wiley & Sons, Hoboken, NJ.

Weese, D. and Burdick, R. K. (2015). Statistical details of analytical similarity for biosimilars: An industry view. Technical report, IABS/FDA Statistical and Data Management Approaches for Biotechnology Drug Development, Rockville, MD.

Welch, B. L. (1947). The generalisation of student's problems when several different population variances are involved. *Biometrika*, 34(1–2):28–35.

Wheeler, D. J. (1993). *Understanding Variation: The Key to Managing Chaos.* SPC Press, Knoxville, TN.

Wheeler, D. J. and Chambers, D. S. (1992). *Understanding Statistical Process Control.* SPC Press, Knoxville, TN.

WHO (2011). Guidelines on stability evaluation of vaccines, annex 3, trs no 962. Technical report, World Health Organization.

Wickham, H. (2016). *ggplot2: Elegant Graphics for Data Analysis.* Springer-Verlag, New York.

Wickham, H., Averick, M., Bryan, J., Chang, W., McGowan, L. D., François, R., Grolemund, G., Hayes, A., Henry, L., Hester, J., Kuhn, M., Pedersen, T. L., Miller, E., Bache, S. M., Müller, K., Ooms, J., Robinson, D., Seidel, D. P., Spinu, V., Takahashi, K., Vaughan, D., Wilke, C., Woo, K., and Yutani, H. (2019). Welcome to the tidyverse. *Journal of Open Source Software*, 4(43):1686.

Wickham, H. and Grolemund, G. (2016). *R for Data Science: Import, Tidy, Transform, Visualize, and Model Data.* O'Reilly Media, Inc.

Wolfinger, R. D. (1998). Tolerance intervals for variance component models using Bayesian simulation. *Journal of Quality Technology*, 30(1):18–32.

Wu, C. W. and Lin, T. Y. (2009). A Bayesian procedure for assessing process performance based on the third-generation capability index. *Journal of Applied Statistics*, 36(11):1205–1223.

Wurth, C., Demeule, B., Mahler, H., and Adler, M. (2016). Quality by design approaches to formulation robustness-an antibody case study. *Journal of Pharmaceutical Sciences*, 105(5):1667–1675.

Yang, H. (2017). *Emerging Non-clinical Biostatistics in Biopharmaceutical Development and Manufacturing.* Chapman & Hall, Boca Raton.

Yang, H. (2018). Setting specifications. In Coffey, T. and Yang, H., editors, *Statistics for Biotechnology Process Development*, pages 145–167. CRC Press, Boca Raton.

Yang, H., Burdick, R. K., Cheng, A., and Montes, R. O. (2018). Statistical considerations for demonstration of analytical similarity. In Gutka, H. J., Yang, H., and Kakar, S., editors, *Biosimilars: Regulatory, Clinical, and Biopharmaceutical Development*, pages 431–468. Springer International Publishing, Cham.

Yang, H., Zhang, J., Yu, B., and Zhao, W. (2015). *Statistical Methods for Immunogenicity Assessment.* Chapman & Hall, Boca Raton.

Yang, P. Y., Hui, C. J., Tien, D. J., Snowden, A. W., Derfus, G. E., and Opel, C. F. (2019). Accurate definition of control strategies using cross validated stepwise regression and monte carlo simulation. *Journal of Biotechnology*, 306:1–10.

Yang, H. Novick, S., Burdick, R. K., Cheng, A., and Montes, R. (2016). On statistical approaches for demonstrating analytical similarity in the presence of correlation. *PDA Journal of Pharmaceutical Science and Technology*, 70(6):547–559.

Young, D. S. (2010). tolerance: An R package for estimating tolerance intervals. *Journal of Statistical Software*, 36(5):1–39.

Young, D. S. (2016). Normal tolerance interval procedures in the tolerance package. *The R Journal*, 8(2):200–212.

Yu, B., Zeng, L., and Yang, H. (2017). A risk-based approach to setting acceptance criteria for pharmaceutical process comparability. *Journal of Pharmaceutical Innovation*, 12:357–366.

Yuksel, N., Kanik, A. E., and Baykara, T. (2000). Comparison of in vitro dissolution profiles by ANOVA-based, model-dependent and -independent methods. *International Journal of Pharmaceutics*, 209:57–67.

Zhang, J., Yu, B., Zhang, L., Roskos, L., Richman, L., and Yang, H. (2015). Non-normal random effects models for immunogenicity assay cut point determination. *Journal of Biopharmaceutical Statistics*, 25(2):295–306.

Zhang, L. and Su, C. (2016). Introduction to nonclinical statistics for pharmaceutical and biotechnology industries. In Zhang, L., editor, *Nonclinical Statistics for Pharmaceutical and Biotechnology Industries*, pages 3–17. Springer International Publishing, Cham.

Zhang, L., Zhang, J., Kubiak, R. J., and Yang, H. (2013). Non-normal random effects models for immunogenicity assay cut point determination. *Journal of Immunological Methods*, 389(1–2):79–87.